ANNALS OF THE NEW YORK ACADEMY OF SCIENCES

Volume 649

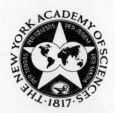

EDITORIAL STAFF

Executive Editor
BILL BOLAND

Managing Editor
JUSTINE CULLINAN

Associate Editor
STEFAN MALMOLI

The New York Academy of Sciences
2 East 63rd Street
New York, New York 10021

BIOLOGICAL EFFECTS AND SAFETY ASPECTS OF NUCLEAR MAGNETIC RESONANCE IMAGING AND SPECTROSCOPY

ANNALS OF THE NEW YORK ACADEMY OF SCIENCES
Volume 649

BIOLOGICAL EFFECTS AND SAFETY ASPECTS OF NUCLEAR MAGNETIC RESONANCE IMAGING AND SPECTROSCOPY

Edited by Richard L. Magin, Robert P. Liburdy, and Bertil Persson

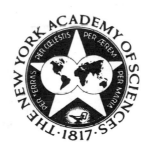

The New York Academy of Sciences
New York, New York
1992

Library of Congress Cataloging-in-Publication Data

Biological effects and safety aspects of nuclear magnetic resonance
    imaging and spectroscopy/edited by Richard L. Magin, Robert P.
    Liburdy, and Bertil Persson.
        p.   cm.—(Annals of the New York Academy of Sciences, ISSN
    0077-8923; v. 649).
        Includes bibliographical references and index.
        ISBN 0-89766-697-6 (cloth: alk. paper).—ISBN 0-89766-698-4
    (paper: alk. paper).
        1. Nuclear magnetic resonance—Health aspects.   2. Nuclear
    magnetic resonance—Physiological effect.   I. Magin, Richard L.
    II. Liburdy, Robert P.   III. Persson, Bertil.   IV. Series.
        [DNLM: 1. Magnetic Resonance Imaging—adverse effects—congresses.
    2. Nuclear Magnetic Resonance—adverse effects—congresses.
    3. Safety—congresses. W1 AN626YL v. 649/WN 445 B6145]
    Q11.N5 vol. 649
    [RC78.7.N83]
    500 s—dc20
    [363.18′9]
    DNLM/DLC
    for Library of Congress
                                                                                    92-1409
                                                                                    CIP

SP
Printed in the United States of America
ISBN 0-89766-697-6 (cloth)
ISBN 0-89766-698-4 (paper)
ISSN 0077-8923

ANNALS OF THE NEW YORK ACADEMY OF SCIENCES

Volume 649
March 31, 1992

BIOLOGICAL EFFECTS AND SAFETY ASPECTS OF NUCLEAR MAGNETIC RESONANCE IMAGING AND SPECTROSCOPY[a]

Editors and Conference Organizers
RICHARD L. MAGIN, ROBERT P. LIBURDY, and BERTIL PERSSON

CONTENTS

Introduction. *By* RICHARD L. MAGIN ix

Emerging Nuclear Magnetic Resonance Technologies: Health and Safety. *By* THOMAS F. BUDINGER 1

Session I. Ultra High Static Magnetic Fields

Interactions between Electromagnetic Fields and Biological Systems. *By* CARL H. DURNEY 19

Molecular and Cellular Responses to Orientation Effects in Static and Homogeneous Ultra High Magnetic Fields. *By* J. D. DE CERTAINES, ... 35

Extremely Low Frequency Magnetic Field Exposure from MRI/MRS Procedures: Implications for Patients (Acute Exposures) and Operational Personnel (Chronic Exposures). *By* FRANK S. PRATO, MARTIN KAVALIERS, KLAUS-PETER OSSENKOPP, JEFFREY J. L. CARSON, DICK J. DROST, and J. ROGER H. FRAPPIER 44

Human Interactions with Ultra High Fields. *By* U. W. BUETTNER 59

Session I Summary. *By* ROBERT P. LIBURDY 67

Session II. Ultra Fast Switched Magnetic Fields

A Theoretical Basis for Coupling via Induced Currents to Biological Systems for Ultra Fast Switched Magnetic Fields. *By* FRANK S. BARNES 69

Biological Interactions of Cellular Systems with Time-varying Magnetic Fields. *By* ROBERT P. LIBURDY 74

Principles of Nerve and Heart Excitation by Time-varying Magnetic Fields. *By* J. PATRICK REILLY 96

Stimulation by Time-varying Magnetic Fields. *By* MICHAEL L. ROHAN and RICHARD R. RZEDZIAN 118

Session II Summary. *By* STEPHEN R. THOMAS 129

[a]This volume is the result of a conference entitled Biological Effects and Safety Aspects of Nuclear Magnetic Resonance Imaging and Spectroscopy, which was sponsored by the New York Academy of Sciences, the National Cancer Institute, and the Food and Drug Administration and held on May 15–17, 1991, in Bethesda, Maryland.

Session III. High Power, Pulsed Radio-Frequency Fields

Absorption and Distribution Patterns of RF Fields. *By* OM P. GANDHI and JIN-YUAN CHEN 131

Homogeneous Tissue Model Estimates of RF Power Deposition in Human NMR Studies: Local Elevations Predicted in Surface Coil Decoupling. *By* PAUL A. BOTTOMLEY and PETER B. ROEMER 144

Increased Radio-Frequency Power Absorption in Human Tissue due to Coupling between Body Coil and Surface Coil. *By* PETER BOESIGER, RETO BUCHLI, MARTIN SANER, and DIETER MEIER 160

Effects of RF Power Absorption in Mammalian Cells. *By* STEPHEN F. CLEARY, LI-MING LIU, and GUANGHUI CAO 166

Spatial Distribution of RF Power in Critical Organs during Magnetic Resonance Imaging. *By* M. GRANDOLFO, A. POLICHETTI, P. VECCHIA, and O. P. GANDHI 176

Predicted Thermophysiological Responses of Humans to MRI Fields. *By* ELEANOR R. ADAIR and LARRY G. BERGLUND 188

Session III Summary. *By* W. GREGORY LOTZ 201

Session IV. Personnel Exposure Levels and Dosimetry of Fields Associated with MR Imaging and Spectroscopy

An Overview of Electromagnetic Safety Considerations Associated with Magnetic Resonance Imaging. *By* EMANUEL KANAL 204

Dosimetry and Effects of MR Exposure to RF and Switched Magnetic Fields. *By* DANIEL J. SCHAEFER 225

Development of Dosimetry Monitors for MRI Staff and Patients. *By* RICHARD G. OLSEN 237

Current FDA Guidance for MR Patient Exposure and Considerations for the Future. *By* T. WHIT ATHEY 242

Session IV Summary. *By* JOHN C. MONAHAN and JEFFREY C. WEINREB 258

Session V. Patient Safety during MRI and MRS

Thermal Responses in Human Subjects Exposed to Magnetic Resonance Imaging. *By* FRANK G. SHELLOCK 260

Local and Global Thermoregulatory Responses to MRI Fields. *By* CHRISTOPHER J. GORDON 273

Health and Physiological Effects of Human Exposure to Whole-Body Four-Tesla Magnetic Fields during MRI. *By* JOHN F. SCHENCK 285

Safety of Patients with Medical Devices during Application of Magnetic Resonance Methods. *By* GERALD M. POHOST, GERALD G. BLACKWELL, and FRANK G. SHELLOCK 302

The Design of RF Systems for Patient Safety. *By* JEFFREY R. FITZSIMMONS 313

Development of Contrast Media for Magnetic Resonance Imaging. *By* H. A. GOLDSTEIN, J. R. WIGGINS, and F. KASHANIAN 322

Clinical Indications for MRI. *By* DAVID D. STARK 332

Session V Summary. *By* ROBERT S. BALABAN 335

Closing Remarks. *By* BERTIL PERSSON 338

Poster Presentations

Comparison of the Effect of ELF on c-myc Oncogene Expression in Normal and Transformed Human Cells. *By* EWA CZERSKA, JON CASAMENTO, JOHN NING, MAYS SWICORD, HEBA AL-BARAZI, CHRISTOPHER DAVIS, and EDWARD ELSON 340

MRI Can Cause Focal Heating. *By* PETER L. DAVIS, YULIN SHANG, and LALITH TALAGALA 343

Permeability of the Blood-Brain Barrier of the Rat Is Not Significantly Altered by NMR Exposure. *By* R. P. LIBURDY, D. J. DE MANINCOR, M. S. ROOS, and K. M. BRENNAN 345

The Effects of a Single Intraoperative Immersion in Various Chemical Agents and Electromagnetic Field Exposure on Onlay Bone Grafts to the Facial Skeleton. *By* JOHN T. NING and ISAAC L. WORNOM III 350

Comparison of the Effect of ELF on Total RNA Content in Normal and Transformed Human Cells. *By* JOHN NING, JON CASAMENTO, EWA CZERSKA, MAYS SWICORD, HEBA AL-BARAZI, CHRISTOPHER DAVIS, and EDWARD ELSON 353

Increased Permeability of the Blood-Brain Barrier Induced by Magnetic and Electromagnetic Fields. *By* BERTIL R. R. PERSSON, LEIF G. SALFORD, ARNE BRUN, JACOB L. EBERHARDT, and LARS MALMGREN 356

Potential Health Risk due to Cardiac Applications of Echo Planar Imaging. *By* MICHAEL B. SMITH, ROSALIE F. TASSONE, and TIMOTHY J. MOSHER 359

Magnetic Resonance Imaging and X-ray Effects on Eye Development in C57BL/6J Mice. *By* D. A. TYNDALL 363

Magnetic Stimulation of the Human Brain. *By* S. UENO and T. MATSUDA 366

Safety Problems of dB/dt Associated with Echo Planar Imaging. *By* S. UENO, O. HIWAKI, T. MATSUDA, H. YAMAGATA, S. KUHARA, Y. SEO, K. SATO, and T. TANOUE 369

Appendix

Principles for the Protection of Patients and Volunteers during Clinical Magnetic Resonance Diagnostic Procedures. *By* THE NATIONAL RADIOLOGICAL PROTECTION BOARD 372

Limits on Patient and Volunteer Exposure during Clinical Magnetic Resonance Diagnostic Procedures: Recommendations for the Practical Application of the Board's Statement. *By* THE NATIONAL RADIOLOGICAL PROTECTION BOARD 376

FDA Safety Parameter Action Levels. *By* THE FOOD AND DRUG ADMINISTRATION 399

Index of Contributors 401

Financial assistance was received from:

Supporter
- NATIONAL CANCER INSTITUTE/NIH (GRANT NO. 1 R13 CA54368)

Contributors
- BERLEX LABORATORIES, INC.
- BRISTOL-MYERS SQUIBB PHARMACEUTICAL RESEARCH INSTITUTE
- SOCIETY FOR MAGNETIC RESONANCE IMAGING

Introduction

Magnetic resonance imaging (MRI) is experiencing rapid growth as a clinical diagnostic tool with the number of MR systems installed worldwide approaching 5000. Medical use of this technology has resulted in the exposure of an increasing patient and health care worker population to a wide variety of static and time-varying electromagnetic fields. In addition, technical developments such as high field imaging systems, fast cardiac imaging, and localized magnetic resonance spectroscopy (MRS) often establish high intensity electric and magnetic fields in local tissue regions. Even though the present generation of MR imaging systems has an excellent safety record, the scientific understanding of the interaction of radio-frequency and magnetic fields with biological systems is incomplete.

Although individual sessions at previous meetings and workshops have addressed some of the key safety issues associated with MRI and MRS, no scientific conference has been devoted exclusively to the potential health hazards and safety aspects of MR imaging and spectroscopy. The organizers of this conference believe that this developing technology will soon employ electromagnetic field conditions that can generate biological effects that could be hazardous.

These conditions include intense static magnetic fields of 4 T or greater, larger magnetic field gradients such as 100 mT/m or 10 gauss/cm, and higher RF frequencies in the vicinity of 200 MHz. Of particular concern are the rapidly switched magnetic fields that occur during fast imaging sequences and the higher absorption of radio-frequency power that occurs when decoupling pulses and surface coils are used in spectroscopy. These field conditions may produce biological responses not observed in the current generation of imaging systems. An important goal of this conference is to examine the potential hazards to patients and staff associated with such biological effects.

Over the course of this conference, we will examine the biological effects arising from static magnetic fields, rapidly switched magnetic field gradients, and radio-frequency absorption. The scientific presentations are arranged to analyze the interaction of electric and magnetic fields with biological systems, beginning with single cells and extending through animal models to eventual clinical applications. The participants of this conference include NMR researchers from universities, hospitals, industry, and governmental regulatory agencies who have direct knowledge of the capabilities of MR systems and of their potential biological effects. In some cases, this analysis will be augmented by experts from outside the NMR community, with individuals, for example, from fields of research such as bioelectricity, biomagnetics, and bioelectromagnetics. Each participant has been given the task of identifying the current state of knowledge of biological effects as it relates to emerging high field MR systems and the emphasis of each presentation will be on mechanisms of interaction and new results.

We hope that this conference will provide a forum for the interchange of ideas and information between researchers with different perspectives on the issues. The scientific presentations and discussions should lead to the identification of those field conditions where reported biological effects may have hazardous consequences. This knowledge is important because the diagnostic capability of MRI is largely determined by the extent to which advanced imaging and spectroscopy pulse sequences can be safely applied. By the end of this conference, we should have (1) obtained a better understanding of the potential hazards associated with high field NMR systems and (2) identified those field conditions where further study is needed to guarantee the safety of patients, technologists, and radiologists.

DEDICATION

While preparing a written record of this meeting, the organizers were saddened to learn of the death of Solomon M. Michaelson. We wish to take this opportunity to dedicate this volume to his memory. S. Michaelson, "Sol" to his many friends and colleagues, was one of the true pioneers in assessing the biological effects and safety hazards of radio-frequency and microwave fields. In his career, Michaelson established high standards of scientific rigor in the study of bioelectric phenomena, trained and collaborated with a new generation of researchers, and served the general public by active participation in almost 50 years of scientific debate on the still unsolved issue of the safety risks posed by the proliferation of electromagnetic radiation sources in our environment. The development of magnetic resonance imaging was unforeseen when Michaelson began his research on the study of the physiological effects of the microwave emissions from radar transmitters. However, the investigative procedures that he championed for analyzing the basic mechanisms of interaction in terms of physical, chemical, and biological processes are clearly evident in the reports assembled in this volume. One measure of a great scientist is that his or her theories and methods find valid application in fields and domains far beyond those of the initial experimental systems. On this scale, Michaelson's contribution to the study of the biological effects and safety aspects of nuclear magnetic resonance (NMR) imaging and spectroscopy is large indeed.

We can confidently proceed with the development of advanced NMR imaging and spectroscopy systems into the 4-tesla region and beyond knowing that we will be revisiting the frequency ranges where Michaelson first began his career. Thus, in the endeavor to establish the safe operating conditions for the useful medical application of this new diagnostic technology, we will have the opportunity of working once again with Solomon Michaelson on an important and challenging problem in bioelectromagnetics.

ACKNOWLEDGMENTS

The conference organizers wish to extend our sincere appreciation to the staff of the New York Academy of Sciences for their excellent work in making arrangements for the meeting and in preparing the manuscripts for publication. In particular, we wish to thank Sherryl Greenberg, Phyllis Steinberg, and Geraldine Busacco for their efforts in planning a successful conference. In addition, we wish to thank Stefan Malmoli for his excellent work in organizing the submitted papers and editing the manuscripts for publication. Finally, a special thanks should go to Teresa Lyles of the Department of Radiology in the College of Medicine at the University of Florida at

Gainesville and to Sandee Stedwell of the Bioengineering Program at the University of Illinois at Urbana-Champaign for their dedicated assistance in preparing the initial proposal to the Academy and in maintaining the essential communication link between the organizers, the Academy, and the conference participants.

Richard L. Magin

Emerging Nuclear Magnetic Resonance Technologies

Technologies

Health and Safety[a]

THOMAS F. BUDINGER

Lawrence Berkeley Laboratory
University of California
Berkeley, California 94720

INTRODUCTION

Although the inception of the ideas behind magnetic resonance can be dated to 1924 with the Stern-Gerlach experiment, it was not until the mid-1980s that human exposures to high static fields, rapidly changing gradient fields, and radio-frequency (RF) pulses from 16 MHz to 64 MHz became commonplace (TABLE 1). The initial attraction of NMR imaging (known as MRI) can be understood from examination of FIGURE 1, which shows the high contrast and volumetric capabilities of this modality to image the human brain. After the discoveries of Purcell and Bloch in the 1940s, chemists and physicists exploited the unique capabilities of NMR spectroscopy to reveal the chemical composition and physical properties of matter. Thus, instead of test tubes and samples being placed in magnets, the arms, legs, and whole bodies of human subjects were immersed in magnetic fields in the 1980s to evaluate chemical composition with particular emphasis on high energy phosphates and their changes from normalcy during exercise and in disease states (FIGURE 2). Now, in the past few years, there has been a merging of the proton imaging studies and NMR spectroscopy studies to give chemical shift imaging in order to describe the spatial distribution of the chemical composition (FIGURE 3).

Studies of the physiological and health-related effects of human subject exposure to the NMR experimental conditions started in earnest in the late 1970s.[1] At that time, most of the magnets had field strengths of 0.15 T with low RF absorbed power less than 0.1 W/kg and switched fields of less than 3 T/s. During the last few years, comprehensive reviews of the literature appeared in 1987[2] and 1989.[3] However, the field strengths have now increased to 1.5 T and greater. RF pulse sequences being used for many useful imaging techniques have been found to deliver sufficient power to cause measurable body temperature distribution changes, and rapidly switched gradients of about 40 T/s used for fast imaging can induce momentary E-fields near the thresholds of neuromuscular stimulation. Thus, whereas the major problem of potential injury from projectiles of ferromagnetic objects attracted by the field and field gradient has remained the most important health hazard, the potentials of physiological effects of heating and of neuroexcitation have precipitated a reevalua-

[a]This work was supported by the National Institute of Heart, Lung, and Blood and by the Office of Health and Environmental Research of the Department of Energy.

tion of the safety of present-day and near-future NMR imaging and spectroscopic methods. In this discussion, an overview of the human health effects will be presented with perspectives on how advances in MRI and NMR spectroscopic methods might present a potential for health effects.

STATIC MAGNETIC FIELD EFFECTS

The largest epidemiological studies on the effects of static fields have been two analyses of the mortality rates in aluminum-plant workers[4,5] and a study completed eight years ago on the prevalence of disease in workers exposed to static magnetic

TABLE 1. Historic Milestones[a]

•	1924:	Demonstration of nuclear magnetic moment space quantization (Stern & Gerlach)
•	1936:	Unsuccessful attempts to achieve magnetic resonance by calorimetry (Gorter)
•	1937:	Demonstration of nuclear magnetism in solid hydrogen (Lasarew & Schubnikow)
•	1938:	First successful detection of nuclear magnetic resonance using atomic beams (Rabi)
•	1945:	Nuclear magnetic resonance absorption in paraffin (Purcell, Torrey & Pound)
•	1945:	Nuclear induction experiment in water (Bloch, Hansen & Packard)
•	1950:	Pulsed magnetic resonance
•	1950:	Discovery of chemical shift (Proctor & Yu)
•	1951:	Discovery of spin-spin coupling (Gutowski et al., Hahn et al.)
•	1953:	First commercial spectrometer (Varian, Inc.)
•	1964:	First superconducting NMR magnet (Weaver; Varian, Inc.)
•	1966:	Pulse Fourier Transform NMR (Ernst & Anderson)
•	1971:	Observation of increased tissue relaxation times in mammalian tumors (Damadian)
•	1972:	First NMR spectrum of living cells (Moon & Richards)
•	1972:	NMR zeugmatography (Lauterbur)
•	1975:	Two-dimensional Fourier Transform Imaging (Kumar, Welti & Ernst)
•	1977:	First human image (Hinshaw et al.)
•	1977:	Echo planar imaging (Mansfield)
•	1980:	Spin warp and gradient echoes (Edelstein & Hutchinson)
•	1981:	Whole-body clinical imaging (Doyle et al.)
•	1982:	First demonstration of 1.5 T imaging and spectroscopy (Bottomley, Edelstein, Hart, Reddington et al., General Electric Inc.)

[a]Modified from Felix Wehrli.[22]

fields near nuclear particle accelerators and detection devices at United States national laboratories.[6] Using questionnaires, medical charts, and (in some cases) personal interviews for 792 exposed subjects and 792 controls matched for age, race, and socioeconomic status, the occurrences of diseases were recorded in 19 categories. The range of exposures was from 0.5 mT daily over many years to 2 T for durations of a few hours. The numbers of individuals with various diseases are shown for exposed and control populations in FIGURE 4. No significant increase or decrease

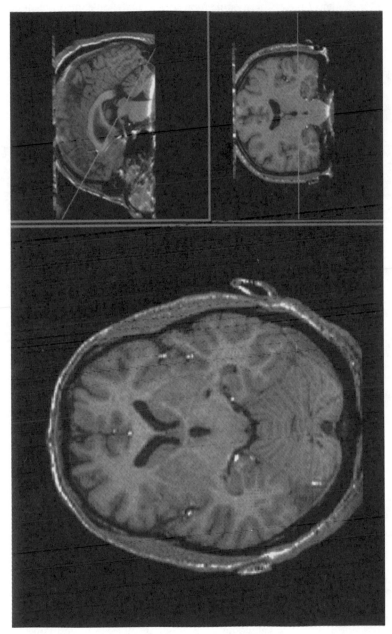

FIGURE 1. Proton NMR at 1.5 T using a three-dimensional echo gradient technique that allows 1-mm resolution in all three directions.

in the prevalence of diseases was found. Of the 792 subjects, 198 had 0.3 T or higher exposures for one hour or longer and no difference was found between this group and the remainder of the exposed populations or the matched controls. There were no trends in the data suggestive of a dose-response.

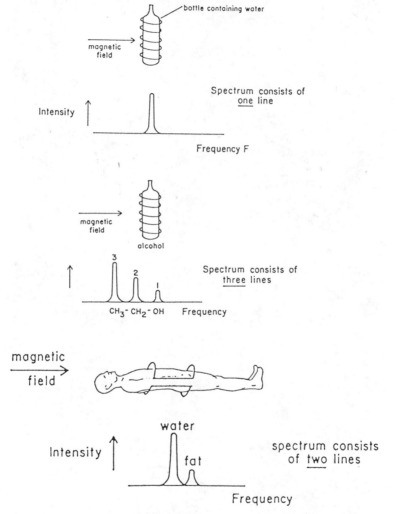

FIGURE 2. Classical NMR spectroscopy has been extended from the test tube to measurements on human subjects (after Andrew[23]).

Even 12 years ago, the known orientation effects *in vitro* of 1 T on retinal rods and sickled red cells from sickle-cell anemia patients were not considered important in limiting human exposures because torques were not significant relative to the viscous forces in the environments of molecular assemblages *in vivo*. The orientation effects

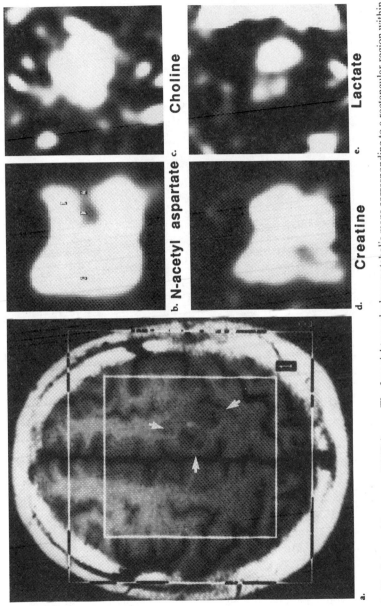

FIGURE 3. The left panel is a proton NMR image. The four right panels show metabolic maps corresponding to a rectangular region within the inner box of the proton image. A tumor region is shown by the arrows (after reference 24).

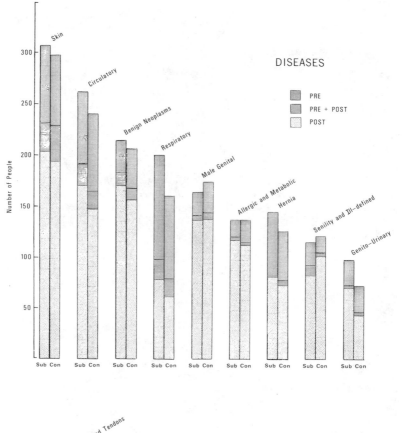

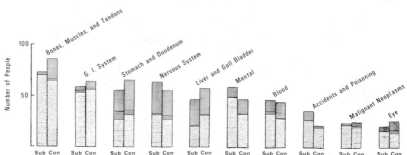

FIGURE 4. Prevalence of disease entities in individuals with occupational exposure to magnetic fields. Controls (Con) were matched for age and general job category.

result from the fact that molecules and some organized cellular structures have magnetic susceptibilities that vary with direction. If this anisotropy in susceptibility is sufficiently large, then a turning torque can be expected. The torque will be proportional to (i) the difference of the susceptibilities, (ii) the orientation of the molecule relative to the field, and (iii) the magnetic field squared, as can be seen from equation 1:

$$W = -\frac{V}{2}(|X_r| + |X_l - X_r| \cos^2[\theta])|B^2|, \tag{1}$$

where $X_l \gg X_r$ and θ is the angle between X_l and B. Note that if n molecules or subcellular units are aligned, the torque will be proportional to the number of coupled units. Indeed, the force of the Earth's magnetic field on a particular species of bacteria is sufficient to orient a chain of 15–20 50-nm magnetite crystals along the local field lines (FIGURE 5).

Today, the majority of imaging is being done at 1.5 T and below. The major reason for the predominant field of 1.5 T for imaging is to improve the signal-to-noise

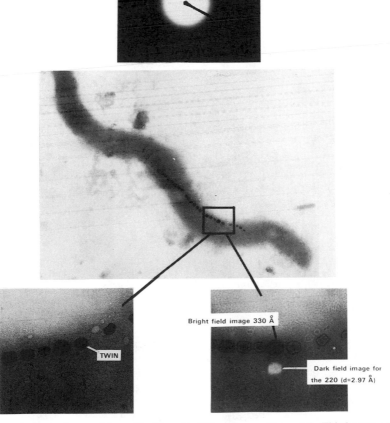

FIGURE 5. Bacteria containing a "backbone" of 50-nm magnetite crystals. This ferromagnetic ensemble provides a mechanism for guiding the bacteria along the Earth's magnetic field lines.

(S/N) and thus reduce the imaging time. This increase in field comes with some loss in intrinsic T_1 contrast.

Recently, magnets of 4 T have become available for human studies. For spectroscopic studies, the field increases give not only an increase in signal-to-noise, but also an increase in spectral dispersion, thus providing greater potentials for measuring tissue chemical composition. Problems ascribed to these high fields are limited to reports of dizziness and nausea by subjects exposed to 4-T fields. These problems have been related to the force on circulating inner ear fluids moving orthogonal to the static magnetic field and are discussed further in this symposium.

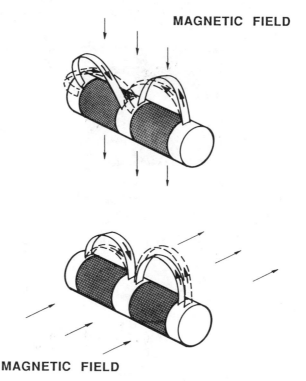

MAGNETIC FIELD

FIGURE 6. Distortion of ion current loops during action potential propagation along a myelinated nerve due to the force from a magnetic field acting on moving charges (after reference 7).

As the proposed static field increases are far beyond 1.5 T even up to 10 T, it has become important to evaluate suspected physiologic effects such as nerve conduction velocity slowing, perturbation of normal electrophysiology, and effects on fluid dynamics. These problems are summarized in the following subsections.

Effects on Nerve Conduction

The theoretic basis for expecting a change in the conduction velocity of nerves is that magnetic fields act on ionic current paths in the same way that they affect an electronic charge moving in a field:

$$F = q(v \times B),\tag{2}$$

where q is the charge, v is the velocity, and B is the magnetic field. This force causes a distortion that is perpendicular to both the magnetic field and the original direction of the ion movement. A magnetic field perpendicular to the current loop pairs associated with the propagation along the nerve will result in a distortion of the current loops (FIGURE 6) and in a consequent reduction in current velocities. Theoretical studies by Wikswo and Barach show that 24 T is required for a 10% reduction in nerve action potential conduction velocity, with the magnitude of the effect depending on the orientation of the axon with respect to the B-field.[7] No effects on action potential, conduction velocity, or refractory period have been found experimentally using the squid grand axon from 2 T to 9 T. In these carefully controlled experiments, it has been learned that a major reason for the previously observed conduction velocity change is probably a lack of adequate temperature control as a 0.2 °C temperature change causes about a 2% change in conduction velocity.

Effects on the Electrocardiogram

An electric potential is produced by a moving conductor such as the flowing blood, beating heart, or respiring lungs in a magnetic field. The induced electrical potentials from this motion are signals superimposed on the normal electrocardiogram[8] and, as expected, these signals increase with field strength (FIGURE 7):

$$\mathscr{E} = v \cdot B \cdot d\tag{3}$$

for a conduction flowing perpendicular to the magnetic field, where $\mathscr{E}$ is the electric potential and d is the diameter of the vessel. The magnitude of the E-field associated with these potential changes is much lower than that needed for electrical excitation of the heart and it was concluded theoretically that the phenomenon is not important physiologically because, even at 10 T, the E-field in the aorta is 10 times less than the theoretical E-field needed for cardiac excitation.

Effects on the Electroencephalogram

Reports in the literature of magnetic field effects on brain waves led to a series of experiments using the cat and implanted electrodes. It appears that the effects are artifacts associated with electrode wire motion in the magnetic field as measured by C. Gaffey and myself (FIGURE 8).

Braking Effect on Flowing Conductors

Consider a pipe of blood flowing with velocity v perpendicular to the magnetic field (B). Once again, note that a force F on the conductors is given by

$$F \propto v \times B.\tag{4}$$

The current of ions associated with this force is related to the conductivity σ. This

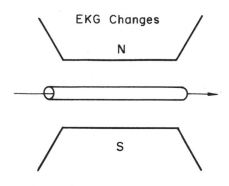

Potential = Field × Velocity × Diameter

(mvolts) = (Tesla)·(cm/sec)·(cm)

FIGURE 7. The magnetohydrodynamic braking force on blood flowing in a high magnetic field is dependent on the diameter of the vessel squared and on the B-field squared.

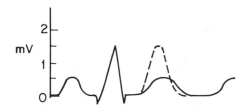

current is also perpendicular to the magnetic field and the flow. The result of the interaction of this current and the static field is another force that is in a direction opposite to the blood velocity (FIGURE 9):

$$-F = \sigma[(v \times B) \times B]. \tag{5}$$

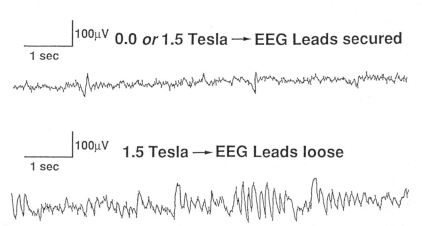

FIGURE 8. The mechanism for distortion of the electrocardiogram due to induced potentials from blood moving in a magnetic field.

An analysis of the magnitude of this retarding force by a number of workers led to the conclusion that the effect might be significant for large vessel flow with an expected requirement of a rise in blood pressure of 28% to maintain constant volume flow in the aorta at 10 T. However, this conclusion was found to be in error experimentally and theoretically.[9] No measurable flow slowing was noted at 4.7 T with flows of 7.0 L/min in tubing of 1.7-cm diameter. An analysis of the mathematical arguments leading to the theoretical conclusion that there should be at least a few percent effect at 4.7 T showed an error in the previous calculation. These new theoretical calculations show that there should be no significant effect on human circulatory dynamics.

Thus, with the exception of dizziness and nausea in some subjects at 4 T and the hazards from projectiles and implanted prostheses, there are no human exposure concerns that can be ascribed to static field effects alone.

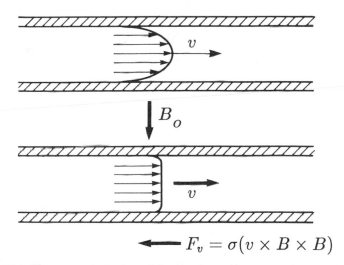

$$F_v = \sigma(v \times B \times B)$$

FIGURE 9. The magnetohydrodynamic braking force of ion currents in a magnetic field.

PHYSIOLOGICAL EFFECTS OF RAPIDLY SWITCHED GRADIENTS

From the early work of Mansfield,[10] it has been recognized that the spatial distribution of the NMR signal could be detected if the spatial gradients in x and y directions were changed very rapidly during a single free induction decay. Twelve years ago, the potential physiological effects were evaluated, which ranged from induction of light flashes (phosphenes) at about 2 T/s to cardiac excitation at a predicted value of 500 T/s. These effects were known to be dependent on the waveform, the B_{max} (rise time), and the duration of the time during which the oscillating gradients were applied (FIGURE 10). As the technique became more developed and was applied in human subjects to acquire images of moving organs (e.g., heart, kidneys, liver),[11] the threshold of neuromuscular excitation was reached at about 60 T/s.[12] Although there are no harmful effects noted at this level or at a

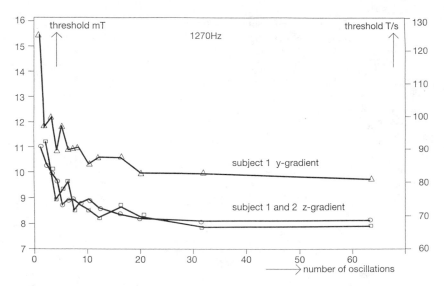

FIGURE 10. The results of experiments to determine the threshold of neuromuscular excitation from sinusoidal fields of different durations. The ordinate gives the maximum field for the oscillating gradient. This value can be converted to the $d\mathrm{B}/dt$ by multiplying by the frequency.

level of about 40 T/s where no sensations are noted in hundreds of studies as reported in this symposium, the human pain threshold is not much above 60 T/s for studies over the torso where the girth of the body gives a loop size for the induction of E-fields near 6 V/m. The value of 6 V/m is the level wherein neuromuscular stimulation is expected.[13] For current loops of smaller diameter (e.g., the heart), the $d\mathrm{B}/dt$ stimulation threshold is proportionally higher. Indeed, the cardiac muscle electrical properties suggest a stimulation threshold much higher than 6 V/m. Studies have now shown that ectopic beat (not fibrillation) can be induced at switched field rates of 600 T/s, but with a wide variability.[14-16] Studies in the ischemic heart and effects of concurrent sympathetic stimulation have not been completed, but it appears that the present level of human exposures is greater than 10 times below that required for human cardiac stimulation.

RF HEATING MEASUREMENT

Temperature elevation due to the absorbed energy associated with the RF power is the major measurable physiological effect of present and future NMR imaging and human spectroscopy studies. The absorbed power is generally given as watts per kilogram (SAR) and the physical characteristics of the SAR are discussed by Durney in this symposium. The mean temperature elevation can be determined from

$$\Delta T \ (^\circ\mathrm{C}) = \frac{\mathrm{SAR} \cdot \mathrm{time}}{\mathrm{specific\ heat}}. \tag{6}$$

For a specific absorbed power of 4 W/kg for 10 min, the maximum temperature rise is equal to 0.7 °C using the soft-tissue specific heat of 0.83 kcal/kg/°C (3.5 kJ/kg/°C).

The urge to go beyond 1.5 T is based on the need of spectroscopy and chemical shift imaging for higher signal-to-noise in order to measure the chemical composition of normal and pathological tissues using ^{1}H and ^{13}C spectroscopic techniques.[17] [31]P spectroscopy (which reveals the bioenergetic state, pH, and some lipid membrane signals) continues to be extensively investigated in the search for patterns of disease and clinical utility with good signal-to-noise at 1.5 T. This appears not to be the case for proton spectroscopy and carbon-13 spectroscopy, wherein signal-to-noise increases are needed to realize fully their potentials. The expected increase in signal-to-noise with field or frequency increases is shown in FIGURE 11.

RF HEATING CONSIDERATIONS AT 4–10 T (160 MHz)

Recent theoretical and experimental phantom studies[18] on a homogeneous sphere simulating the human head show the increase in absorbed power with frequency (FIGURE 12). Corroborating studies using a realistic layered model[19] show that the SAR increases quadratically with f below 200 MHz and linearly above 250 MHz. At 10 T, a 30°, 2-ms sinc pulse with 10 zero-crossings can be applied as fast as once every 13 ms for ^{1}H and once every 26 ms for ^{31}P and [23]Na without exceeding the FDA guidelines.

Fast imaging of the head with soft RF pulses can be performed at field strengths as high as 10 T. Localized spectroscopic studies of ^{1}H, ^{31}P, [23]Na, and ^{13}C with surface coils are feasible up to 10 T.

PROTON SPECTROSCOPY

Recently, proton spectroscopy has revealed rather specific patterns in prostate cancer, multiple sclerosis, and tumors of the central nervous system. The interesting

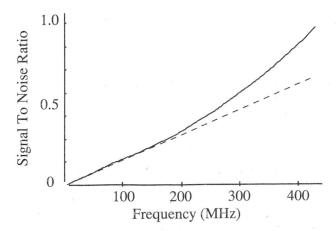

FIGURE 11. Signal-to-noise increases with frequency linearly up to about 80 MHz (about 2 T). Theoretical predictions show that, for the human head, there will be quadratic dependency between signal-to-noise and frequency above 80 MHz.[18]

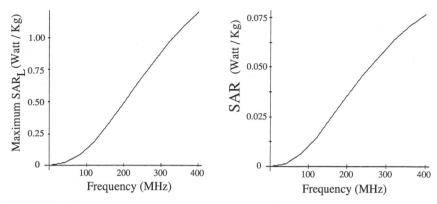

FIGURE 12. The maximum SAR$_L$ and the SAR are plotted versus frequency for a 20-cm-diameter sphere with appropriate frequency-dependent conductivity and dielectric properties. The data are for a 12-cm-diameter coil displaced 2 cm from the sphere. The RF for these studies was a 75-μm pulse with a repetition every 400 ms and with an amplitude to give a 35° tip in a volume element 5 cm into a sphere.[18]

findings of increased spectral peaks in regions for citrate in prostate cancer and for lactate and alanine in brain tumors are presently very active areas of medical science research. These results appear to have more promise than the ^{31}P studies and have led to enthusiasm to proceed with studies at fields higher than 1.5 T.

CARBON-13 SPECTROSCOPY

The body's capability to dissipate heat is particularly important for surface coil spectroscopy of metabolite content wherein proton decoupling is used in carbon-13 spectroscopy. Single frequency proton decoupling above 64 MHz is severely limited by the maximum LSAR. It can be shown that the normal heat conduction of muscle and fat will allow local absorption of as much as 20 W/kg in 2-cm-diameter regions with a local temperature elevation of only 1 °C. With normal circulation, there should be no appreciable temperature elevation. An example of proton-decoupled C-13 spectroscopy of the human calf is shown in FIGURE 13. In this case, the decoupling was broadband and an estimate of the deposited power in watts per kilogram per average power delivered by the surface coil was 1.16.[20] It is possible to significantly reduce the power deposition using other decoupling techniques (single shot), which have allowed studies on infants.[21]

HIGH RESOLUTION PROTON IMAGING

The discovery of new pulse sequences using reduced flip angles and gradient echoes led to fast scan methods enabling higher resolution and true three-dimensional imaging methods. These methods make practical submillimeter resolutions as shown in FIGURE 14 and quantitative three-dimensional studies as shown in

FIGURE 15. However, the methods come at some expense of an increase in average absorbed power due to the increase in the duty cycle. Thus, continual surveillance is required to avoid exceeding safe heat deposition levels.

SUMMARY

NMR imaging (MRI) and spectroscopy have been applied to an increasing number of patients and volunteers for 10 years. The field strength has increased by a factor of 10 since 1979 and the switched gradients have increased by over a factor of 10 since 1980. RF absorbed power has increased by almost a factor of 10 in many studies due to both the increase in frequency and the increase in duty cycle associated with new RF pulse protocols. Even with these increases, all available evidence argues that the clinical procedures offer no hazards to human subjects. Known hazards associated with flying ferromagnetic objects, internal prostheses, and wires or metal objects in contact with the skin of patients can be avoided.

Although hazards are not expected for the present procedures, emerging methods using fast scan strategies and higher frequency RF of the higher fields will

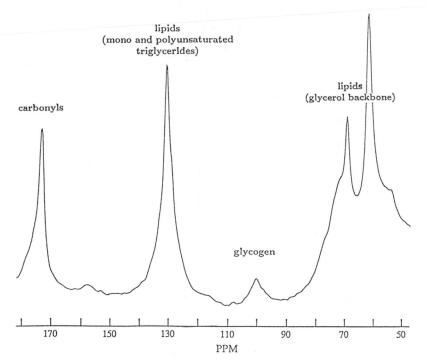

FIGURE 13. Glycogen ^{13}C spectra from the human calf detected by natural abundance ^{13}C (proton decoupled at 2.3 T using a doubly tuned surface coil and 20 min of acquisition—20,000 scans).

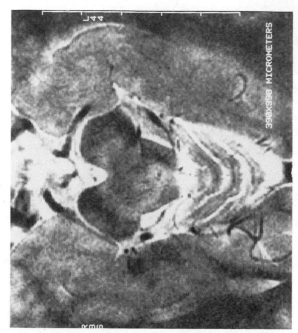

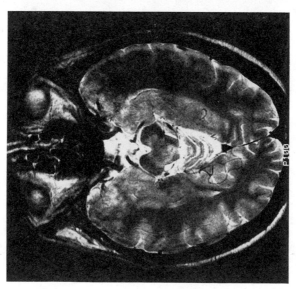

FIGURE 14. High resolution images showing the human hippocampus in a living subject with an in-plane resolution of 0.4 mm for a slice thickness of 1.5 mm.

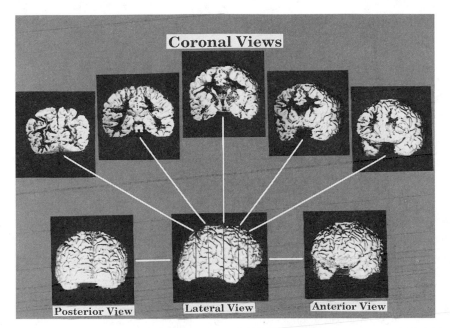

FIGURE 15. Three-dimensional volumetric techniques of NMR allow the acquisition of human brain data with the resolution of 1 mm and with the capability of separating the brain from the scalp and the white matter from the gray matter for quantitative studies of brain architecture.[25] Only 15 minutes of patient time was required in 1991 (compared to more than 2 hours to acquire similar information in 1980).

require a closer vigilance and will demand continuing experimental and theoretical work such as detailed in this symposium.

ACKNOWLEDGMENTS

The collaborators on the unreferenced work presented here to illustrate NMR advances are Felix Wehrli, Paul Lauterbur, Richard Newmark, and Cornelius Gaffey. The manuscript was prepared by Judy Blair.

REFERENCES

1. BUDINGER, T. F. 1979. IEEE Trans. Nucl. Sci. **NS26:** 2821–2825.
2. TENFORDE, T. S. & T. F. BUDINGER. 1987. Biological effects and physical safety aspects of NMR imaging and *in vivo* spectroscopy. *In* NMR in Medicine: The Instrumentation and Clinical Applications. Med. Phys. Monogr. Volume 14. S. R. Thomas & R. L. Dixon, Eds.: 493–548. AIP. New York.
3. PERSSON, B. R. R. & F. STAHLBERG. 1989. Health and Safety of Clinical NMR Examinations. CRC Press. Boca Raton, Florida.
4. MILHAM, S., JR. 1979. J. Occup. Med. **21:** 475–480.
5. ROCKETT, H. E. & V. C. ARENA. 1983. J. Occup. Med. **25:** 549–557.

6. BUDINGER, T. F., K. S. BRISTOL, C. K. YEN & P. WONG. 1984. Abstracts, Third Annual Meeting, Society of Magnetic Resonance in Medicine (New York, August 13–17), p. 113.
7. WIKSWO, J. P., JR. & J. P. BARACH. 1980. IEEE Trans. Biomed. Eng. **27:** 722.
8. GAFFEY, C. T., T. S. TENFORDE & E. E. DEAN. 1980. Bioelectromagnetics **1:** 209.
9. KELTNER, J. R., M. S. ROOS, P. R. BRAKEMAN & T. F. BUDINGER. 1990. Magn. Reson. Med. **16:** 139–149.
10. MANSFIELD, P. 1977. J. Phys. **C10:** L55–L58.
11. COHEN, M. S. & R. M. WEISSKOFF. 1991. Magn. Reson. Imag. **9:** 1–37.
12. BUDINGER, T. F., H. FISCHER, D. HENTSCHEL, H. E. REINFELDER & F. SCHMITT. 1991. J. Comput. Assist. Tomogr. In press.
13. REILLY, J. P. 1989. Med. Biol. Eng. Comput. **27:** 101–110.
14. SILNY, J. 1986. The influence of threshold of the time-varying magnetic field in the human organism. *In* Biological Effects of Static and Extremely Low Frequency Magnetic Fields. J. H. Bernhardt, Ed.: 105–112. M. M. Verlag. Munich.
15. BOURLAND, J. D., J. A. NYENHUIS, G. A. MOUCHAWAR, L. A. GEDDES, D. J. SCHAEFER & M. E. RIEHL. 1991. Abstracts, Tenth Annual Meeting, Society of Magnetic Resonance in Medicine (San Francisco, August 10–16), p. 969.
16. BUDINGER, T. F., K. N. BRENNAN, J. C. GILBERT, M. S. ROOS, S. T. WONG, F. SCHMITT & D. HENTSCHEL. 1991. Abstracts, Seventy-seventh Scientific Assembly and Annual Meeting of the Radiological Society of North America (Chicago, December 1–6).
17. COHEN, S. M., Ed. 1987. Ann. N.Y. Acad. Sci. Volume 508.
18. KELTNER, J. R., J. W. CARLSON, M. S. ROOS, S. T. S. WONG, T. L. WONG & T. F. BUDINGER. 1991. Magn. Reson. Med. In press.
19. WONG, S. T. S., J. R. KELTNER & M. S. ROOS. 1991. Abstracts, Tenth Annual Meeting, Society of Magnetic Resonance in Medicine (San Francisco, August 10–16), p. 971.
20. ALGER, J. F. 1987. Ann. N.Y. Acad. Sci. **508:** 414–416.
21. MOONEN, C. T., R. J. DIMAND & K. L. COX. 1988. Magn. Reson. Med. **6:** 140–157.
22. WEHRLI, F. W. 1991. Past, present, and future of magnetic resonance. *In* Clinical CT and MRI. D. Buthiau, Ed.: 111–126. Frison Roche. Paris.
23. ANDREW, E. R. 1986. NMR spectroscopy principles. *In* Medical Magnetic Resonance Imaging and Spectroscopy—A Primer. T. F. Budinger & A. R. Margulis, Eds.: 71–80. Society of Magnetic Resonance in Medicine. Berkeley, California.
24. LUYTEN, P. R., A. J. H. MARIEN, W. HEINDEL, P. H. J. VAN GERWEN, K. HERHOLZ, J. A. DEN HOLLANDER, G. FRIEDMANN & W-D. HEISS. 1990. Radiology **176:** 791–799.
25. BUDINGER, T. F., F. W. WEHRLI, H. W. CHUNG & S. J. ZINREICH. 1991. Abstracts, Tenth Annual Meeting, Society of Magnetic Resonance in Medicine (San Francisco, August 10–16), p. 751.

Interactions between Electromagnetic Fields and Biological Systems

CARL H. DURNEY

Electrical Engineering Department
and
Bioengineering Department
University of Utah
Salt Lake City, Utah 84112

INTRODUCTION

Because of their effectiveness in diagnostic medicine, magnetic resonance imaging (MRI) systems are routinely used in virtually every major hospital in the world. As more and more patients are being exposed to the electromagnetic (EM) fields produced by MRI systems, questions about patient safety are becoming more and more pressing. As MRI systems are improved, patients will be exposed to stronger static magnetic fields, to more intense, higher-frequency radio-frequency (rf) electromagnetic fields, and to more rapidly switched magnetic field gradients. The importance of studying the effects of these EM fields on patients and operating personnel to identify possible hazards and to ensure safety is obvious.

The complex problem of evaluating the effects of EM fields on the human body can be divided into two parts. One part is determining the EM fields inside the body, that is, the internal EM fields. These internal fields are usually found using macroscopic models of body tissue. The other part is using macroscopic and microscopic models of the body tissue to determine the effect of the internal EM fields on the tissue. It goes without saying that the interaction between systems that produce EM fields and the human body is complicated.

MRI systems typically generate three kinds of EM fields: (1) a static magnetic field, (2) switched (time-varying) magnetic field gradients, and (3) rf electric and magnetic fields. Finding the internal static magnetic field produced by the static magnetic field of the MRI system is easy because the human body is essentially transparent to static magnetic fields. Finding the internal EM fields produced by both the switched gradients and the rf fields is often difficult because the human body interacts strongly with the generating system (typically, the MRI gradient and rf magnetic field coils). The interaction includes effects such as near-field coupling and mutual coupling between sources and the body.

Internal EM fields cause two main effects on body tissue: (1) thermal effects, which are due to EM heating of tissue, and (2) more direct EM field effects, such as nerve and muscle stimulation and cellular effects. Because the biological system of the human body is highly electrical in nature, applied electromagnetic fields might be expected to affect that system drastically. Fortunately, however, the body in most cases seems to be well protected against external EM fields and is able to minimize their effects.

The purpose of this discussion is to review the basic principles of EM fields

19

needed to understand how EM fields affect the human body and to summarize characteristics and behaviors relevant to the effects of MRI systems on the human body.

SOME BASIC PRINCIPLES OF ELECTROMAGNETIC FIELD THEORY

Coulomb's Force Law

It is fascinating that all of classical electromagnetic field theory is based on the basic physical phenomenon that charges exert forces on each other. This force of attraction or repulsion is described by the familiar Coulomb's law,

$$F_1 = \frac{Q_1 Q_2}{4\pi\epsilon_0 R^2},\qquad(1)$$

where F_1 is the force on the charge Q_1 due to the presence of Q_2, as indicated in FIGURE 1, and ϵ_0 is the permittivity of free space. Because keeping track of forces on individual charges is too difficult, a force field called an electric field is defined to account for these interactions.

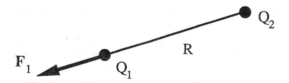

FIGURE 1. Force on charge Q_1 due to the presence of charge Q_2 (Coulomb's force law).

Definition of Electric and Magnetic Fields

The electric field at a given point in space is defined in terms of the force exerted on an infinitesimally small test charge Q placed at that point. The electric field strength at a point is defined as

$$E = F/Q,\qquad(2)$$

where F is the vector force on the test charge Q at that point (vectors are designated by boldface type). The units of electric field strength are volts/meter in the SI system of units, which is used throughout this discussion.

Another kind of force is exerted on moving charges. This force is accounted for by defining a magnetic flux density vector field as

$$B = F/Qv,$$

where F is the magnitude of the force on the test charge Q and v is the magnitude of the velocity of Q. In terms of vectors, the relationship between the magnetic flux density vector **B** and the force **F** is

$$F = Q(v \times B).\qquad(3)$$

Lorentz Force Equation

From these definitions of electric and magnetic fields, it follows that the force on a charge q in the presence of both an **E** and a **B** field is

$$\mathbf{F} = q(\mathbf{E} + \mathbf{v} \times \mathbf{B}). \tag{4}$$

This relationship is called the Lorentz force equation. It describes how the electric and magnetic fields affect charges.

An energy transfer relation can be derived from the Lorentz force equation to show how the internal **E** and **B** generated by MRI systems affect the human body. Multiplying **v** on both sides of equation 4 gives

$$P = \mathbf{v} \cdot \mathbf{F} = q(\mathbf{v} \cdot \mathbf{E} + \mathbf{v} \cdot \mathbf{v} \times \mathbf{B}) = q(\mathbf{v} \cdot \mathbf{E}) \tag{5}$$

because P, the rate of energy transfer (power), is the dot product of force and velocity and because $\mathbf{v} \cdot \mathbf{v} \times \mathbf{B} = 0$. From equation 5, it is clear that only the internal **E** field transfers energy to charges in the body and **B** does not transfer any energy. Thus, if an rf **B** could be generated without an accompanying **E**, the MRI fields would not heat the body. As explained later, an **E** is generated by a time-changing **B** and, except possibly at very low frequencies, it is not possible to produce the desired **B** without it inducing an **E**.

The Lorentz force equation is one of the basic EM field equations. Others are Maxwell's equations (reviewed next). For a person in an MRI system, the Lorentz force equation describes how the EM fields generated by the MRI system affect charges in the body. Maxwell's equations describe how charges generate EM fields, both the charges in the MRI coils, for example, and the charges in the patient's body. To find the interaction between the MRI systems and the human body, both sets of equations must be solved simultaneously.

Maxwell's Equations

Both the curl and the divergence of a vector are required to define the vector. Thus, the curl and divergence have come to be interpreted as sources of vectors. The defining equations in both point form and integral form for the electric field strength are

$$\nabla \times \mathbf{E} = -\partial \mathbf{B}/\partial t, \tag{6}$$

$$\oint \mathbf{E} \cdot d\mathbf{l} = -\int (\partial \mathbf{B}/\partial t) \cdot d\mathbf{S}, \tag{7}$$

$$\nabla \cdot \mathbf{E} = \rho/\epsilon_0, \tag{8}$$

$$\oint \mathbf{E} \cdot d\mathbf{S} = \int (\rho/\epsilon_0)\, d\mathbf{V}, \tag{9}$$

where ρ is the charge density. The first of these equations states that a time-varying **B** is a source (curl-type) of **E** and that the **E** field lines encircle the $-\partial \mathbf{B}/\partial t$ lines. These induced **E** fields cause currents in conducting material that are characteristically called eddy currents. In MRI systems, the rf **B** induces eddy-like **E** fields according to equation 6. Equation 7, which is the integral form of equation 6, means that the integral of **E** (potential difference at low frequencies) around any closed path is equal to the total magnetic flux passing through any surface bounded by that path. At low frequencies, this magnetic flux is described in terms of inductance. Thus, at low frequencies, equation 7 is equivalent to Kirchhoff's voltage law.

Equation 8 means that charge is also a source (divergence-type) of **E** and that **E** field lines begin and end on charge. Equation 9, which is the integral form of equation 8, means that the total electric flux passing out through any closed surface is proportional to the total charge enclosed within the surface (Gauss's law). In MRI systems, any accumulation of charge, at some point on a coil, for example, will generate an **E**.

The defining equations in point form and integral form for **B** are

$$\nabla \times \mathbf{B} = \mu_0(\mathbf{J} + \epsilon_0 \partial \mathbf{E}/\partial t), \tag{10}$$

$$\oint \mathbf{B} \cdot d\mathbf{l} = \mu_0 \int [\mathbf{J} + \epsilon_0(\partial \mathbf{E}/\partial t) \cdot d\mathbf{S}], \tag{11}$$

$$\nabla \cdot \mathbf{B} = 0, \tag{12}$$

$$\oint \mathbf{B} \cdot d\mathbf{S} = 0, \tag{13}$$

where μ_0 is the permeability of free space. Equation 10 means that current is a curl-type source of **B**. The current consists of two kinds—movement of charge and time-changing **E**. The latter kind of current is called displacement current. According to equation 10, the **B** field lines encircle the total current lines. Equation 11, which is the integral form of equation 10, means that the integral of **B** around any closed path is proportional to the total current passing through any surface bounded by that path. At low frequencies, the current on the right-hand side of equation 11 could correspond to conduction plus displacement current in a capacitor.

Equation 12 states that there are no divergence-type sources of **B**. Thus, according to equations 10 and 12, **B** field lines are always closed, unlike **E** field lines, which can begin and end on the charge.

Current Continuity Equation

Expressed in both point form and integral form, the current continuity relation is

$$\nabla \cdot \mathbf{J} = -\partial\rho/\partial t, \tag{14}$$

$$\oint \mathbf{J} \cdot d\mathbf{S} = \int(-\partial\rho/\partial t)\, d\mathbf{V}. \tag{15}$$

Equation 14 means that changing charge is a source of current. Equation 15 states that the total current passing out through any closed surface is equal to the time rate of change of the total charge within the surface; that is, charge is conserved.

GENERATION OF ELECTROMAGNETIC FIELDS

In this section, the characteristics of EM field sources, without interaction with the body, are reviewed.

Field Behavior as a Function of Frequency

Because the nature of EM fields is characteristically a strong function of frequency, much insight can be gained by considering field behavior as a function of frequency. It is interesting to note that the relatively concise EM equations reviewed earlier apply over a surprisingly wide range of frequencies—from zero all the way to the X-ray range. However, finding a general solution that is valid over this entire range is not practical. Consequently, special techniques that apply in limited frequency ranges have been developed.

Let L be the largest dimension of a system and let λ be the free-space wavelength of the EM fields. Then, field behavior can be characterized as follows:

$\lambda \gg L$ quasi-static field theory applies
             E, B are weakly coupled
             circuit theory is a valid approximation to EM field theory

$\lambda \sim L$ EM field theory must be used (microwave theory)
             E, B are strongly coupled

$\lambda \ll L$ optics and ray theory apply.

For wavelengths long compared to the size of the system, Maxwell's equations may be approximated by the simpler electric circuit theory. Quasi-static field theory also applies. An important feature of field behavior in this range is that the electric and magnetic fields are only weakly coupled. This can be seen from equations 6 and 10. At low frequencies, the time rate of change is small enough that the time derivatives on the right can sometimes be neglected. This is important in MRI systems because it means that, in this frequency range, an rf **B** can be generated with only a very weak accompanying **E**. Because, as explained earlier, only the internal **E** generates heat in the body, body heating can therefore be minimized by minimizing the rf **E**. In addition, when **B** is essentially uncoupled from **E**, it is much easier to obtain a uniform **B** field inside the body for imaging. Because the body is approximately nonmagnetic, it does not directly perturb the generated **B**. However, the body has strong dielectric properties and therefore greatly perturbs **E**. Hence, if the **B** is linked to an **E**, the body's effect on **E** will also affect **B**.

In the second range listed, circuit theory is not valid and Maxwell's equations must be solved without the low-frequency approximations that are so useful in the lower-frequency ranges. Furthermore, in this range, **E** and **B** are strongly coupled. One cannot be generated without the other. In MRI systems, therefore, it may be impossible in this range to reduce the internal **E** field enough to avoid substantial body heating.

In the third range, field behavior is usually most conveniently characterized in terms of rays and beams using appropriate optical or ray techniques.

Quasi-static Field Generation

In the range where the quasi-static field approximation is valid, sources of **E** and **B** can be typified as E-type, B-type, and combinations of these two.

E-type sources are those in which charge is the dominant source, and equation 8

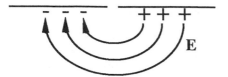

FIGURE 2. Example of an E-type source (capacitor plates).

describes the generation of **E**. The **B** fields generated are very weak because they are produced by time-varying **E**, which in the quasi-static case is not strong. A simple coplanar capacitor is shown in FIGURE 2 as a typical example of an E-type source. Charge accumulates on the plates and the E-field lines begin and end on the charge. In MRI systems, charge can accumulate at any two points between which there exists a potential difference. This charge will then produce an **E** field, which in MRI systems is usually undesirable.

B-type sources are those in which charge is negligible and current is the dominant source, for which equation 10 describes the generation of **B**. A time-changing **B** then generates an **E**, as described by equation 6. This secondarily generated **E** is often negligible in the quasi-static case, depending on how slowly **B** is changing with time. The simple current loop shown in FIGURE 3 is an example of a B-type source. Because the current is uniform, $\nabla \cdot \mathbf{J} = 0$ and there is no charge density to generate a primary **E**. The **B**-field lines encircle the current. The characteristic secondary **E** circulating around **B** produces eddy currents in conducting media. In MRI systems operating in the quasi-static range, it is this kind of **E** that typically causes heating in the human body. Because these eddy fields are generated by the time-varying **B**, they are impossible to eliminate. The higher the frequency, the stronger these eddy fields are and the more serious problem they can pose.

FIGURE 4 shows an example of a combination of E-type and B-type sources. The gap in the current loop causes an accumulation of charge, which then produces a primary **E**. The current in the loop also produces a **B**, which in turn generates a secondary **E**. The resultant **E** is a combination of these two. In the quasi-static case, experience indicates that the primary **E** produced by the charge is frequently much

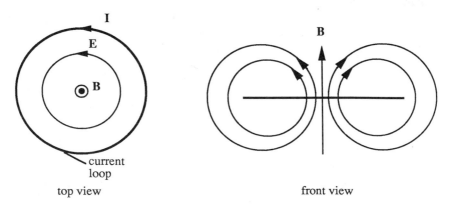

FIGURE 3. Example of a B-type source (current loop).

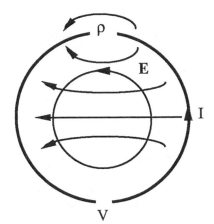

FIGURE 4. Example of a combination of E-type and B-type sources.

stronger than the secondary **E**. Avoiding any accumulation of charge will reduce **E** by avoiding primary generation of **E**.

Higher-Frequency Field Generation

At frequencies in the second range, where the quasi-static field theory does not apply, sources are not easily categorized as either E-type or B-type. FIGURE 5 shows an example of how a current loop can generate both primary **E** and **B**, even though it does not contain a gap like the one in FIGURE 4. In this case, the current reverses direction halfway around the loop because the frequency is high. Consequently, the divergence of **J** is no longer zero, charge accumulates even though there is no gap, and this charge generates a primary **E**. Calculations show that this primary **E** dominates over the secondary **E** so that the resultant **E** is like that shown in the figure.

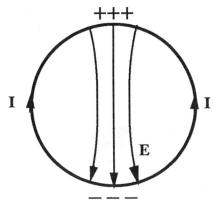

FIGURE 5. Electric field produced by a current loop at higher frequencies.

At higher frequencies, **E** and **B** are strongly coupled and one cannot be generated without the other. One consequence of this is that the human body, even though it is largely nonmagnetic, will strongly affect **B** through its dielectric effect on **E**.

Near Fields, Far Fields

The fields generated by sources are often characterized as near fields or far fields. Near fields, as the name implies, are those fields in regions near the source. These fields typically contain terms like $1/r^3$, $1/r^2$, and $1/r$, where r is the distance from the source. Near fields usually vary more rapidly with space than those farther from the source. Far fields are those fields in regions farther away from the source. Far fields typically vary as $1/r$. Far fields are usually simpler mathematically and conceptually. Analysis of near fields is usually much more difficult than analysis of far fields.

MACROSCOPIC TISSUE MODEL

This section describes a model that accounts for the interaction of source fields and tissue on a macroscopic scale.

Permittivity and Permeability

The complicated system of charges in materials interacts with applied EM fields in two basic ways. First, the applied **E** and **B** exert forces on the charges in the material, which produce a new pattern of charges. This new charge pattern acts as a source of **E** and **B** and produces additional EM fields to those originally applied. The combination of these two effects produces net EM fields and charge patterns different from those that would exist without the interaction. These effects on the charges in the material and the generation of fields by the altered charge patterns can both be accounted for by combining the current resulting from the forces on charges with equation 10. The current produced in the material by the applied fields is

$$\mathbf{J}_m = \sigma\mathbf{E} + \epsilon_0\chi\partial\mathbf{E}/\partial t + \nabla \times \mathbf{M}, \qquad (16)$$

where σ is conductivity, χ is electric susceptibility, and **M** is magnetization. The σ accounts for the drift of conduction charges. The χ accounts for two kinds of polarization. One is the separation of charge produced by the applied **E**, which is called induced polarization. The other is orientation of electric dipoles in the material by the applied **E**. In the absence of the applied **E**, the electric dipoles in the material are randomly oriented because of thermal excitation. The applied **E** causes a slight orientation of these dipoles, which produces a net polarization. Similarly, the magnetic dipoles are randomly oriented in the absence of applied fields because of thermal excitation. The slight orientation of each dipole by the applied magnetic field creates an average orientation that is called the magnetization **M**.

Adding the material current of equation 16 to the current in equation 10 results in

$$\nabla \times \mathbf{B} = \mu_0[\mathbf{J} + \sigma\mathbf{E} + \epsilon_0(\chi + 1)\partial\mathbf{E}/\partial t + \nabla \times \mathbf{M}].$$

Collecting terms gives

$$\nabla \times (\mathbf{B}/\mu_0 - \mathbf{M}) = \mathbf{J} + \sigma\mathbf{E} + \epsilon_0\chi\partial\mathbf{E}/\partial t.$$

With the following definitions,

$$\mathbf{B}/\mu_0 - \mathbf{M} = \mathbf{H}, \tag{17}$$

$$\epsilon = \epsilon_0(1 + \chi), \tag{18}$$

$$\mathbf{M} = \chi_m\mathbf{H}, \tag{19}$$

and

$$\mu = \mu_0(1 + \chi_m), \tag{20}$$

the results are

$$\nabla \times \mathbf{H} = \mathbf{J} + \sigma\mathbf{E} + \epsilon\partial\mathbf{E}/\partial t \tag{21}$$

and

$$\mathbf{B} = \mu\mathbf{H}. \tag{22}$$

Here, $\mathbf{H}$ is defined as magnetic field intensity, ϵ is permittivity, χ_m is magnetic susceptibility, μ_0 is the permeability of free space, and μ is the permeability of a material. The units of $\mathbf{H}$ are amperes/meter. Because the human body is largely nonmagnetic, $\mu = \mu_0$ for body tissue and $\mathbf{B} = \mu_0\mathbf{H}$ both inside the body and out. The definition, $\mathbf{D} = \epsilon\mathbf{E}$, where $\mathbf{D}$ is displacement flux density, is also made.

For the sinusoidal steady-state case, a complex permittivity is defined as

$$\epsilon = \epsilon_0(1 + \chi + \sigma/j\omega\epsilon_0) = \epsilon_0(\epsilon' - j\epsilon''), \tag{23}$$

where $j = \sqrt{-1}$. Relative permittivity is defined as $\epsilon_r = \epsilon/\epsilon_0$; $\epsilon' - j\epsilon''$ is the complex relative permittivity.

In this macroscopic model, the conductivity, permittivity, and permeability account for all the interactions between the applied EM fields and the material. It is fortunate that such a complex interaction can be modeled in this relatively simple way.

The permittivity of tissue varies strongly with frequency, as indicated by FIGURES 6 and 7, which show the average values of measured results for muscle tissue as compiled by William Hurt.[1] In the frequency range of typical MRI systems, though, neither the conductivity nor the permittivity is changing rapidly. The values for other tissues can be significantly different from those of muscle. For example, at 100 MHz, the conductivity of fat is about one-tenth of that of muscle and the permittivity of fat is about one-seventh of that of muscle.

Energy Absorption

Energy absorption in tissue is described by

$$P = \omega\epsilon_0\epsilon''|\mathbf{E}|^2 = \sigma|\mathbf{E}|^2 \quad [\text{W/m}^3], \tag{24}$$

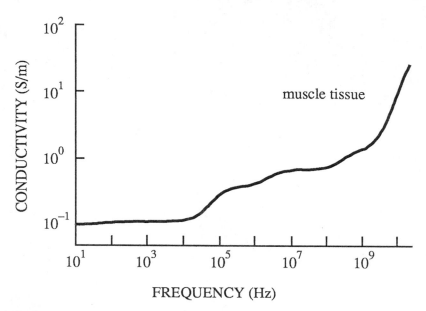

FIGURE 6. Average conductivity of muscle tissue as a function of frequency (after William Hurt[1]).

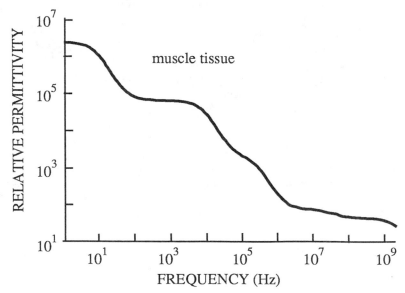

FIGURE 7. Average relative permittivity of muscle tissue as a function of frequency (after William Hurt[1]).

where P is the density of the rate of energy absorption or the density of power absorption and $\mathbf{E}$ is the rms electric field strength. The σ and ϵ'' describe the lossiness of the material. The loss tangent or dissipation factor is defined as $\tan \delta = \epsilon''/\epsilon'$. Generally speaking, the wetter a tissue is, the greater the σ and ϵ'' and the greater the power absorption for a given $\mathbf{E}$.

The bioelectromagnetics community has adopted the term specific absorption rate (SAR) defined by

$$ \text{SAR} = P/\rho_m = \omega\epsilon_0\epsilon''|\mathbf{E}|^2/\rho_m = \sigma|\mathbf{E}|^2/\rho_m, \tag{25} $$

where ρ_m is the mass density in kg/m^3. "Specific" refers to the normalization to mass density and "absorption rate" refers to the rate of energy absorption.

INTERACTIONS BETWEEN FIELD SOURCES AND THE HUMAN BODY

Near-Field, Mutual Coupling

As explained previously, electric and magnetic fields are generated by charge and currents, such as those in MRI coils. The generated EM fields interact with the charges in the body, as described by the macroscopic tissue model. This interaction includes the effect of the charges in the body back on the generated fields. Thus, the calculation of the fields inside the body must include the effect of the fields on the body and the effect of the body back on the fields; that is, the presence of the body changes the current in the coils. This two-way interaction is described in terms of mutual coupling. When the body is far enough away from the field-generating sources, mutual coupling can usually be neglected, which simplifies the analysis. When the body is close to the field-generating system, as it usually is in MRI systems, mutual coupling cannot be neglected and the determination of the internal fields is much more complicated than without mutual coupling.

When the body is close to the field-generating sources, it is in the near-field region, as explained earlier. This also makes the determination of the internal body fields more complicated because commonly used far-field simplifying approximations cannot be used and far-field characteristics may not apply. For example, skin depth is defined as the depth from the surface of an object at which the $\mathbf{E}$ has decayed to e^{-1} of its value at the surface. The concept of skin depth is useful because it describes how fields penetrate objects. The skin depth for a plane wave incident on a lossy dielectric planar half-space is easily calculated. A plot of skin depth for a half-space with permittivity equal to two-thirds of that of muscle is shown in FIGURE 8. The permittivity is taken to be two-thirds of that of muscle because that is approximately the average permittivity of the human body. FIGURE 8 shows that the skin depth decreases rapidly with frequency, indicating that it is difficult to get fields to penetrate the human body at higher frequencies. Although this trend probably applies to near-field interactions, the calculated results for the plane wave (far-field) case shown in FIGURE 8 certainly do not apply to MRI systems where the body is very close to the field-generating system, and there is little resemblance to plane wave propagation.

Similarly, the whole-body average SAR shown in FIGURE 9 indicates how plane wave absorption in models of the human body in free space varies with frequency. Although this might again give some useful information about absorption trends, it certainly does not apply to MRI systems.

Effects of Body Inhomogeneities

In the quasi-static frequency range, body structure has little direct effect on the internal magnetic fields because the body is nonmagnetic. However, the body structure has a large effect on the electric field because the permittivity of tissue is

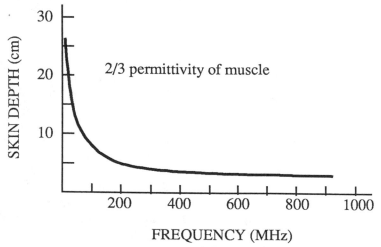

FIGURE 8. Skin depth as a function of frequency for a plane wave incident on a lossy dielectric half-space with a permittivity equal to two-thirds of that of muscle tissue.

relatively high. When the magnetic field is strongly coupled to the electric field, the magnetic field will also be affected by inhomogeneities in the body.

Insight into the effects of body structure can be gained from the boundary conditions for electric fields, which are summarized in FIGURE 10. Because the tangential components of **E** must be continuous at a boundary between tissues of two different permittivities, the presence of the boundary does not disrupt the tangential components. However, the boundary disrupts the normal components significantly because the normal components must be discontinuous by the ratio of the permittivities. Thus, in any configuration containing dielectric boundaries normal to the **E** fields produced by the source, inhomogeneities will have a great effect on the internal field distribution. This may mean, for example, that internal field distributions produced by a given source will vary greatly from one patient to the next.

Some rf sources may also overheat the fat in some patients, as is well known

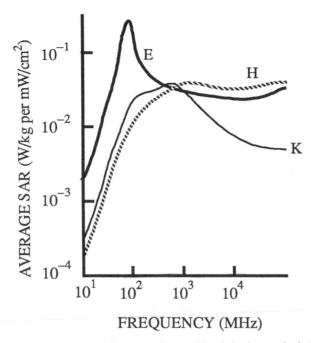

FREQUENCY (MHz)

FIGURE 9. SAR as a function of frequency for models of the human body in free space, irradiated by a plane wave: E stands for E polarization (incident **E** parallel to the long axis of the body), H stands for H polarization (incident **H** parallel to the long axis of the body), K stands for K polarization (propagation vector parallel to the long axis of the body).

among those who design electromagnetic applicators to produce hyperthermia for cancer therapy. When **E** is normal to a fat-muscle interface, the **E** in the fat can be much greater than in the muscle because the permittivity of fat is roughly ten times less than that of muscle. The reason for the fat overheating is illustrated in FIGURE 11 for the simple case of planar layers in which **E** is constant. At 100 MHz, the relative permittivity for fat is approximately $\epsilon_f = 10 - j10.79$. For muscle, it is

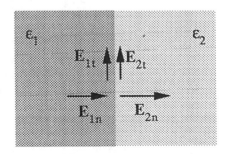

FIGURE 10. Boundary conditions on an electric field.

$$\mathbf{E}_{1t} = \mathbf{E}_{2t} \qquad \epsilon_1 \mathbf{E}_{1n} = \epsilon_2 \mathbf{E}_{2n}$$

approximately $\epsilon_m = 70 - j107.85$. From equation 24, the ratio of the P in the fat to the P in the muscle is given by

$$P_f/P_m = \epsilon_f''|E_f|^2/\epsilon_m''|E_m|^2. \qquad (26)$$

Because the boundary conditions require $\epsilon_f E_f = \epsilon_m E_m$, equation 26 becomes

$$P_f/P_m = \epsilon_f''|\epsilon_m|^2/\epsilon_m''|\epsilon_f|^2 = 7.64. \qquad (27)$$

Thus, the fat will be heated much more than the muscle. This simple analysis for a planar model illustrates the more general characteristic that normal **E** tends to overheat fat at a fat-muscle interface. Surface coils, in particular, should be checked to see whether they produce normal **E** fields strong enough to cause the fat to heat excessively.

Methods of Calculating Internal Fields

As MRI systems are developed for operation at higher and higher frequencies, design and analysis become more and more complicated. When quasi-static tech-

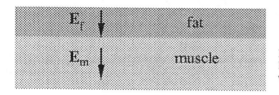

FIGURE 11. Electric fields in planar layers of fat and muscle illustrating why fat overheats.

niques no longer apply, other methods are needed. Because the calculations must include near-field mutual coupling, analytical mathematical techniques probably cannot be used for a detailed analysis that includes a moderately realistic representation of the human body and numerical EM techniques must be used.

Significant advances in computing power have led to ever more powerful numerical EM techniques that could be used for evaluating patient safety in MRI systems. Although a detailed description of numerical EM techniques is beyond the scope of this discussion, some general comments about the field may provide some perspective about how numerical techniques can be useful.

Numerical EM techniques can be classified as numerical methods for solving Maxwell's equations in either (1) the finite-difference approximation of partial differential equations or (2) a discrete approximation to integral equations. The finite-difference time-domain (FDTD) technique, the finite-element analysis, the transmission-line method (TLM), and the method of moments are some of the more well-known and commonly used techniques.

Numerical EM techniques all have some common limitations. They require a lot of computer memory and computation time. In addition, some of them are limited in the degree to which the models represent the structure being analyzed. Finite-difference techniques, for example, are usually based on rectangular mathematical cells, which do not represent curved objects very well. Nonetheless, these numerical methods are powerful and could be useful for analyzing and designing MRI systems.

MRI SYSTEM CHARACTERISTICS

The previous sections reviewed some of the fundamentals of EM theory important for understanding how MRI systems can affect patients. In this section, some of the characteristics of the MRI system are discussed in terms of these concepts.

The categorization of system behavior in terms of the wavelength ranges given earlier is approximate, of course, and the transition between the ranges is very gradual. Some numbers for wavelength as a function of frequency will help put these characteristic field behaviors in perspective for MRI systems:

Frequency (MHz)	Wavelength (meters)
1	300
10	30
100	3
200	1.5
300	1

First, it is obvious that MRI systems will never fall into the third category where the size of the system is very large compared to a wavelength. MRI systems operating near 1 MHz could probably be safely categorized in the long wavelength range, but those operating at and above 100 MHz could not. Advancements in MRI systems that require operation at higher frequencies are pushing the systems from the quasi-static range into the middle range, where some of the advantages of quasi-static operation are lost.

The increased complexity of operation in the middle wavelength range can be illustrated by considering the approximate equivalent circuit of a simple one-turn surface coil shown in FIGURE 12. The capacitances represent the distributed capacitance between various parts of the coil. At low frequencies, these small capacitances can be neglected, the coil looks inductive, and the current is uniform around the coil. A secondary **E** will be generated by the time-changing **B**, but there will be no primary **E** generated. At higher frequencies where the capacitive reactances are not negligible, a much different behavior can result. The current through the capacitances will cause the current to not be uniform around the coil, there will be potential differences between various points of the coil, and the resulting accumulation of charge will generate primary **E** fields, perhaps strong ones. Additional capacitances, not shown in the figure, will couple the fields to the body. The coupled **E** normal to the fat-muscle interface could heat the fat excessively.

One of the main advantages lost in going from the quasi-static range to the middle range is the weak coupling between **B** and **E**. Designers of advanced MRI systems operating at higher frequencies face two major problems stemming from the closer coupling between **E** and **B**: (1) the permittivity of the body will make **E** very inhomogeneous inside the body and the strong coupling between **E** and **B** will cause

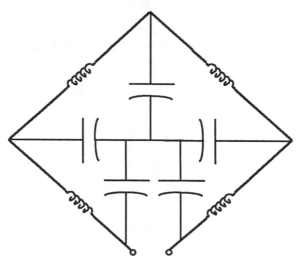

FIGURE 12. Approximate equivalent circuit of a surface coil.

B also to be inhomogeneous; (2) unavoidably stronger **E** fields will be generated inside the patients. The first problem is related primarily to proper operation of the MRI system. The second problem is one of patient safety. Will the greater heating produced by the stronger internal **E** fields be hazardous to the patient? Will the stronger internal **E** fields produce other undesirable effects, such as nerve stimulation? These questions need to be answered by both calculations and measurements. The numerical EM techniques discussed earlier should be implemented to help provide the answers.

REFERENCE

1. Durney, C. H., H. Massoudi & M. F. Iskander. 1986. Radiofrequency Radiation Dosimetry Handbook. Fourth edition, p. 4.52–4.53. USAFSAM-TR-85-73. USAF School of Aerospace Medicine, Aerospace Medical Division (AFSC), Brooks Air Force Base, Texas 78235-5301.

Molecular and Cellular Responses to Orientation Effects in Static and Homogeneous Ultra High Magnetic Fields

J. D. DE CERTAINES

Laboratoire de Résonance Magnétique en Biologie et Médecine
Faculté de Médecine
Université de Rennes
and
Centre Anti-Cancéreux Eugène Marquis
35043 Rennes, France

INTRODUCTION

The biological effects of magnetic fields have stimulated the curiosity of the human species since the beginning of time. This very old, yet very new, subject has led to a multitude of observations, but until quite recently scientific evidence has been hidden in a cloud of magic and even deliberate fraud.[1] Most of the work in this field is relatively recent; according to T. S. Tenforde, nearly 90% of the work published in the twentieth century has been reported since 1960.[2] Unfortunately, all of these reports cannot be used to establish a solid basis of knowledge due to insufficient rigor in the methodology (for review, see references 3 and 4). Scientific analysis is hindered both by wide variability in the characteristics of magnetic fields (intensity, stability, uniformity) and by overly complex biological models, often involving whole animals. This makes it impossible to distinguish among the large number of potential sites and mechanisms of action and retroaction. Consequently, very little of the huge mass of contradictory data can be used to ascertain what truly is a cause of potential effects on the living organism. If progress is to be made in this field, work must be based on subcellular and cellular systems. Investigations using well-known nonbiological models, for example, liquid crystals, can provide information necessary for understanding the effects of magnetic fields on the ordered arrangements of biomolecules.

Macroscopic theories explaining the effects of magnetic fields deal mainly with the orientation effect, the concentration in a field gradient, magnetohydrodynamics, and nervous conduction. Microscopic theories (spin-exclusion mechanism), proposed despite the absence to date of any convincing experimental data to explain the effect on chemical reactions,[5,6] shall not be discussed here. The major concern shall be centered on the orientation effects that a constant uniform field produces on organized multiple molecular systems. These effects are based on well-documented experimental results and open perspectives for a wide range of potential applications in medicine.

PRINCIPLES OF THE ORIENTATION EFFECT IN A CONSTANT AND UNIFORM FIELD: EXAMPLE OF LIQUID CRYSTALS

Orientation Energy of an Isolated Molecule

The energy of interaction between a field B and a diamagnetic molecule is defined by the equation,

$$U = -\frac{1}{2} \int_v X B^2 \, dv,$$

where X is the magnetic susceptibility tensor, v is the volume of the biological structure, and B is the magnetic field applied. Thus, the energy in an MRS magnet at 3 T is nine times greater than that in an MRI magnet at 1 T.

Particles or molecules with magnetic anisotropy properties are oriented under the effect of a constant and uniform external magnetic field. If anisotropy susceptibility is great enough, one can expect to observe a turning torque proportional to the difference $(X_1 - X_r)$ between the axial and the radial principal volume susceptibilities, the effective volume V of the molecule, the angle a between the anisotropic axis of the molecule and the external field B, and the square of the magnetic field:

$$U = -(1/2)V B^2 (X_1 - X_r) \cos^2 a.$$

The magnetic potential energy at $a = 90°$ has been conveniently assigned as the zero reference. When a particle or molecule has diamagnetic anisotropy and $(X_{axial} - X_{radial}) > 0$, it will orient parallel to the applied field in order to reach a minimum level of magnetic potential energy. It will orient perpendicular to the applied field if $(X_{axial} - X_{radial}) < 0$.

Because the diamagnetic anisotropy of isolated molecules is generally so small, until now only very sensitive techniques, for instance, birefringence,[7,8] could detect the resulting orientation in magnetic fields.

In a single alpha-helical segment containing 25 peptide bonds, for example, the diamagnetic anisotropy is of the same order of magnitude as the diamagnetic anisotropy of a single aromatic residue. According to the calculation made by Chabre,[9] the orientation energy for a single alpha-helical segment is $10^{-28} \cdot B^2$, where B is the external field (in gauss). Even without accounting for possible interaction forces, the orientation energy must be greater than the thermal energy ($kT = 4.1 \times 10^{-14}$ ergs at 25 °C), which would require extremely high fields. Conversely, one can estimate the number of parallel alpha-helical peptides required to produce significant orientation in a field of 1 T for a protein assembly carrying only parallel alpha helices, that is, 10^7 peptides.

Large molecules such as biopolymers (actin, collagen, fibrin, etc.) can be oriented when placed in a strong magnetic field.[10-14] Conditions for an effect on large molecules have been calculated by Dorfman.[15] In general, strong fields of 1 to 10 T are required for such an orientation to develop.

Orientation of Multiple Molecular Systems: Example of Liquid Crystals

The orientability of large ordered systems, for example, liquid crystals or their biological analogues, can be increased by adding the effects on each component molecule. Orientation can be obtained with fields of 1 T or even less.

The major axis of a nematic system tends to orient along the lines of an external field B. However, a nematic system is not an isolated molecule, but rather a very large assembly of ordered molecules, approximately 10^{20}, all turning together. Thus, the coupling energy is no longer that of an isolated molecule, that is, 5×10^{-21}, but rather 0.5 ergs[16] and therefore much greater than kT, making it possible for the multiple molecular system to turn as a unit in B.

Many workers have investigated these orientation effects in liquid crystals.[17] For example, a field B parallel to the free surface of a nematic liquid crystal creates a structure of crests and valleys if the component molecules are arranged perpendicularly to the surface. If the molecules are arranged parallel to the free surface, applying a field B perpendicular to this surface creates a network of hills and funnels. As early as the late 1960s, such theoretical structures were verified experimentally with fields as weak as 0.3 T.

Early observations were also made of changes in the L period of the helicoidal structure of a cholesteric system and of subsequent unwinding of the helix leading to a transition cholesteric-nematic system above a certain field intensity. For cholesteric systems having a large period, approximately 10 microns, transition towards a nematic structure occurs in a field of about 1 T. The characteristic times of magnetical orientation of such systems depend both on the field intensity and on the parameters of the systems themselves: size, viscosity, rigidity, and anisotropy of magnetic susceptibility.

These phenomena have interested physicists because weak structural transitions can greatly modify optical properties. Biologists have been interested because of analogies between membrane structures and liquid crystal structures.[18,19] Spin probe studies of multilayered lipid membranes have shown that phospholipid molecules orient in a constant magnetic field.[20,21] Furthermore, liquid crystal structures in biological systems apparently involve more than membranes (nucleic acids, proteins), offering perspectives for the study of the effects of magnetic fields on the organization of subcellular structures. For instance, it has been demonstrated that solutions of rodlike virus particles, which become lyotropic liquid crystals at concentrations above 1%, can be kept macroscopically aligned in a field of about 6 T.[22] Such an effect at less than 1 T has been observed by anisotropic absorption of ultrasonic waves.[23]

ORIENTATION EFFECTS IN MEMBRANE MODELS: RESULTS OBTAINED WITH RED BLOOD CELLS

Membrane Models and Possible Action of a Magnetic Field

Keeping in mind the example of liquid crystals, it would be interesting to analyze classical models of biological membranes, examining their potential susceptibility to the orientation action of a magnetic field.

It is impossible to act on a system that is too rigid, that is, rich in strong intermolecular bonds. This means that certain models cannot be used, for example, the model described in 1943 by Danielli and Davson based on electrostatic bonds between phospholipids and proteins forming a coherent, physically stable structure. In the 1950s, Parpart and Ballentine investigated the extraction of lipids bound to erythrocyte membranes. Their work led to early micellar models based on masses of globular protein scattered throughout a layer of phospholipid, with more than half of the bonds holding the lipids together being weak hydrophobic bonds. This conception suggests much greater membrane flexibility because the threshold of energy required for membrane deformation would be much lower.

Later, in 1964, Lucy and Glavert produced a model of cell membranes formed by a central layer of lipid formed by spherical micellae lying within a surrounding layer of protein. Although the possibility of membrane distortion from the Parpart and Ballentine model was retained, this newer micellar model also distinguished between the protein and lipid portions of the membrane. In 1966, Green proposed an assembly of lipoprotein subunits binding the protein structure more closely to the lipid configuration. Kavanau,[24] investigating the work of Luzzati and Reiss-Husson[19] on an artificial phospholipid-water model, emphasized that structural phases could undergo modifications depending upon the site on the membrane and upon the functional status of the cell. In this model, the structural conformation of the membrane results from the phospholipid elements that, by inducing transconformation of the protein portion, can act on the functional element.

In order to better understand the effects of magnetic fields, the analysis of experimental data should be based on certain characteristics of these models: (i) the presence of weak bonds proposed by Parpart and Ballentine refuting the rigid model of Danielli and Davson, (ii) the more intimate relationship between protein structure and lipid configuration as introduced by Green, and (iii) the more dynamic conception of the membrane structure as formulated by Kavanau from the work of Luzzati.[25]

Now, a model proposed by Bothorel and Lussan[26-28] that satisfies these three requirements shall be discussed. This model considers that (i) the lipid-protein bonds are essentially hydrophobic, (ii) the polar groups of the lipids are on the surface and the proteins lie within the membrane, and (iii) there can be two configurations, "open" and "closed", corresponding to different states of permeability and enzyme activity. In the closed configuration, each phospholipid opens up, interlinking the proteins and rendering the membrane as impermeable as possible. In the open configuration, the lipid chains form intramolecular and intermolecular bonds and tend to fold up on themselves, thus favoring membrane permeability. In this model, phospholipids take on two different orientations depending on the membrane configuration phase. They are perpendicular to the plane of the membrane in the open configuration and they tend toward a position tangent to the surface in the closed configuration. Depending upon the orientation of these molecules in relation to the magnetic field, their orientation could either be reinforced or modified, or at least facilitated, during transition between the two configurations. According to Lussan and Bothorel, membrane pores are dynamic and not static structures. Therefore, the probability of their existing could be increased by a magnetic field.

In the open configuration, membrane permeability is greatest and phospholipids are aligned in their most regular configuration. The degree of regularity could be enhanced by the action of a magnetic field. Increased membrane permeability has indeed been observed under the action of a magnetic field in work reported by Bresler and Bresler,[29,30] Aoki et al.,[31] Piruzyan and Kuznetsov,[32] Simonov et al.,[33] Pierron,[34] and Chalazonitis et al.[35]

Changes in the configuration of proteins positioned within the membrane depend upon interactions with the lipid molecules and could be associated with modified activity. Bothorel and Lussan explain the regulation of membrane enzyme activity by the following process of ionic action: (i) variation in the composition of the aqueous medium, (ii) reorientation of the lipid chains, (iii) modification of the tertiary structure of the enzyme trapped in the membrane, and (iv) triggering of enzyme activity dependent on the protein's tertiary structure. The orientation effect of a constant magnetic field on the lipid chains could induce reorientation independently of variations in the composition of the aqueous medium.

Another question to discuss is whether the effect of a magnetic field is sufficient to induce reorientation of a biological system or if it simply acts as a catalyzer during transition in a system about to change its configuration phase. Does the magnetic field act as an inducer or is it simply a catalyzer?

Based on work with multiple laminar vesicles at temperatures close to the critical temperature T_c for phase transition, Liburdy and Tenforde[36] believe that the effect of a moderate field would be insufficient to break the chemical bonds and could only be effective near the T_c. In their liposome model at 40.5 °C, the calculated threshold for obtaining an orientation effect (as a function of Boltzmann thermal energy) is 12 mT, not accounting for stabilization forces of the membrane phospholipids: intergroup bonds, van der Waals forces, and the excluded volume effect.

Experimental Results on Red Blood Cells

The red blood cell provides a simple and well-known model for testing this orientation effect on membranes. After exposing erythrocyte sediments to a 0.79-T field, there was no cellular lysis, but the number of cells having a deformed aspect was nearly four times greater than that for control cells.[37] Scan electron microscopy showed that the deformed cells were essentially discocrenated forms and more rarely spherocrenated forms, which are different from prelytic forms occurring in an irreversible process.[25] In a 1.2-T field, Pierron[34] showed that these deformations occurred after 20 to 25 minutes of exposure. Under these conditions, potassium leakage, increased ATP production, and more remarkable specific antibody reactions have been observed. These variations are reversible and the normal situation is reestablished within 30 minutes after removing the field.

If one considers the red blood cell membrane as a liquid crystal structure,[38] the hypotheses suggested earlier could explain the observed results. The transconfiguration of the membrane receptor sites could explain the modification in antibody sensitivity.

The same hypothesis applied to mitochondrial membranes could explain the increased ATP production observed by Pierron. The model of Bothorel and Lussan, cited earlier, can be applied to mitochondria[39] in which deformations have been observed after exposure to a magnetic field.[40] In addition, a functional relationship has been demonstrated between mitochondrial ultrastructure and activity: the "condensed" state, analogous to that observed under the effect of a magnetic field, corresponding to an active phase and the steady state corresponding to a phase of lesser activity.[41]

Another example of an orientation effect on red blood cells has been seen in sickle-cell anemia where packed fibers of deoxyhemoglobin distort the red cells that take on an elongated shape. Such cells can be oriented in a magnetic field.[42]

OTHER EXPERIMENTAL RESULTS ON MEMBRANE SYSTEMS

The frog retinal rod outer segment, with its regular quasi-crystalline structure and well-known biochemical composition, was the first natural membrane system in which a quantitative analysis of magnetic orientation was attempted.

The outer segments of the frog retinal rod are microscopic elongated cell fragments that orient in parallel to the lines of a constant and uniform field in a physiologic suspension.[43] It would appear that the paraffin chains of the double lipid layer are the most orientable molecules that could add their molecular anisotropies to produce a macroscopic anisotropy sufficiently powerful to orient the cell. However, Hong et al.[44] have demonstrated that the diamagnetic anisotropy of the paraffin chain should orient perpendicularly to the field, that is, in a plane parallel to the field and with the greater axis of the retinal rod outer segment perpendicular to the field. This does not coincide with experimental results. Thus, the overall diamagnetic anisotropy cannot result from the lipids, but rather from the proteins in the membrane, especially from rhodopsin, which comprises more than 80% of the protein fraction.[45,46]

Using a special device with which the electromagnet can be rotated 90°, thus changing the axis of the field in relation to the sample, Chagneux and Chalazonitis have studied the speed of orientation in these systems in a homogeneous field. The orientation time was about 2 seconds at 2 T and 10 seconds at 1 T, but more than 20 seconds at 0.5 T.[47]

Unicellular green alga *Chlorella*, which has only one chloroplast, is another classical model for studying orientation effects. In a magnetic field of 1 T or greater, the whole alga orients and modifies its fluorescence intensity.[44,48-51] An analogous effect has been obtained with the spinach chloroplast and other photosynthesis systems.[52,53]

Using this model, Geacintov et al.[48] studied the effect of medium viscosity on the orientation effect. Indeed, the velocity of orientation decreased with increasing viscosity. This would mean that in a complex biological medium, which is more viscous than a suspension of green algae, the time of orientation should be significantly increased for a given field intensity and a given diamagnetic anisotropy.

CONCLUSION AND PERSPECTIVES

The theoretical calculations and experimental results presented here show the following: (i) the orientation effects of a constant and uniform magnetic field can be obtained at intensities of a few teslas, or tens of teslas, as long as the organized multimolecular system is large enough; (ii) the threshold level of action is determined by the ratio between the magnetic orientation energy and the thermal energy kT; (iii) there is a relationship between the square of the orienting field intensity and the duration of exposure required to obtain an effect, due to internal resistance of the media; and (iv) taking into consideration these prerequisites, a moderate intensity field probably acts most often as a transition activator in states close to phase changes.

The potential risks involved in short duration exposures to fields of 1 to 3 T, levels used in MRS in clinical medicine, if they exist, probably do not result from an orientation effect because of the following: (i) the orientation effect requires a constant field direction in relation to the object being oriented, a requirement obviously not met for blood cells circulating *in vivo* and which is attenuated in certain other tissues by internal movements; (ii) the exposure duration/field intensity ratio is near the threshold levels required to observe an effect; (iii) if the effect acts as a catalyzer and not as an inducer, it can accelerate biological processes already under way, but cannot trigger them; and (iv) the experimental results strongly suggest that the orientation effects are reversible during a period comparable to the time required to obtain an effect. Nevertheless, these observations do not exclude the possibility of starting a long-term process at the time of the reversible effect.

Although further study should be conducted to better establish the field intensity thresholds and exposure durations, it does not appear that these potential orientation effects should be considered to constitute contraindications for high intensity MRS investigations.

On the other hand, under optimal conditions for observing an effect (high intensity field, longer exposure, immobilization of the structures during exposure), these effects could be used as positive activators for cells *in vitro*. This, for example, is the question raised by adoptive immunotherapy of cancer.[54] Three methods of immunotherapy by autotransfusion of activated cells have been proposed using LAK (lymphokine-activated killer) cells,[55] TIL (tumor infiltrating lymphocytes),[56] and MAK (macrophage adoptive killers).[57] In light of the principles described herein, activation, or amplification of activation, by *in vitro* action of a constant and uniform magnetic field on LAK, TIL, or MAK cell membranes appears quite feasible.

This possibility is based on experimental evidence from *in vitro* studies involving immunity regulation. Earlier, the modifications in the reaction of certain antibodies as observed by Pierron[34] after a 20-minute exposure to a 1.2-T field were cited. The tetrazolium nitroblue reduction test that reflects NADH-oxidase activity during phagocytosis is modified by exposure to a 0.5-T field for two hours in a cell population considered to be preactivated.[58] Secretion of MIF (migration inhibiting factor) by phytohemagglutinin (PHA)–stimulated lymphocytes is modified after two hours of exposure to a 0.4-T field.[25] *In vitro* leukocyte cytotoxicity for primary liver cancer cells is increased after exposure for three hours at 0.5 T.[59] These findings via *in vitro* tests have led to preliminary immunotherapy trials using autotransfusion of leukocytes exposed *in vitro* to a constant magnetic field. Several cases showing promising results have been reported in patients with advanced stage primary liver cancer.[60] For further research, attempts should be made to use the magnetic field, not as an activating agent alone, but rather in combination with the LAK, TIL, and MAK methods now under evaluation.

ACKNOWLEDGMENTS

I wish to thank A. Bellossi (Department of Biophysics, Rennes Cancer Institute) and L. Toujas (Department of Immunology and Immunotherapy, Rennes Cancer Institute) for reviewing this discussion.

REFERENCES

1. DE CERTAINES, J. D. 1976. Recherche **65**(7): 286.
2. TENFORDE, T. S. 1979. Magnetic Field Effects on Biological Systems. Plenum. New York.
3. GROSS, L. 1964. *In* Biological Effects of Magnetic Fields. M. F. Barnothy, Ed.: 297. Plenum. New York.
4. DAVIS, L. D., K. PAPPAJOHN & I. M. PLAVNIEKS. 1962. Fed. Proc. Fed. Am. Soc. Exp. Biol. **21:** 1.
5. BUCHACHENKO, A. L., R. Z. SAGDEEV & K. M. SALIKHOV. 1978. Magnetic and Spin Effects in Chemical Reactions (in Russian). Nauka. Moscow.
6. VANAG, K. & A. N. KUZNETSOV. 1988. Izv. Akad. Nauk SSSR (Biol.) **2:** 215.
7. WEILL, G. 1986. *In* Biophysical Effects of Steady Magnetic Fields. G. Maret *et al.*, Eds.: 2–6. Springer-Verlag. Berlin/New York.
8. MARET, G. & K. DRANSFELD. 1985. *In* Strong and Ultrastrong Magnetic Fields and Their Applications. Top. Appl. Phys., vol. 57. Springer-Verlag. Berlin/New York.
9. CHABRE, M. 1986. *In* Biophysical Effects of Steady Magnetic Fields. G. Maret *et al.*, Eds.: 28. Springer-Verlag. Berlin/New York.
10. TORBET, J. & M. J. DICKENS. 1984. FEBS Lett. **173:** 403.
11. TORBET, J. & M. C. RONZIERE. 1984. Biochem. J. **219:** 1057.
12. MURPHY, N. S. 1984. Biopolymers **23:** 1261.
13. TORBET, J., J. M. FREYSSINET & G. HUDRY-CLERGEON. 1981. Nature **289:** 91.
14. FREYSSINET, J. M., J. TORBET, G. HUDRY-CLERGEON & G. MARET. 1983. Proc. Natl. Acad. Sci. U.S.A. **80:** 1616.
15. DORFMAN, A. G. 1962. Biofizika (USSR) **7**(6): 733.
16. GR. DES CRISTAUX LIQUIDES D'ORSAY. 1971. Recherche **12:** 433.
17. DE GENNES, P. G. 1974. Physics of Liquid Crystals. Oxford University Press (Clarendon). London/New York.
18. CHAPMAN, D. 1968. Ann. N.Y. Acad. Sci. **137:** 745.
19. LUZZATI, V. & F. REISS-HUSSON. 1962. J. Cell Biol. **12:** 207.
20. GAFFNEY, B. J. & H. M. MACCONNEL. 1974. Chem. Phys. Lett. **24:** 310.
21. MIEROVITCH, E. & J. H. FREED. 1980. J. Phys. Chem. **84**(24): 3295.
22. MARET, G., N. BOCCARA & J. KIEPENHEUER. 1986. Biophysical Effects of Steady Magnetic Fields. Springer-Verlag. Berlin/New York.
23. DRANSFELD, K., Z-M. SUN & V. UHLENDORF. 1986. *In* Biophysical Effects of Steady Magnetic Fields. G. Maret *et al.*, Eds.: 7. Springer-Verlag. Berlin/New York.
24. KAVANAU, J. L. 1965. Structure and Function in Biological Membranes. Holden–Day. San Francisco.
25. DE CERTAINES, J. D. 1977. Ph.D. thesis. Rennes University, France.
26. BOTHOREL, P. & C. LUSSAN. 1968. C. R. Acad. Sci. (Paris) **266D:** 2492.
27. BOTHOREL, P. & C. LUSSAN. 1970. C. R. Acad. Sci. (Paris) **271D:** 680.
28. LUSSAN, C. & P. BOTHOREL. 1969. C. R. Acad. Sci. (Paris) **269D:** 1118.
29. BRESLER, S. E. & V. M. BRESLER. 1974. Dakl. Akad. Nauk SSSR **214**(4): 936.
30. BRESLER, S. E. & V. M. BRESLER. 1978. Dakl. Akad. Nauk SSSR **242**(2): 465.
31. AOKI, H., H. YAMAZAKI, T. YOSHINO & T. AKAGI. 1990. Res. Commun. Chem. Pathol. Pharmacol. **69**(1): 103.
32. PIRUZYAN, L. A. & A. N. KUZNETSOV. 1983. Izv. Akad. Nauk SSSR (Biol.) **6:** 805.
33. SIMONOV, A. N., V. A. LIVSSHITS *et al.* 1986. Biofizika **31**.
34. PIERRON, N. 1970. DEA thesis. University of Nancy, France.
35. CHALAZONITIS, N., R. CHAGNEUX & A. ARVANITAKI. 1964. C. R. Soc. Biol. **158**(10): 1902.
36. LIBURDY, R. P. & T. S. TENFORDE. 1986. *In* Biophysical Effects of Steady Magnetic Fields. G. Maret *et al.*, Eds.: 44. Springer-Verlag. Berlin/New York.
37. BELLOSSI, A., Y. BRESSON & J. D. DE CERTAINES. 1971. C. R. Soc. Biol. **169**(6): 1503.
38. DINTENFASS, L. 1969. Mol. Cryst. Liq. Cryst. **8:** 101.
39. LUSSAN, C. & P. BOTHOREL. 1969. C. R. Acad. Sci. (Paris) **269D:** 792.
40. STREKOVA, V. Y. & G. A. TARAKANOVA. 1972. Elektron. Obrab. Mater. (USSR) **2:** 77.
41. HACKENBROCK, C. R. 1966. J. Cell Biol. **30:** 269.

42. COSTA RIBEIRO, P., M. A. DAVIDOVITCH, E. WAJNBERG, G. BEMSKI & M. KISCHINEVSKY. 1981. Biophys. J. **36:** 443.
43. CHALAZONITIS, N., R. CHAGNEUX & A. ARVANITAKI. 1970. C. R. Acad. Sci. (Paris) **271D:** 130.
44. HONG, F. T., D. MAUZERALL & A. MAURO. 1971. Proc. Natl. Acad. Sci. U.S.A. **68:** 1283.
45. WORCESTER, D. L. 1978. Proc. Natl. Acad. Sci. U.S.A. **75:** 5475.
46. FABRE, M. 1986. *In* Biophysical Effects of Steady Magnetic Fields. G. Maret *et al.*, Eds.: 28. Springer-Verlag. Berlin/New York.
47. CHAGNEUX, R. & N. CHALAZONITIS. 1972. C. R. Acad. Sci. (Paris) **274D:** 317.
48. GEACINTOV, N. E., F. VAN NOSTRAND, J. F. BECKER & J. B. TRINKEL. 1972. Biochim. Biophys. Acta **226:** 486.
49. BECKER, J., M. MICHEL-VILLAZ & G. PAILLOTIN. 1973. Biochim. Biophys. Acta **314:** 42.
50. BRETON, J., J. F. BECKER & N. E. GEACINTOV. 1973. Biochem. Biophys. Res. Commun. **54:** 1403.
51. BECKER, J., J. BRETON, N. E. GEACINTOV & F. TRENTACOSTI. 1974. Biochim. Biophys. Acta **440:** 531.
52. BRETON, J., M. MICHEL-VILLAZ & G. PAILLOTIN. 1973. Biochim. Biophys. Acta **314:** 42.
53. GEACINTOV, N. E., F. VAN NOSTRAND, J. F. BECKER & J. B. TRINKEL. 1972. Biochim. Biophys. Acta **267:** 65.
54. ROSENBERG, S. A. 1984. Cancer Treat. Rep. **68:** 233.
55. ROSENBERG, S. A., B. PACKARD, P. M. ACHERSOLD *et al.* 1985. N. Engl. J. Med. **316:** 1676.
56. ROSENBERG, S. A., P. SPIESS & R. LAFRENIERE. 1986. Sciences **233:** 1318.
57. ANDREESEN, R., C. SCHEINBENBOGEN, W. BRUGGER *et al.* 1990. Cancer Res. **50:** 7450.
58. BELLOSSI, A., J. D. DE CERTAINES & J. P. TOUJAS. 1976. Wadley Med. Bull. **6**(1): 17.
59. BELLOSSI, A., M. RIOCHE & A. ABONDO. 1975. Ouest Med. **28**(6): 365.
60. BELLOSSI, A. & J. D. DE CERTAINES. 1979 (August). Fifth Int. Conf. Med. Phys., Jerusalem.

Extremely Low Frequency Magnetic Field Exposure from MRI/MRS Procedures

Implications for Patients (Acute Exposures) and Operational Personnel (Chronic Exposures)[a]

FRANK S. PRATO,[b] MARTIN KAVALIERS,[c]
KLAUS-PETER OSSENKOPP,[d] JEFFREY J. L. CARSON,[b,e]
DICK J. DROST,[b] AND J. ROGER H. FRAPPIER[b]

[b]Bioelectromagnetics Western
and
Department of Nuclear Medicine and Magnetic Resonance
and
Lawson Research Institute
St. Joseph's Health Center
London, Ontario, Canada N6A 4V2

[c]Bioelectromagnetics Western
and
Division of Oral Biology
Faculty of Dentistry
University of Western Ontario
London, Ontario, Canada N6A 5C1

[d]Bioelectromagnetics Western
and
Department of Psychology
University of Western Ontario
London, Ontario, Canada N6A 5C2

INTRODUCTION

This report addresses the question of risk associated with (a) acute exposure to magnetic fields associated with magnetic resonance imaging/magnetic resonance spectroscopy (MRI/MRS) (i.e., a patient examination) and (b) chronic exposure to stray fields (i.e., operational personnel). Certain risks exist and are well defined, such as risks from flying projectiles and cardiac pacemaker malfunction due to the static magnetic field (B_0)[1,2] and risks of tissue heating and burns due to the radio-frequency (rf) field.[3–5] Many of these nonstochastic risks can be easily minimized. However, the

[a]This work was supported by a grant (No. MA9981) from the Medical Research Council of Canada and by a grant (No. UNLP 5026) from UpJohn London Neurosciences Program.
[e]J. J. L. Carson was supported by the Medical Research Council of Canada through a training award.

question remains as to whether or not nonthermal risks exist that would be analogous to the stochastic risks produced by low doses of ionizing radiation in X-ray and nuclear medicine imaging.[6]

In a series of experiments since 1982 investigating nonthermal effects, we have determined that there are no measurable effects for acute MRI exposures or chronic exposures of up to two years on the following: (1) anxiety (humans[7] and rats[8]); (2) spatial memory (humans[7] and rats[9]); (3) long-term memory (humans[7] and rats[8]); (4) intelligence quotient (humans[7]); (5) visual acuity and reaction time (humans[7]); and (6) acute changes in serum melatonin levels (humans[10]) or long-term stress (rats[11]). However, we have determined that exposure to MR imaging procedures does produce small, but measurable effects such as increases in the blood-brain permeability in rats,[12,13] increases in proline incorporation into the predentin collagen matrix in mice,[14] attenuation of morphine-induced[15] and fentanyl-induced[16] analgesia in mice, and increases in the cytosolic free calcium concentration in HL60 cells.[17] Evidence in our laboratory increasingly suggests that, when a nonthermal biological response is observed, it is due to exposure to the extremely low frequency magnetic fields (ELFMF) that are produced by the positional encoding gradients in MRI (which, of course, are also used in some MRS applications).

The stochastic risks (e.g., cancer mortality) associated with radiologic and nuclear medicine imaging procedures are extrapolated from studies of large populations exposed to ionizing radiation invariably given at much higher doses and at different dose rates. The risks obtained from these epidemiological studies, that is, 4×10^{-5} mSv^{-1},[18] indicate that the danger from the dose of ionizing radiation given to a patient from a radiological procedure (e.g., 2 mSv[19]) or that received by operational personnel (approximately 3 mSv[18]) is extremely small. In fact, this risk could never be proven, that is, the exposure groups and control groups needed would be far too large to be feasible, as literally millions of individuals would have to be followed for decades. Nevertheless, even though such risk can never be proven (i.e., remains hypothetical), it is inferred based on the epidemiological studies. Unfortunately, like it or not, we face the same dilemma in MRI/MRS because (a) epidemiological studies of populations chronically exposed (or thought to be exposed) to extremely low frequency (ELF) magnetic fields (MF) have shown a small increase in cancer risk[20-25] (approximately 10^{-4}) and (b) ELF magnetic fields occur during MRI/MRS. Therefore, we have undertaken to investigate the possible biological effects of acute exposures to the ELFMF accompanying MRI/MRS procedures. In addition, we have done ELF magnetic field measurements and compared them to field levels in the epidemiological studies to determine whether or not MRI/MRS workers should be concerned regarding chronic exposures.

In 1984, Kavaliers, Ossenkopp, and Hirst[26] reported that acute exposures (90 min) to ELF magnetic fields reduced the enhanced analgesic response to morphine in mice. In 1985, we demonstrated that exposure to an MRI procedure (22.5 min, TE = 30, TR = 1030, 23 slice) at 0.15 T also reduced morphine-induced analgesia[15] and, in 1987, we reported that this effect on the mouse opioid system was primarily due to the ELFMF produced by the gradient coils rather than the static field or amplitude-modulated 6.25-MHz rf field.[27] Also, in 1987, Ossenkopp and Kavaliers reported that the inhibition of morphine-induced analgesia by 60-Hz magnetic fields was a function of magnetic field intensity with a threshold of approximately 0.1 mT.[28]

In addition, unpublished results from our laboratory of exposure of morphine-injected snails to a pulsed magnetic field produced by a bone healing device that contained magnetic field frequencies up to 3000 Hz also reduced the antinociception effect.

Because exposure of this animal model to ELFMF demonstrated a reproducible and biological important response, it was decided to further use this model to investigate (a) the physical characteristics of the ELF field that elicits this response, (b) whether or not the ELFMF effect is reversible, (c) whether the ELF interaction is with the opiate (i.e., morphine) or with the animal's opioid system, (d) whether or not there is a dose response, and (e) whether or not the antinociceptive effects of ELFMF occur in other animals considerably removed from rodents, that is, mollusks.

NOCICEPTION AND ANALGESIA (ANTINOCICEPTION)

Because nociception is being used as a probe to evaluate the importance of acute MRI/MRS procedures, a short description of this important physiological system is warranted. All animals encounter threats to their physical integrity in the environment and defensive responses to noxious stimuli are found in all major animal phyla.[29,30] The ability of animals to recognize and physically react to aversive or noxious stimuli that can compromise their integrity is described by the term nociception.[31] Nociception can be used to provide an index of an animal's sensitivity to aversive environmental conditions and thus can allow for the determination of the capacity to execute adaptive behavior. In rodents, laboratory measures of nociception include recording of limb flexion or withdrawal [lifting a foot off an aversive, usually thermal, surface (often called a "hot plate")], active avoidance, and removal of the tail ("tail flick") from a thermal stimulus.

Nociceptive responses have been similarly observed and recorded in invertebrates.[29] For example, within a few seconds after the land snail, *Cepaea nemoralis*, is placed on a surface warmed to 40 °C, the snail lifts the anterior portion of its fully extended foot from the aversive surface.[32] This "foot-lifting" behavior is not observed in snails that are exposed to temperatures normally present in their natural habitats, but becomes increasingly evident as the temperature is raised to 40 °C. This nociceptive response of *Cepaea* and other gastropod mollusks is comparable to the foot-lifting response exhibited by rodents when placed on a warmed surface.

Measurements of alterations in nociceptive responses (decreases in sensitivity, antinociception, or analgesia when considered in terms of pain) are widely used to determine the behavioral and physiological status of animals following exposure to aversive or potentially aversive stimuli. Antinociception has been widely documented in animals following exposure to diverse environmental stimuli with both opioid and nonopioid mechanisms being implicated.[29] In vertebrates, the tonic activity of endogenous opioid systems can be increased by a range of environmental stimuli. In rodents, this "stress" or environmentally induced analgesia[33] can be recorded as an increased latency of a foot-lift or tail-flick response. Administration of either endogenous opioid peptides, such as enkephalin, or exogenous opiate agonists, such as the prototypic opiate agonist morphine, produces similar antinociceptive (analgesic) effects. Prototypic exogenous opiate antagonists, such as naloxone, can reverse or attenuate these analgesic effects and, in certain cases, reduce nociceptive responses.[34]

Similar evidence for opioid involvement in the mediation of antinociception or analgesia and nociception is present for mollusks. Morphine, as well as endogenous opioid peptides, can enhance the latency of response of the snail *Cepaea* to a warmed surface.[32] As in rodents, this morphine-induced antinociception or analgesia is dose-dependent and naloxone-reversible.

Exposure to various magnetic stimuli, including weak 60-Hz magnetic fields, has significant inhibitory effects on exogenous and endogenous opioid-mediated antinociceptive responses in both rodents and *Cepaea*.[32] These similar effects in *Cepaea* and rodents raise the possibility of a fundamental similarity and phylogenetic continuity in the effects of magnetic fields on opioid-mediated biological responses.

METHODS

Mice

Mice (20–25 g, CF-1, Charles River, Quebec) were kept on a 12-h-light/12-h-dark cycle at 22 ± 1 °C. At the mid-dark period and while maintained under a low-intensity red light, groups of five mice in Plexiglas holders were exposed to the ELFMF produced by the gradient coils of the MR imager; or they were exposed to a sham procedure by being placed in the MR imager, but with all fields (B_0, rf, and gradient) off; or they were left in their home cages and used as controls. The exposure was of variable length (4.7, 11.6, or 23.2 min) and was given either before or after an intraperitoneal (ip) injection of morphine (10 mg/kg per 10 mL saline). Thirty minutes after injection, the nociceptive responses of individual mice were determined. Nociception was measured as the latency of a foot-lifting response to an aversive thermal stimulus [50 ± 0.5 °C, analgesiometer ("hot plate"), Technilab, New Jersey[35]]. Each mouse was removed from the heated surface following the response and was returned to its home cage. A cutoff time of 150 s was used.

The nociceptive measures have no other evident behavioral effects in mice. In addition, histological examinations of the feet of rodents exposed to higher temperatures (60 °C) for longer time periods have shown no evidence of tissue damage.[36]

Snails

Snails were kept on a 12-h-light/12-h-dark cycle at 22 °C. During the light cycle, the basal nociceptive response of fully hydrated snails was determined prior to experimental treatment. The same animals were then injected with morphine (10 μg/2.0 μL saline, equivalent to 10 mg/kg) and were exposed for 23.2 min to one of four conditions: (1) a complete MRI procedure, (2) a sham MRI procedure, (3) the ELFMF produced by the MR gradient coils, and (4) a sham ELFMF. After exposure, the nociceptive responses of hydrated snails were again determined. Nociception (i.e., analgesia) was measured as the latency of response ("foot-lifting" response) to a warmed thermal surface (38.5 ± 0.5 °C). The behavioral endpoint was the time at which the foot reached its readily discernible maximum elevation. After displaying this avoidance response, individual snails were quickly removed from the thermal surface. Solutions were injected with a 5.0-μL microsyringe (#75, Hamilton, Nevada) either into the foot or in the mantle cavity into the hemocoel. Results of previous studies had established that magnetic stimuli had no evident effects on the motoric abilities of the mice or snails. In addition, the testing surfaces were confirmed not to generate any measurable spurious time-varying magnetic fields.

Animal Exposure Conditions

The animal exposures including complete imaging, sham imaging, gradient fields, and sham gradient fields were all performed on a Teslacon 0.15-T resistive system (Technicare Corporation, Cleveland, Ohio). For the sham exposures, there was a residual static magnetic field between 0.2 and 0.4 mT. (For the sham exposures that were controls for a complete MRI procedure, the sound of the imaging was recorded and then played back through audio speakers to replicate the sound intensities.[37]) The center of the Plexiglas mouse cage or snail holder was offset 32 cm from the magnetic center of the imager along the bore of the magnet (i.e., along the z-axis) in order to ensure adequate exposure of the mice to the time-varying fields associated with positional encoding. The imaging procedure was a 23.2-min, 22-slice, 0.75-cm-slice-thickness transverse spin echo sequence with a repetition time (TR) of 1030 ms and an echo time (TE) of 30 ms. A complete description of the gradient exposures appears elsewhere.[17,37] In brief, the z-gradient (Gz) was approximately 1.9 mT m^{-1} and the y- and x-gradients (Gy and Gx) were approximately 1.4 mT m^{-1}. The rise times were of the order of 2–3 ms and the magnitude Fourier transform of the gradient waveforms indicated that almost all of the frequency components were less than 300 Hz, very much in the ELF range.

Statistical Analysis

Data analysis consisted of analysis of variance procedures and the post hoc comparisons were orthogonal tests. The minimum significance level used for hypothesis testing was the 0.05 level.

Gradient Magnetic Field Measurement and Analysis

Magnetic Resonance Imager and Pulse Sequence

All measurements were made on a 0–2 tesla rampable magnetic resonance imaging/spectroscopy unit (Magnetom 63SP, Siemens, Erlangen, Germany). All measurements were made with the main static magnetic field ramped down to zero gauss. (A remnant static magnetic field of between 4 and 12 gauss was measured.) Measurements were made during a 21-slice spin echo imaging sequence (TR = 1050 ms, TE = 30 ms). The slice select (Z) gradients were in the z-direction (parallel to the main magnetic field). The phase-encode (Y) gradient was in the y-direction (vertical) and was turned off. The frequency-encode (X) gradient was in the x-direction (horizontal).

Magnetic Field Measurement and Frequency Analysis

The method of field measurement and analysis was similar to the method published previously.[17] The magnetic field generated by the magnetic resonance imager was measured with a gaussmeter (model 9200; axial probe model FAB92-0915, bandwidth dc to 5 kHz; F. W. Bell, Orlando, Florida). The z-directed magnetic field was detected at a location on the axis of the main magnet (z-axis) 27.5 cm in the z-direction from the magnetic center (the point within the magnetic resonance imager where all three gradient magnetic fields are zero). The magnetic field waveform (see FIGURE 5A later) was periodic (50-ms repetition rate). Twenty waveforms were digitized at 33.50 kHz with 10 bit resolution and then they were averaged (APC computer, NEC Information Systems, Lexington, Massachusetts; Innotech Computers digitizing board, London, Ontario, Canada). This resulted in an array of 1675 points that was subsequently converted to an array of 1024 points using linear interpolation. The 1024-point array was then transformed into the frequency domain (see FIGURE 5B later) using a Fast Fourier Transform algorithm (MathCAD 2.5 software, Mathsoft Incorporated, Cambridge, Massachusetts).

Magnetic Field along the z-Axis

Measurements of the z-directed magnetic field on the axis of the main magnet were made at various locations ranging from −20 cm to +300 cm from the magnetic center. The maximum height of the gradient waveform (spoiler gradient at 41–50 ms, see FIGURE 5A later) was measured at each location (see FIGURE 6 later). Spoiler values above 0.01 mT were measured with the gaussmeter (FIGURE 6, closed circles). Smaller spoiler values were measured with a search coil (FIGURE 6B, open circles) (built in our laboratory, 8 turns 28 AWG, 0.293-m diameter), which was connected to an instrumentation amplifier (built in our laboratory, gain adjustable 1–100,000 x's, bandwidth > 10 kHz). Both the gaussmeter and the instrumentation amplifier were connected to a digital storage oscilloscope (model 468, Tektronix, Beaverton, Oregon), which allowed waveform averaging when required. The magnetic field was estimated from the search coil waveform by assuming that the rise time on the leading edge of the spoiler gradient was independent of position and to first-order linear. Based on this assumption, the height of the rectangular pulse representing the time derivative of the rising edge of the spoiler gradient was proportional to the magnitude of the magnetic field. The constant of proportionality was determined by comparing the height of the rectangular pulse from the search coil to a known spoiler value as measured with the gaussmeter.

RESULTS

FIGURE 1 demonstrates that the ELF magnetic fields generated by the Gz field are primarily responsible for the antinociception effect. Fourier analysis of the ELFMF produced by each of the three gradients[17] indicated that the amplitudes of the ELF components produced by Gz were approximately 0.1 mT from dc to 100 Hz,

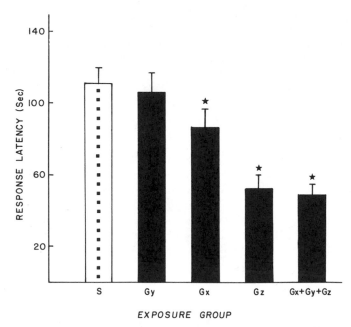

FIGURE 1. Separate effects of the three time-varying magnetic field gradients on morphine-induced analgesia in mice. Mice were exposed for 23.2 min, then removed and injected with morphine, and then exposed for another 23.2 min. Error bars correspond to one standard error of the mean with a minimum of 20 mice/experiment, except for Gx+Gy+Gz, where 10 mice were used. Stars indicate a statistically significant ($p < 0.001$) depression. Gz was significantly different ($p < 0.001$) from Gx, but not different from Gx+Gy+Gz.

whereas the amplitude from Gy varied from 0 to 0.04 mT and the amplitude from Gx fell in between the other two.

FIGURE 2 suggests that the ELFMF antinociception effect is temporary with complete recovery by 24 hours.

FIGURE 3 shows that the attenuating effect of the magnetic field is also increased as the ELF exposure time is increased. This figure also shows that the ELF effect on the opioid system is dependent on whether or not the exposure occurred immediately prior to the injection or after the injection. Exposure to the ELFMF prior to injection produced a significant attenuation of the morphine-induced analgesia after only 4 min of exposure. In contrast, exposure for 4 min after the injection had no significant effects.

FIGURE 4 shows the snail data. It confirms the results previously obtained with mice, demonstrating again that exposure to ELFMF produced by MR gradient coils attenuates morphine-induced antinociception (analgesia).

FIGURE 5 shows the waveform and corresponding magnitude Fourier transform of the Gz plus Gx field. The ELF magnetic fields produced by the other two physical gradients (Gx and Gy) are lower than those due to Gz. FIGURE 6 shows the change in ELFMF intensity for the Gz spoiler pulse as a function of distance from the center of the MR imager. The spoiler gradient had a value of 7 mT m^{-1} within the field of view of the imager and a nominal rise time of 1 ms.

DISCUSSION

FIGURE 2 demonstrates that the effect of ELFMF is temporary because normal opioid response to an exogenous opiate is restored within 24 h after the exposure.

FIGURE 3 indicates that there is a form of dose response: when the gradient field exposure is increased from 4.6 min to 23.2 min, the attenuation of morphine-induced analgesia is increased. Furthermore, the effects of the fields do not have a direct effect on the morphine or on its interaction with the receptors because postinjection exposure was not as effective as preinjection exposure in producing an inhibition of the levels of analgesia. The ability of preinjection exposure to reduce analgesia when fentanyl is used in place of morphine has also been established.[16]

FIGURE 4 demonstrates that the magnetic field attenuation of morphine-induced analgesia also occurs in snails as well as mice and that, in both cases, the primary

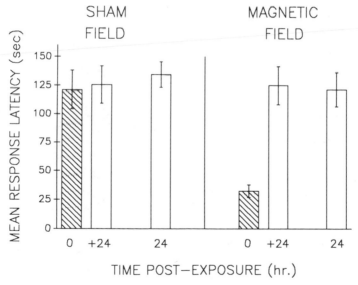

FIGURE 2. Four groups of 10 mice per group were exposed to sham (on the left) or gradient field (on the right) conditions for 23.2 min and then they were injected with morphine. The mice were then put back in the MRI machine and were exposed to the same preinjection experimental condition for another 23.2 min. Finally, approximately 7 min after this second exposure, two groups of mice (hatched bars labeled 0) were tested on the hot plate, that is, approximately 30 min after they were injected. Twenty-four hours later, these animals were injected with morphine and, 30 min later, they were tested (clear bars marked +24). Note that only the ELFMF-exposed group was significantly different from all the other groups ($p < 0.01$). The other two groups were not initially tested, but were subsequently injected and tested 24 h later (clear bars marked +24). This was done to control for any learned behavior of the mice for the hot plate. The error bars correspond to one standard error of the mean.

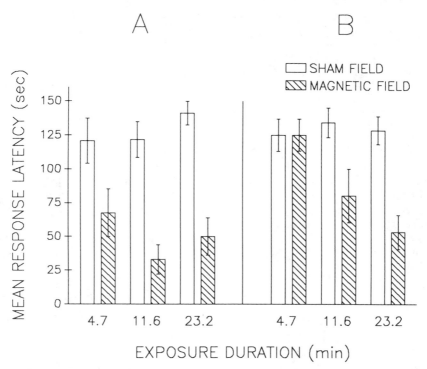

FIGURE 3. Effect of exposure duration (4.7, 11.6, and 23.2 min) before (A) and after (B) morphine injection. Mice were sham exposed or ELFMF exposed either before or after morphine injection. Preexposure was more effective in reducing analgesia and no dose-response relationship was observed (A). In contrast, a dose-response relationship was seen in the postexposure group (B). Each bar corresponds to a minimum of 10 mice and error bars correspond to one standard error of the mean.

effect is due to the ELFMF produced by the gradient fields. This broad phylogenetic continuity in the effects of magnetic stimuli on opioid-induced antinociception raises the possibility of ELFMF interactions with the opioid system in humans. This possibility is under investigation.

As can be seen from FIGURE 5, the major frequency component of the gradient fields is less than 300 Hz, which corresponds to the ELF range that is being extensively investigated by those concerned with magnetic fields produced by electric power distribution and use. Interestingly enough, the major frequency components of bone healing devices also have components in the ELF range with frequency analysis indicating values from 0 to approximately 2000–3000 Hz.[38]

FIGURE 6 shows the change in ELFMF intensity for Gz as a function of distance from the center of the MR imager. FIGURE 6 indicates that MRI/MRS operational personnel would spend most of their time in ELF fields below 0.1 μT if they were working around a heavily shielded 1.5-T magnet. However, the situation for unshielded magnets and unshielded gradients may not be so favorable. We have calculated the magnetic field falloff from a Maxwell pair[39] with a radius of 0.45 m (separation of coils was 0.78 m) to stimulate a Gz gradient coil for a whole-body 1-m bore magnet without magnet or gradient shielding and normalized to 2.5 mT at $z = 0.475$ m (see FIGURE 6). In this case, the field does not drop to the 0.1-μT level until z equals 9 m. Although this calculation represents a worst case scenario because even an unshielded magnet will increase the magnetic field drop-off with distance from the coil, it does imply that further measurements on shielded gradients and unshielded magnets should be made.

Kavaliers and Ossenkopp have indirect evidence that the site of interaction of ELFMF is associated with the mechanisms that maintain the intracellular free calcium concentration. They have implicated the calcium channel with experiments done in mice demonstrating that ELFMF effects were reduced/eliminated by intracerebroventricular (ICV) injection of the calcium channel antagonists nifedipine, diltiazem, and verapamil. Conversely, they showed that the ELFMF effects could be increased by injection of the calcium channel agonist BAY K 8644.[40] They have shown that ELFMF effects were increased if the Ca^{2+} ionophore A21387 was injected into the cerebral ventricles and that the effects were reduced if the ionophore was replaced by the chelator EGTA.[41] In separate experiments, they showed that morphine-induced analgesia was reduced/eliminated by ICV injection of Ca^{2+}, but not Ba^{2+}, in a dose-dependent manner.[41]

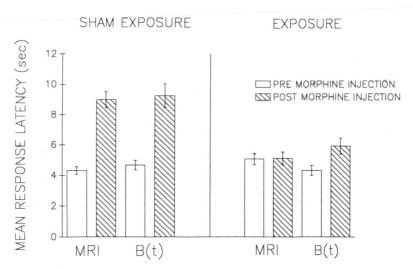

FIGURE 4. Effects of exposure to a complete MRI procedure or just to the ELFMF produced by the gradient field exposure on morphine-induced analgesia in snails. The left panel corresponds to the sham-exposed group and the right panel corresponds to the exposed group. In the sham group, nociceptive response latency was significantly increased twofold by the injection of morphine ($p < 0.001$). This analgesia was completely (significantly, $p < 0.001$) eliminated when the snails were exposed to a complete 23.2-min imaging procedure between the morphine injection and the hot-plate testing. Exposure to just the gradient fields also significantly reduced the analgesia ($p < 0.001$). Snail numbers for MRI sham exposure, gradient field–only sham exposure, MR imaging procedure exposure, and gradient field–only exposure were 17, 19, 21, and 20, respectively, and the error bars correspond to one standard error of the mean.

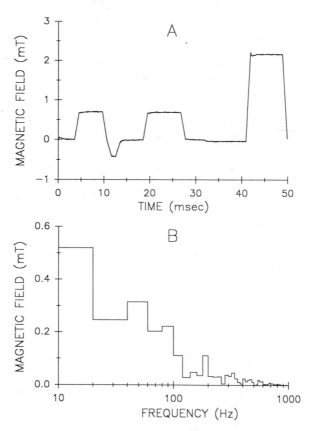

FIGURE 5. Typical spin echo gradient waveform (A) and corresponding magnitude Fourier transform (B) measured in the center of the bore of the magnet, but offset 27.5 cm from the magnet center and towards the magnet front end, that is, $x = 0$ cm, $y = 0$ cm, $z = +27.5$ cm. The Gz gradient was set at approximately 2 mT m^{-1} for slice selection and 7 mT m^{-1} for spoiling; rise times were a nominal 1 ms. The phase-encode (Gy) gradient was turned off because it was relatively small and variable. The frequency-encode (Gx) gradient was small and corresponds to the small negative step seen in panel A just prior to the spoiler gradient.

This evidence indirectly implicates intracellular free calcium ($[Ca^{2+}]_i$) as a target of ELFMF exposure during an MR imaging procedure. We tested this hypothesis directly using a fluorescence technique and showed that exposure to a 23.2-min MR imaging procedure increased $[Ca^{2+}]_i$ in HL60 cells by approximately 20%.[17] We also confirmed that it was the gradient field exposure that produced these changes and not the static or rf fields.[17] More recent studies on snails by Kavaliers and Ossenkopp have now shown that the ELFMF effects on the opioid system are reduced by protein kinase C inhibitors and are enhanced by a protein kinase C activator.[42] Further control experiments have demonstrated that morphine-induced analgesia is reduced by a protein kinase C activator.[42] Of course, even if the site of interaction of ELFMF in the calcium regulatory pathway is demonstrated, it is not self-evident that it is the only site affected or whether or not such effects are harmless. Considerable further work is needed to determine the time course and recovery of such $[Ca^{2+}]_i$ changes and what physical characteristics of the ELFMF are important to elicit these changes. (Continuous exposures in the land snail for 120 h to a 60-Hz, 0.1-mT magnetic field reduced analgesia to sham levels,[43] but, perhaps more importantly, increased mortality two weeks after the end of the exposure period from less than 10% for the sham group to over 40% for the exposed group.[44]) Nevertheless, it is reasonable to suggest that the MR-induced changes from an acute exposure are small and probably reversible. However, prolonged alterations in $[Ca^{2+}]_i$ due to chronic exposure may be deleterious. Of course, until the time course is known, it is impossible to judge the possible deleterious effects of a chronic exposure.

Given the uncertainty in the time course of the $[Ca^{2+}]_i$ changes and the literature correlating ELFMF exposure to increased incidence of certain malignancies, it would seem prudent to reduce chronic ELFMF exposure until more is known. FIGURE 6 demonstrates that such a reduction should not be difficult to achieve in practice and probably is in effect at most MRI/MRS sites. The ELF magnetic fields produced by the gradients fall off considerably faster than the static field. Therefore, most operators have been serendipitously protected in the past because the operator consoles are usually in static fields below 1 mT and, consequently, the amplitude of the ELFMF is below 0.1 μT. This may be important because the epidemiological studies implicate increases in malignancies if the amplitude of the 60-Hz magnetic field exposure is at least 0.1 μT.[24,25]

Although the move to faster switched gradients for fast imaging procedures may

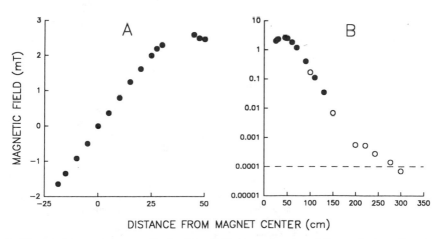

DISTANCE FROM MAGNET CENTER (cm)

FIGURE 6. The maximum amplitude of the ELFMF as a function of distance in the *z*-direction from the center of the magnet measured for a Gz value of 7 mT m⁻¹ and a nominal rise time of 1 ms. On the left (A) are values within the magnet; on the right (B), the values extend outward 3 m from the magnet center. The dashed horizontal line above the abscissa corresponds to the lower limit of the ELFMF amplitude thought to increase cancer incidence, that is, 0.1 μT. These data were collected on a rampable 2-T MR imaging system with 35,000 kg of passive iron shielding. The point at which the amplitude falls below 0.1 μT will depend on the gradient coil design (shielded gradients may fall off more quickly) and on the magnet shielding (unshielded magnets may result in a slower falloff).

be of concern for induced current densities in tissue, it may not be a concern for the effects being discussed in this report. We expect that such gradients may produce smaller effects on the opioid system. First, these gradients have lower peak values and have a shift in frequency content to higher values. Unreported work in our laboratory and that of others suggest that as the frequency is shifted higher, that is, from 100 to 2000 Hz, cellular effects of ELFMF may be reduced.[38,45–47]

In conclusion, given the present concern regarding the possible harmful effects of chronic ELFMF exposures, it is important to address whether or not such exposures are of any concern in MRI/MRS. Even if ELFMF chronic exposures are harmful, evidence from our laboratory suggests that acute exposures experienced by the patient should not be a concern. Such brief exposure to ELFMF produces small effects that appear to be reversible. However, at this time, it would be prudent to limit chronic exposure to strong ELFMF. From our assessment, the ELF magnetic fields from MR systems drop off more quickly than the static magnetic fields. Consequently, the MRI/MRS operator may be protected from significant ELFMF exposure. Of course, considerably more research work must be done to firm up these suggestions. The time course and recovery of the $[Ca^{2+}]_i$ changes as a function of ELFMF exposure must be determined and additional measurements of the ELFMF falloff distances from the magnet must be made, particularly for the combination of unshielded magnets with unshielded gradient coils.

ACKNOWLEDGMENTS

We thank John Parr for the preparation of the manuscript and Mark Hamon for the preparation of the figures.

REFERENCES

1. NEW, P. F. J., B. R. ROSEN, T. J. BRADY, F. S. BUONANNO, J. P. KISTLER, C. T. BURT, W. S. HINSHAW, J. H. NEWHOUSE, G. M. POHOST & J. M. TAVERAS. 1983. Potential hazards and artifacts of ferromagnetic and nonferromagnetic surgical and dental materials and devices in nuclear magnetic resonance imaging. Radiology 147: 139–148.
2. PAVLICEK, W., M. GEISINGER, L. CASTLE, G. P. BOROKOWSKI, T. F. MEANEY, B. L. BREAM & J. H. GALLAGHER. 1983. The effect of nuclear magnetic resonance on patients with cardiac pacemakers. Radiology 147: 149–153.
3. SHELLOCK, F. G., D. J. SCHAEFER & J. V. CRUES. 1989. Alterations in body and skin temperatures caused by magnetic resonance imaging: is the recommended exposure for radiofrequency radiation too conservative? Br. J. Radiol. 62: 904–909.
4. SHELLOCK, F. G. 1989. Biological effects and safety aspects of magnetic resonance imaging. Magn. Reson. Q. 5: 243–261.
5. SHELLOCK, F. G. & G. L. SLIMP. 1989. Severe burn of the finger caused by using a pulse oximeter during MR imaging. Am. J. Roentgenol. 153: 1105.
6. BEERS, G. J. 1989. Biological effects of weak electromagnetic fields from 0 Hz to 200 Hz: a survey of the literature with special emphasis on possible magnetic resonance effects. Magn. Reson. Imag. 7: 309–331.
7. SWEETLAND, J., A. KERTESZ, F. S. PRATO & K. NANTAU. 1987. The effect of magnetic resonance imaging on human cognition. Magn. Reson. Imag. 5: 129–135.
8. OSSENKOPP, K. P., N. K. INNIS, F. S. PRATO & E. A. SESTINI. 1986. Behavioral effects of

exposure to nuclear magnetic resonance imaging. I: Open-field behavior and passive avoidance learning in rats. Magn. Reson. Imag. **4:** 275–280.

9. INNIS, N. K., K. P. OSSENKOPP, F. S. PRATO & E. A. SESTINI. 1986. Behavioral effects of exposure to nuclear magnetic resonance imaging. II: Spatial memory tests. Magn. Reson. Imag. **4:** 281–284.

10. PRATO, F. S., K. P. OSSENKOPP, M. KAVALIERS, P. UKSIK, R. L. NICHOLSON, D. J. DROST & E. A. SESTINI. 1988/1989. Effects of exposure to magnetic resonance imaging on nocturnal serum melatonin and other hormone levels in adult males: preliminary findings. J. Bioelectricity **7:** 169–180.

11. TESKEY, G. C., K. P. OSSENKOPP, F. S. PRATO & E. A. SESTINI. 1987. Survivability and long-term stress reactivity levels following repeated exposure to nuclear magnetic resonance imaging procedure in rats. Physiol. Chem. Phys. Med. NMR **19:** 43–49.

12. SHIVERS, R. R., M. KAVALIERS, G. C. TESKEY, F. S. PRATO & R. M. PELLETIER. 1987. Magnetic resonance imaging temporarily alters blood-brain barrier permeability in the rat. Neurosci. Lett. **76:** 25–31.

13. PRATO, F. S., J. R. H. FRAPPIER, R. R. SHIVERS, M. KAVALIERS, P. ZABEL, D. J. DROST & T. Y. LEE. 1990. Magnetic resonance imaging increases the blood-brain barrier permeability to 153-gadolinium diethylenetriaminepentaacetic acid in rats. Brain Res. **523:** 301–304.

14. KWONG-HING, A., H. S. SANDHU, F. S. PRATO, J. R. H. FRAPPIER & M. KAVALIERS. 1989. Effects of magnetic resonance imaging (MRI) on the formation of mouse dentin and bone. J. Exp. Zool. **251:** 53–59.

15. OSSENKOPP, K. P., M. KAVALIERS, F. S. PRATO, G. C. TESKEY, E. SESTINI & M. HIRST. 1985. Exposure to nuclear magnetic resonance imaging procedure attenuates morphine-induced analgesia in mice. Life Sci. **37:** 1507–1514.

16. TESKEY, G. C., F. S. PRATO, K. P. OSSENKOPP & M. KAVALIERS. 1988. Exposure to time-varying magnetic fields associated with magnetic resonance imaging reduces fentanyl-induced analgesia in mice. Bioelectromagnetics **9:** 167–174.

17. CARSON, J. J. L., F. S. PRATO, D. J. DROST, L. D. DIESBOURG & S. J. DIXON. 1990. Time-varying electromagnetic fields increase cytosolic free Ca^{2+} in HL60 cells. Am. J. Physiol. **259** (Cell Physiol. **28**): C687–C692.

18. INTERNATIONAL COMMISSION ON RADIOLOGICAL PROTECTION. 1991. 1990 Recommendations of the International Commission on Radiological Protection. Publication No. 60. Pergamon. Elmsford, New York.

19. INTERNATIONAL COMMISSION ON RADIOLOGICAL PROTECTION. 1987. Radiation Dose to Patients from Radiopharmaceuticals. Publication No. 53. Volume **18:** 1–4. Pergamon. Elmsford, New York.

20. WERTHEIMER, N. & E. LEEPER. 1979. Electrical wiring configurations and childhood cancer. Am. J. Epidemiol. **109:** 273–284.

21. LIN, R. S., P. C. DISCHINGER, J. CONDE & K. P. FARRELL. 1985. Occupational exposure to electromagnetic fields and the occurrence of brain tumors. J. Occup. Med. **27:** 413–419.

22. PRESTON-MARTIN, S., W. MACK & B. E. HENDERSON. 1989. Risk factors for gliomas and meningiomas in males in Los Angeles county. Cancer Res. **49:** 6137–6143.

23. SAVITZ, D. A., H. WACHTEL, F. A. BARNES, E. M. JOHN & J. G. TURDIK. 1988. Case-control study of childhood cancer and exposure to 60-hertz electric and magnetic fields. Am. J. Epidemiol. **128:** 10–20.

24. AHLBOM, A. 1988. A review of the epidemiologic literature on magnetic fields and cancer. Scand. J. Work Environ. Health **14:** 337–343.

25. AHLBOM, A., E. N. ALBERT & A. C. FRASER-SMITH. 1987. Biological effects of power line fields. New York State Power Lines Project Scientific Advisory Panel Final Report, p. 72–82.

26. KAVALIERS, M., K. P. OSSENKOPP & M. HIRST. 1984. Magnetic fields abolish the enhanced nocturnal analgesic response to morphine in mice. Physiol. Behav. **32:** 261–264.

27. PRATO, F. S., K. P. OSSENKOPP, M. KAVALIERS, E. SESTINI & G. C. TESKEY. 1987. Attenuation of morphine-induced analgesia in mice by exposure to magnetic resonance imaging: separate effects of the static, radiofrequency, and time-varying magnetic fields. Magn. Reson. Imag. **5:** 9–14.

28. OSSENKOPP, K. P. & M. KAVALIERS. 1987. Morphine-induced analgesia and exposure to 60 Hz magnetic field: inhibition of nocturnal analgesia is a function of magnetic field intensity. Brain Res. **418:** 356–360.
29. KAVALIERS, M. 1988. Evolutionary and comparative aspects of nociception. Brain Res. Bull. **21:** 923–931.
30. WOOLF, C. J. & E. T. WALTERS. 1991. Common patterns of plasticity contributing to nociceptive sensitization in mammals and *Aplysia.* Trends Neurosci. **14:** 74–78.
31. SHERRINGTON, C. S. 1906. The Integrative Action of the Nervous System. Yale University Press. New Haven, Connecticut.
32. KAVALIERS, M. & K. P. OSSENKOPP. 1991. Opioid systems and magnetic field effects in the land snail, *Cepaea nemoralis.* Biol. Bull. **180:** 301–309.
33. AMIT, Z. & G. H. GALINA. 1986. Stress-induced analgesia: adaptive pain suppression. Physiol. Rev. **66:** 1091–1120.
34. MARTIN, W. R. 1984. Pharmacology of opioids. Pharmacol. Rev. **35:** 283–323.
35. HUNSKARR, S., O. G. BERGE & K. HOLE. 1986. A modified hot-plate sensitive to mild analgesics. Behav. Brain Res. **21:** 101–108.
36. ANKIER, S. I. 1974. New hotplate tests to quantify antinociceptive and narcotic antagonist activities. Eur. J. Pharmacol. **27:** 1–4.
37. PRATO, F. S., K. P. OSSENKOPP, M. KAVALIERS, G. C. TESKEY & D. J. DROST. 1987. MRI exposure attenuates morphine-induced analgesia in mice: separate effects of the three time-varying magnetic fields. Sixth Annu. Meet. Soc. Magn. Reson. Med. **17–21/08:** 398.
38. MADRONERO, A. 1990. Influence of magnetic fields on calcium salts crystal formation: an explanation of the "pulsed electromagnetic field" technique for bone healing. J. Biomed. Eng. **12:** 410–414.
39. MANSFIELD, P. & P. G. MORRIS. 1982. NMR Imaging in Biomedicine, p. 322. Academic Press. New York.
40. KAVALIERS, M. & K. P. OSSENKOPP. 1987. Calcium channel involvement in magnetic field inhibition of morphine-induced analgesia. Arch. Pharmacol. **336:** 308–315.
41. KAVALIERS, M. & K. P. OSSENKOPP. 1986. Magnetic field inhibition of morphine-induced analgesia and behavioral activity in mice: evidence for involvement of calcium ions. Brain Res. **379:** 30–38.
42. KAVALIERS, M., K. P. OSSENKOPP & D. M. TYSDALE. 1991. Evidence for the involvement of protein kinase C in the modulation of morphine-induced "analgesia" and the inhibitory effects of exposure to 60 Hz magnetic fields in the snail, *Cepaea nemoralis.* Brain Res. **554:** 65–71.
43. KAVALIERS, M., K. P. OSSENKOPP & S. M. LIPA. 1990. Day-night rhythms in the inhibitory effects of 60 Hz magnetic fields on opiate-mediated "analgesia" behaviors of the land snail, *Cepaea nemoralis.* Brain Res. **517:** 276–282.
44. OSSENKOPP, K. P., M. KAVALIERS & S. LIPA. 1990. Increased mortality in land snails (*Cepaea nemoralis*) exposed to power line (60 Hz) magnetic fields and effects of the light-dark cycle. Neurosci. Lett. **114:** 89–94.
45. GOODMAN, R. & A. S. HENDERSON. 1988. Exposure of salivary gland cells to low-frequency electromagnetic fields alters polypeptide synthesis. Proc. Natl. Acad. Sci. U.S.A. **85:** 3928–3932.
46. GOODMAN, R., L. X. WEI, J. C. XU & A. HENDERSON. 1990. Quantitative changes in transcripts result from varying signal amplitude. Twelfth Annu. Meet. BEMS **10–14/06:** 11.
47. GREENE, J. J., W. J. SKOWRONSKI, J. M. MULLINS, R. M. NARDONE, M. PENAFIEL & R. MEISTER. 1991. Delineation of electric and magnetic field effects of extremely low frequency electromagnetic radiation on transcription. Biochem. Biophys. Res. Commun. **174:** 742–749.

Human Interactions with Ultra High Fields

U. W. BUETTNER

Department of Neurology
Eberhard-Karls-University
D-7400 Tübingen, Germany

INTRODUCTION

There is a large body of evidence that static magnetic fields at currently used strengths up to 2 T in clinical application are safe and that possible interactions are harmless. This is one major conclusion of more than ten years of routine application of MRI in institutions all over the world. With the advent of technological progress and additional practical clinical and scientific demands (spectroscopy), MRI devices have been developed with field strengths up to 7 and more tesla.[1,2] Therefore, it is wise and necessary to continue research to explore the possible biologic and human interactions. TABLE 1 gives a list of possible human interactions with magnetic fields and shows the crucial points of current discussion. For a conservative approach, it is essential to take the recommendations of the different national authorities into consideration.[3,4] For static magnetic fields, the limits were set at 2.5 and 2 T, respectively.

The perspective of this contribution is to review the literature with special concern to MRI static magnetic fields and human interactions and to stress results from our own clinic[5] with respect to static magnetic field effects on auditory and somatosensory evoked potentials of patients, which were very recently extended to include controls with an examination time immediately following exposure to the field. This is only one possible access to the investigation of magnetic field effects that might outlast the exposure time.

METHODS

Twenty-five patients (13 women, 12 men; aged 23 to 72 years) were submitted to MRI investigation for diagnostical purposes. Most of them suffered from brain tumors, syringomyelia, and different diagnostically obscure diseases. The histories and diagnoses are not critical for the present investigation; therefore, they are not further described. After a first examination with brain stem auditory (BAEP) and somatosensory (SEP) evoked potentials, the MRI was performed with a superconducting system operating at 1.5-T field strength (Magnetom, Siemens) corresponding to a resonance frequency for protons of about 63 MHz. Body and head coils with a diameter of 500 mm and 300 mm, respectively, served as the transmitter and receiver coils. A gradient magnitude of 3 mT/m was available with a gradient rise time of 1 ms. Generally, the following sequences were used: T_1-weighted multislice single echo

59

TABLE 1. Possible Human Interactions with the Magnetic Field

Site of Action or Mechanism	Possible Sequelae[a]
(1) Thermal effects	cataract, change of metabolism
(2) Heart	arrhythmia
(3) Implants (e.g., clips, pacemakers)	damage to tissue, dysfunction of pacemaker
(4) Pregnancy	?
(5) Human metabolism	?
(6) Pulse generation	peripheral and central nervous system disorder
(7) Brain activity (EEG)	focal neurological and neuropsychological disorders
(8) Psychogenic (nonspecific)	claustrophobia

technique (TR of 400 ms, TE of 30 ms, two averages); T_2-weighted multislice double echo sequences (TR of 1600 ms, TE of 60 and 120 ms); CPGM (Carr-Purcell-Gill-Meibom) sequence of 8 or 16 echoes (TR of 2000 ms, TE of 30–480 ms). The power absorption for the radio frequencies used for the "worst case" in a patient weighing 81 kg is shown in TABLE 2. The time that elapsed between the MRI measurements and the evoked potential recordings was about 20 minutes up to 3 hours in the former investigation, whereas, in recent experiments on another 5 patients, it took about 5 minutes between magnetic field exposure and the first recordings. The full recording session for BAEP and SEP took about 30 minutes.

Median nerve SEPs were recorded following stimulation of either the median or ulnar nerve at the wrist with 0.2-ms square-wave pulses adjusted to 4 mA above the motor threshold. Recording was done either simultaneously from different points of the somatosensory afference (Erb's point, C7, C2, and C'_3/C'_4) or from the contralateral scalp alone (C'_3/C'_4, respectively) against an F_z-reference electrode. A total of 27 recordings were evaluated. BAEPs were routinely recorded simultaneously from both mastoids against a C_z-reference (platinum needles) following rarefaction click stimulation with pulses of 100 μV delivered monaurally over shielded earphones (70 dB SL at 11.9 Hz). Normal values for latencies, interpeak latencies, side differences, and the amplitude relation IV/V versus I were derived from our own laboratory data.[6] A total of 38 recordings could be quantitatively evaluated. FIGURE 1 illustrates the sites where BAEPs are generated within the brain stem and stresses the intraindividual constancy of these potentials. FIGURE 2 is a scheme of the stimulation and recording sites of a median nerve SEP.

TABLE 2. Human Power Absorption by MRI Radio-Frequency Exposure[a]

	Body Coil	Head Coil
SE/400 ms/30 ms	0.103 W/kg	0.009 W/kg
SE/1600 ms/60 ms, 120 ms	0.161 W/kg	0.014 W/kg
SE/2000 ms/30–480 ms	0.121 W/kg	0.011 W/kg

[a]SE = spin echo.

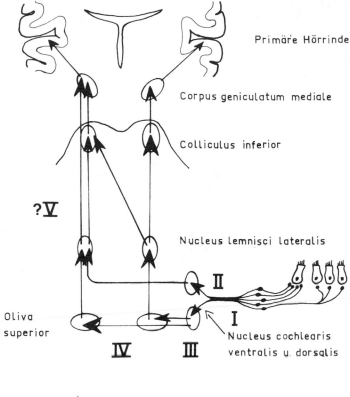

Primäre Hörrinde

Corpus geniculatum mediale

Colliculus inferior

?V

Nucleus lemnisci lateralis

II

Oliva superior

I

IV III

Nucleus cochlearis
ventralis u. dorsalis

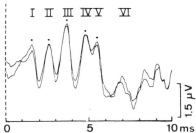

FIGURE 1. Illustration of the auditory pathway with location of the assumed generators of the waves of the BAEP. The normal waveform is shown in the bottom part of the figure. The waves with unknown origin are indicated by a question mark. (From reference 7, with permission.)

RESULTS

Brain Stem Auditory Evoked Potentials

BAEPs originate in the auditory nerve and in the ascending auditory pathway and are generally believed to monitor brain stem function. Although there are several anatomical and physiological restrictions to this notion, we agree that BAEPs may represent a good indicator of brain stem function because numerous synapses are involved in the transmission of sensory information. The example of FIGURE 3 is representative and shows a high intraindividual constancy of the latencies and shapes of the curves across the MRI session. TABLE 3 gives the results of 38 measurements for latencies and interpeak latencies (IPL). Because latency differences were very small and near the limits of visual analysis, we defined changes smaller than 0.2 ms as

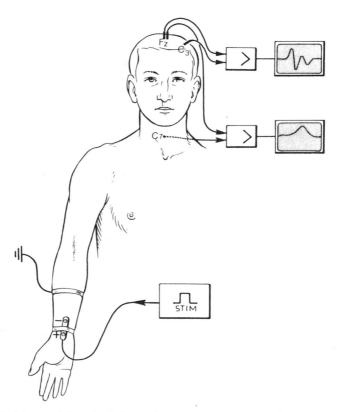

FIGURE 2. Scheme of the stimulation and recording device for median nerve SEP. (From reference 7, with permission.)

"no change". Changes of latency or IPL occurred only in a few instances, clearly within the limits of our normal collective.[6] Amplitudes are difficult to evaluate with BAEPs. There is broad agreement that, for clinical evaluation, only the latency relation IV/V versus I should be used because all other amplitude parameters are variable and dependent on slight changes of the state of the patient and methods. The amplitude relation as defined here was normal in all instances.

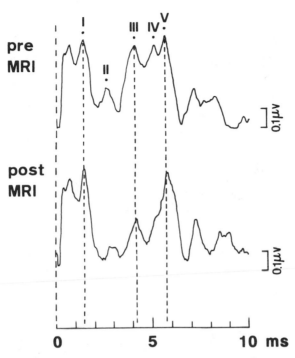

right ear

FIGURE 3. BAEP from a patient subjected to a diagnostic MRI with brain stem angioma. The latencies and amplitudes are quite similar, but the curves show a pathology with a prolonged interpeak I–III latency pointing to a brain stem process.

Somatosensory Evoked Potentials

Median nerve SEPs either recorded simultaneously from different sites of the somatosensory afference or only from above the contralateral scalp reliably monitor the function of the peripheral and central pathway. FIGURE 4 shows a typical cortical record with a clearly structured N 20 (postcentral generator) and the preceding wavelets in the ascending side of the potential, which are attributed to subcortical

TABLE 3. Latency Changes of BAEP Post versus Prior MRI ($n = 38$)[a]

	Peak			IPL		
	I	III	IV/V	I–III	III–V	I–V
no change (<0.2 ms)	38	35	35	33	35	36
0.2 ms	—	3	3	5	2	2
0.3 ms	—	—	—	—	1	—

[a]There was no change in the amplitude relation IV/V versus I; IPL = interpeak latency.

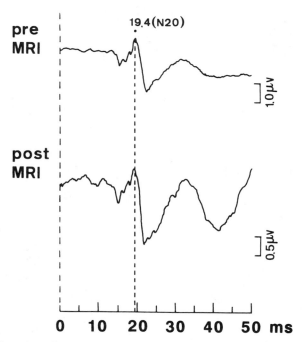

FIGURE 4. Normal median nerve SEP with nicely reproduced waves across the diagnostic MRI exposure.

generators. The origin of the late negative wave at about 32 ms is not really understood. This is a quasi-arbitrary example of pre- and post-MRI recordings demonstrating the constancy of these potentials. TABLE 4 is the quantification for all recordings. The maximum latency change among all recordings was 0.9 ms. Latency increases and decreases were nonsystematically distributed.[5] For the normal values in our laboratory, intraindividual side differences of up to 1.6 ms are regarded as normal. Although the figure of 1.6 ms does not correspond to the variability of intraindividual repetition, this value together with TABLE 4 suggests that the laten-

TABLE 4. Latencies and Amplitudes of SEP Post versus Prior MRI ($n = 27$)

	No Change (< 0.2 ms)	0.2–0.4 ms	> 0.4 ms
N 20 latency	8	13	6 (max. 0.9 ms)
	No Change (< 33%)	33–50%	> 50%
N 20 amplitude [difference (%)]	20	4	3 (max. 400%)

cies in the present study represent a normal intraindividual repetition variability. A factor that might influence the repeated recordings is the stress that the patients experience after several hours of examinations and transports. This might be reflected in the amplitude values of N 20, where only in a few instances larger differences occurred.

DISCUSSION

Recent reviews[8,9] and a basic paper on the health effects of MRI[10] should be consulted for a more complete and general overview on the subject.

Evoked Potentials

The present study proves that the somatosensory afference and the auditory brain stem pathway do not show any lasting effects of static magnetic field exposure. This is in agreement with several other studies that used similar field strengths and that recorded somatosensory[11] and visual and somatosensory evoked potentials[12] without any changes of latency or amplitude during exposure to the field. These findings challenge the results of von Klitzing,[13] who (in a series of mostly German-language papers) described changes of BAEP, SEP, and EEG. At least some of the data rely on interpretations of obvious artifacts. The negative finding with respect to detectable neurophysiologic changes due to magnetic field influence does not imply that changes do not occur. It must be expected that impulse propagation and synaptic processes might be affected at least by much stronger fields.[14]

EEG and Cognition

Several groups investigated the EEG, including power spectra, and applied several neuropsychological tests to assess cognitive deficiencies without finding any support for field-induced changes.[15-17]

Miscellanea

Two issues deserve special attention, namely, static field effects on the cardiac rhythm[18] and the corneal temperature changes during exposure to strong static and radio-frequency fields.[19] The cardiac cycle length was reported to increase by 17% during field exposure and the corneal temperature was significantly elevated by 0.5 °C on average (0–1.8 °C). Both changes were measured at field strengths of 2 T and 1.5 T, respectively. These changes are thought to be harmless, but have to be taken into consideration when stronger fields are applied.

ACKNOWLEDGMENTS

Special thanks are due to Ms. Winkler, who performed the neurophysiological recordings and completed part of the figures with high proficiency. The help of

Professor Voight (Department of Neuroradiology, University of Tübingen) is greatly appreciated.

REFERENCES

1. ORTENDAHL, D. A. 1988. Whole-body MR imaging and spectroscopy at 4 T: where do we go from here? Radiology 169: 864–865.
2. BARFUSS, H., H. FISCHER, D. HENTSCHEL, R. LADEBECK & J. VETTER. 1988. Whole-body MR imaging and spectroscopy with a 4-T system. Radiology 169: 811–816.
3. NRPB. 1983. Revised guidance on acceptable limits of exposure during nuclear magnetic resonance clinical imaging. Br. J. Radiol. 56: 974–977.
4. BGA. 1984. Empfehlungen zur Vermeidung gesundheitlicher Risiken verursacht durch magnetische und hochfrequente elektromagnetische Felder bei der NMR-Tomographie und in-vivo-NMR-Spektroskopie. Bundesgesundheitsblatt 27: 92–96.
5. NIEMANN, G., G. SCHROTH, U. KLOSE & U. W. BUETTNER. 1988. Influence of magnetic resonance imaging on somatosensory and brain-stem auditory evoked potentials in man. J. Neurol. 235: 462–465.
6. BUETTNER, U. W., M. STÖHR & E. KOLETZKI. 1983. Brain stem auditory evoked potential abnormalities in vascular malformations of the posterior fossa. J. Neurol. 229: 247–254.
7. STÖHR, M., J. DICHGANS, H. C. DIENER & U. W. BUETTNER, Eds. 1989. Evozierte Potentiale. (Second edition.) Springer-Verlag. Berlin/New York.
8. BEERS, G. J. 1989. Biological effects of weak electromagnetic fields from 0 Hz to 200 MHz: a survey of the literature with special emphasis on possible magnetic resonance effects. Magn. Reson. Imag. 7: 309–331.
9. SHELLOCK, F. G. 1989. Biological effects and safety aspects of magnetic resonance imaging. Magn. Reson. Q. 5: 243–261.
10. BUDINGER, T. F. 1981. Nuclear magnetic resonance (NMR) in vivo studies: known thresholds for health effects. J. Comput. Assist. Tomogr. 5: 800–811.
11. HONG, C-Z. & F. G. SHELLOCK. 1990. Short-term exposure to a 1.5 tesla static magnetic field does not affect somatosensory-evoked potentials in man. Magn. Reson. Imag. 8: 65–69.
12. VOGL, T., W. PAULUS, A. FUCHS, K. KRIMMEL & S. KRAFCZYK. 1988. Einfluß der in-vivo-Kernspintomographie auf somatosensorisch und visuell evozierte Potentiale beim Menschen. Digit. Bilddiagn. 8: 1–6.
13. VON KLITZING, L. 1986. Do static magnetic fields of NMR influence biological signals? Clin. Phys. Physiol. Meas. 7: 157–160.
14. WIKSWO, J. P. & J. P. BARACH. 1980. An estimate of the steady magnetic field strength required to influence nerve conduction. IEEE Trans. Biomed. Eng. (BME.27) 12: 722.
15. BESSON, J., E. I. FOREMAN, L. M. EASTWOOD, F. W. SMITH & G. W. ASHCROFT. 1984. Cognitive evaluation following NMR imaging of the brain. J. Neurol. Neurosurg. Psychiatry 47: 314–316.
16. BARTELS, M., K. MANN, M. MATEJCEK, M. PUTTKAMMER & G. SCHROTH. 1986. Magnetresonanztomographie und Sicherheit. Fortschr. Geb. Röntgenstr. 145: 383–385.
17. SWEETLAND, J., A. KERTESZ, F. S. PRATO & K. NANTAU. 1987. The effect of magnetic resonance imaging on human cognition. Magn. Reson. Imag. 5: 129–135.
18. JEHENSON, P., D. DUBOC, T. LAVERGNE, L. GUIZE, F. GUERIN, M. DEGEORGES & A. SYROTA. 1988. Change in human cardiac rhythm induced by a 2-T static magnetic field. Radiology 166: 227–230.
19. SHELLOCK, F. G. & J. V. CRUES. 1988. Corneal temperature changes induced by high-field-strength MR imaging with a head coil. Radiology 167: 809–811.

Session I Summary

ROBERT P. LIBURDY

Bioelectromagnetics Research Group
Research Medicine and Radiation Biophysics Division
Lawrence Berkeley Laboratory
University of California
Berkeley, California 94720

NMR imaging technology is developing at a rapid rate with special emphasis on achieving greater spatial and temporal resolution to aid the medical practitioner in providing health care. There are associated issues of health and safety of future high-field systems that pertain both to the health-care provider and to the patient, and this is the focus of the present symposium.

The keynote speaker, T. F. Budinger, reviewed the past ten years of available evidence dealing with health and safety as relating to current NMR imaging systems. Static magnetic, switched magnetic, and RF fields have increased significantly in field strength by factors of ten or more during this period and there is no evidence that NMR clinical procedures offer hazards to humans. Budinger pointed out that emerging technologies are being developed that employ fast scan strategies, higher frequency RF, and static magnetic fields that exceed 2.0 tesla. It is critical that these technical developments are matched with continuing experimental and theoretical work that deals with health and safety issues.

An understanding of how NMR fields physically interact with biological systems is central to studying the health and safety of NMR. This understanding must be based on physical principles dealing with forces that interact with charges present in biological systems. C. H. Durney discussed the three kinds of fields unique to the NMR imaging environment: static magnetic, switched magnetic, and RF fields. Understanding the latter two fields in terms of their internal dosimetry in body tissue in the NMR environment is a complex problem because near-field coupling and mutual coupling between sources and the body do exist and because the body is inhomogeneous and comprises layers of tissue of different permittivity. Durney emphasized that time-varying magnetic fields do not impart energy to biological systems, but that they do induce internal electric fields that do. The strength of the internal electric field is a function of the frequency, size, and shape of the field source and of the shape and size of the target tissue. Emerging NMR systems will unavoidably result in larger internal electric fields in tissue and the challenge lies in developing advanced numerical techniques and experimental approaches to accurately quantitate these fields.

J. D. de Certaines, F. S. Prato, and U. W. Buettner discussed the interactions of biological systems with NMR imaging fields at the cellular, animal, and human level, respectively. High strength static magnetic fields of ≥ 4.0 tesla are proposed for future imaging systems and de Certaines presented evidence that orientational effects can occur in large organized structures such as protein assemblies and periodic biopolymers like DNA at such field strengths. Potential risks *in vivo* due to such orientational effects are most likely nonexistent because they would require a constant field direction, which is not met for moving cellular systems *in vivo*. In addition, such changes are expected to be reversible during a time period commensurate with that of the NMR exposure and such changes, if they occur, would take place near the threshold required for the effect.

F. S. Prato presented work that he and colleagues carried out on morphine-induced analgesia responses in whole organisms exposed to NMR imaging fields. They observed antinociception (decreased analgesia) effects that are small and reversible, which represent nonthermal whole animal responses of mice and land snails to NMR imaging exposures using complete fields and switched gradient fields alone. The reversible nature of these small changes suggests that short-term exposures pose no adverse harmful health risks. At the molecular level, such changes in the opioid system may involve calcium (as discussed by Prato) and further work at the cellular level is required to define a possible site of interaction. In this symposium, I present research on calcium signal transduction in thymic lymphocytes that bears on these issues.

How the human responds to NMR imaging fields is a central question to health issues and U. W. Buettner presented research dealing with central nervous system function in human subjects exposed to a 1.5-tesla NMR imaging protocol. Alterations in auditory and somatosensory evoked potentials in a series of 25 patients are not evident to a detectable degree postexposure. This suggests that basic information processing in the brain stem and cortex is unaffected at these field strengths. Buettner cautioned that impulse propagation and synaptic processes might be affected by much stronger fields, and theoretical modeling and experimental animal studies are needed in this area.

A Theoretical Basis for Coupling via Induced Currents to Biological Systems for Ultra Fast Switched Magnetic Fields[a]

FRANK S. BARNES

Department of Electrical and Computer Engineering
University of Colorado
Boulder, Colorado 80309

INTRODUCTION

The development of new fast imaging NMR systems leads to the exposure of a significant fraction of the population to larger transient magnetic fields and thus to larger values of induced currents in the human body than have previously concerned designers of NMR systems. These currents may be as large as or larger than the natural currents that are flowing in the same region of the body. It is important to be able to estimate these currents in order to predict their impact on the biological system. The magnitude, time, and spatial distributions of these currents are all likely to be important in determining the biological impact. In this short report, we will review the basic equations and work out a number of examples that may help to illuminate possible side effects of the large transient magnetic fields.

THE BASIC FIELD EQUATIONS

In calculating the induced currents, it is most convenient to start with Maxwell's equation for the induced electric field, $\vec{E}$, in integral form or[1]

$$\int_{\ell} \vec{E} \cdot d\vec{\ell} = \int_{S} \frac{\partial \vec{B}}{\partial t} \cdot d\vec{S},$$

where ℓ is the length of the enclosed path encircling the area $\vec{S}$, $\vec{B}$ is the magnetic flux density, and t is the time.

For the case of a uniform magnetic field and a homogeneous material, we can obtain the value for the current density, $\vec{J}$, from Ohm's law or

$$\vec{J} = \sigma \vec{E},$$

where σ is the conductivity. In order to get an idea of the maximum values that might be expected, let us consider an approximation for a whole body exposure to a field that is changing with rate such that

$$|\partial \vec{B}/\partial t| = 10 \text{ T/s},$$

[a]This work was financially supported by the University of Colorado.

69

TABLE 1. Conductivities[a] for Some Common Biological Materials[4]

blood	$\sigma = 0.67$ S/m
lung	$\sigma = 0.05$ S/m
liver	$\sigma = 0.14$ S/m
fat	$\sigma = 0.04$ S/m
bone	$\sigma = 0.01$ S/m
cell fluid	$\sigma = 0.5$ S/m
membrane	$\sigma = 10^{-7}$–10^{-5} S/m

[a]These conductivities increase slowly with frequency and vary over a range of about a factor of 10. Different samples may give different results.

where we will approximate the area of the body by rectangle 0.2 m × 2 m so that S = 0.4 m[2] and $\ell = 4.4$ m. If we take a maximum value for $\sigma = 1$ S/m, then J = 0.91 A/m[2]. This current is approximately a factor of 100 larger than the values we found sufficient to change the firing rate of nerve cells taken from the ganglion of an aplysia.[2] More typical values of σ are given in TABLE 1 and the exposure area S is likely to be smaller so that real values of J will be considerably lower. In addition, the conductivity of biological materials is usually anisotropic and inhomogeneous and is a slowly varying function of frequency. For example, muscle tissue is anisotropic and typically varies over a range of 0.08 S/m to 0.6 S/m with angle.[3] Thus, a more favorable value for the maximum current density for whole body exposure is likely to be in the range of 0.40 A/m[2]. If we look at a structure like the head, just inside the skull with a radius of approximately 0.07 m, this reduces to about 0.17 A/m[2]. This value is still large compared to 0.01 A/m[2], which has been found to effect the firing rate of nerve cells.[2]

If we look at this induced current more closely, we find that most of it flows between the cell and only a small fraction of a dc current flows across the membranes as indicated in FIGURE 1. This problem becomes even more complex if we look at the

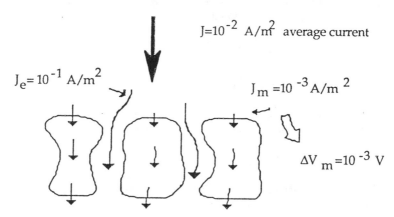

FIGURE 1. Partition of induced 60-Hz currents through and around cells[5] for an average tissue current of $J = 10^{-2}$ A/m[2], where J_e is the current density between the cells and J_m is the current density through the membrane.

variety of fluid, tissue, and bone that may appear in a current path. Another way to view these possible combinations is to calculate the maximum voltage, V, that could be generated or

$$V = -\int_\ell E \cdot d\ell;$$

for the whole body in our rectangular approximation, V = 4 volts and, for the head, V = 0.15 volts. These voltages are clearly large in comparison to the values necessary to perturb a single cell membrane, which may be as low as 10^{-4} volts. Thus, if we have a path enclosing a significant area with most of the path in low resistivity fluids, such as blood, the voltage will be concentrated across the high resistance region. In the worst case, this would be a single membrane.

Still another way to view this process is to ask the following: what is the area required to generate a voltage large enough to cause a given biological change? For the presumed maximum rate of change of B or $|\partial B/\partial t| = 10$ T/s, V = 10 S. This means that it takes approximately a centimeter of area enclosed by a low loss path to generate a millivolt signal that is easily detectable across a cell membrane. Such a situation could occur across a connection between a muscle or nerve cell that may be as long as several centimeters or in a combination of cells connected by gap junctions.

Another situation that can lead to the generation of currents in the body is rapid motion by the patient with respect to the magnetic field. The basic Lorentz equation is

$$\vec{F} = q(\vec{E} + \vec{v} \times \vec{B}).$$

If this equation is viewed as a means for finding the velocity, $\vec{v}$, this is equivalent to a value of an externally generated electric field, $\vec{E}$. This value of $\vec{E}$ can then be used for estimating the possible biological effects. If we ignore the vector properties of this equation and look only at the maximum values, then

$$|v| = |B/E|$$

and, for B = 4 T and E = 10^{-2} V/m, v = 4×10^{-6} m/s or 4 μm/s. This is clearly a very slow velocity that is required to get an easily detectable current pulse. A more likely velocity, such as a few centimeters per second, leads to fields on the order of 100 V/m, which could lead to the firing of a nerve cell 500 μm long with an induced transmembrane potential of 50 mV. In any case, this equation gives a clear warning that patients should be moved slowly in large magnetic fields in order to avoid undesirable shifts in cell membrane potentials.

An additional mechanism for interaction is the induced electric field gradients, ∇E, with dipole moments. The force on a dipole is given by $\vec{F} = (\vec{P} \cdot \nabla \vec{E})$, where $\vec{P}$ is the permanent dipole moment. For an induced dipole, the force is given by $\vec{F}_i = \alpha V (\vec{E} \cdot \nabla \vec{E})$, where α is the tensor polarizability and V is the volume. For low levels of fields, these forces are small. In order to get forces on dipoles of a single charge that are equal to those on singly charged ions, we need gradients of the fields that are on the order of the length of the molecule, d, multiplied by the field or $|\vec{F}_{dipole}/\vec{F}_{ion}| = |d\nabla\vec{E}/\vec{E}|$. Reasonable values of d are 10^{-9} to 10^{-8} m. Gradients of the field that are large enough to be important most likely occur near membrane surfaces and may be significant in orienting and moving large molecules.

It has recently been discovered that brain tissue from the human brain has a residual magnetic moment that implies the existence of particles of magnetite or Fe_2O_3.[6] The force on a magnetic dipole is given by

$$\vec{F} = \vec{m}\nabla\vec{B},$$

where $\vec{m}$ is the magnetic dipole moment and $\nabla\vec{B}$ is the gradient of the magnetic flux density. Inside, the solenoid magnetic field is relatively uniform and these forces should be small. However, these forces may be significant in the transition region when the patient is entering the magnet. These magnetic particles are from 20 to 50 nm on a side and are arranged in chains approximately 1 μm long in homing pigeons, salmon, and some other animals. In these animals, the magnetite particles are used as a compass. If similar chains of magnetite particles exist in humans, a dc magnetic field would exert a torque on the combination of particles:

$$\vec{T} = \vec{m}\vec{H} \sin \Theta,$$

where H is the magnetic field, Θ is the angle between H and m, and $B = \mu H$, with μ being the magnetic permeability. At magnetic fields of 1.5 to 4 T, the peak torques exerted by these fields would be more than 30,000 times the torques exerted by the Earth's magnetic fields and it would not be a surprise if they caused some problems, although to our knowledge none have been observed.

CONCLUSIONS

In conclusion, we have reviewed some of the mechanisms by which magnetic fields can interact with biological systems. Sample calculations indicate that the induced currents or voltages from the movement of the patient even at moderate speeds may be large enough for the patient to detect and that rapid motions should be avoided. Similarly, rapid changes in the magnetic field with respect to time will lead to induced currents and voltages that may be larger than those that occur during normal cell processes. There is a possibility that these induced currents could interfere with normal body functions. It is too early to access the possible importance of magnetite particles. However, when the distribution of these particles is known and their function understood, it will be very interesting to see what the large fields of an NMR magnet do to the related biological systems. In this review, we have not covered the possible effects of the RF fields. The physical effects of RF fields on biological systems are reviewed in reference 7.

REFERENCES

1. JOHNK, C. 1975. Engineering Electromagnetic Fields and Waves. Wiley. New York.
2. BARNES, F. S., A. SMOLLER & A. SHEPPARD. 1986. Proceedings of the Ninth Annual Conference of the IEEE Engineering in Medicine and Biology Society.

3. EPSTEIN, B. R. & K. R. FOSTER. 1983. Anisotropy in the dielectric properties of skeletal muscle. Med. Biol. Eng. Comput. **21:** 51–55.
4. BARNES, F. S. 1986. Interaction of dc electric fields with living matter. *In* Handbook of Biological Effects of Electromagnetic Fields. C. Polk & E. Postow, Eds. CRC Press. Boca Raton, Florida.
5. WACHTEL, H. Private communication.
6. KIRSCHVINK, J. L., A. K. KIRSCHVINK & B. WOODFORD. 1990. Human brain magnetic and squid magnetometry. Abstr. Annu. Int. Conf. IEEE Eng. Med. Biol. Soc. **12:** 3.
7. BARNES, F. S. 1989. Radio-microwave interactions with biological materials. Health Phys. **56**(5): 759–766.

Biological Interactions of Cellular Systems with Time-varying Magnetic Fields[a]

ROBERT P. LIBURDY

Bioelectromagnetics Research Group
Research Medicine and Radiation Biophysics Division
Lawrence Berkeley Laboratory
University of California
Berkeley, California 94720

INTRODUCTION

The interaction of time-varying magnetic fields with biological systems, both at the tissue and at the whole organism level, has been authoritatively reviewed by C. Polk and T. S. Tenforde, who contributed to the *CRC Handbook of Biological Effects of Electromagnetic Fields*.[1] In addition, the special case of NMR field interactions with biological tissue and with whole animals is discussed by T. F. Budinger in this symposium and in an excellent review,[2] as well as by B. R. R. Persson and F. Stahlberg[3] and by G. J. Beers.[4] Other specialists have conducted important research directly relevant to NMR fields and are contributors to the present publication.

The research reviewed here covers new investigations being conducted in our laboratory dealing specifically with cellular interactions with time-varying magnetic fields. We are engaged in studies using the lymphocyte as a model system to investigate field interactions with signal transduction events at the cell surface. Signal transduction in the T-lymphocyte is well characterized and it represents an excellent model for investigating field effects that occur at the cell surface and within the cell membrane.[5,6] Our working hypothesis is that cell surface events involved in signaling due to receptor binding and subsequent cell membrane biochemical events triggered by ligand-receptor complex formation may be influenced by magnetic fields. This approach is characterized by two features:[5] first, it focuses on the cell membrane as a substrate for magnetic field interactions; second, because its emphasis is signal transduction, it deals with early events responsible for a wide variety of important cellular processes such as RNA, DNA, and protein synthesis, which depend on calcium signaling.

The research presented here will first deal with 60-Hz sinusoidal fields that are relevant to environmental and occupational exposures that individuals may encounter in the home or workplace, respectively. Next, we will present recent research from our laboratory dealing with high-field NMR. Although these two electromag-

[a]This research was supported by the Office of Health and Environmental Research and the Office of Energy Management, Utilities System Division, United States Department of Energy, under Contract No. DE-AC-3-76SF00098. Support was also provided by the NIH under Grant No. CA53711 from the NCI to Robert P. Liburdy.

netic environments are significantly different in terms of their field composition (NMR fields comprise static, RF, and switched magnetic fields) and in terms of their accessibility for human exposure, they are worth comparing. This follows from our demonstration here that an important link between these two different electromagnetic environments is the switched gradient field, which contains ELF components. For example, we will show that a Fourier analysis of the switched waveform used in our NMR exposures reveals a 20-Hz fundamental frequency, with significant components at 40 and 60 Hz.

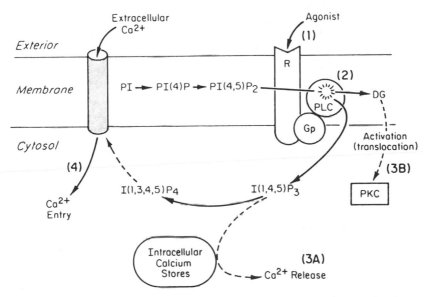

FIGURE 1. Molecular events during receptor-mediated signal transduction in T-lymphocytes: Ligand binding to the T-cell receptor complex [R] initiates events in the phosphatidylinositol [PI] pathway.[19] Phospholipase C [PLC] is activated via a G-protein complex and hydrolyzes phosphorylated PI to generate IP$_3$. IP$_3$ is water-soluble and acts as an endogenous ionophore to release calcium from intracellular stores into the cytosol; it also results in the opening of a specialized voltage-independent membrane channel to allow extracellular calcium to enter the cell. Both extracellular and intracellular calcium participate in T-cell activation.

EXPERIMENTAL PROCEDURES

Signal Transduction in T-Cell Activation

The model system employed in these studies is the activated lymphocyte. Mitogen activation of the T-lymphocyte is one of the best-characterized cellular systems for signal transduction studies.[6,7] FIGURE 1 depicts the molecular events that are triggered following the binding of mitogen, or ligand, to the T-cell receptor complex [R]. Once ligand binds to the receptor complex, activation of the coupled

G-protein complex occurs, which activates phospholipase C [PLC]. PLC splits phosphatidylinositol 4,5-bisphosphate [PI(4,5)P$_2$] in the membrane bilayer to yield diacylglycerol [DAG], which remains in the plane of the bilayer and activates protein kinase C [PKC], and to yield inositol 1,4,5-trisphosphate [IP$_3$], which is soluble and enters the cytosol. IP$_3$ acts as an intracellular ionophore to release calcium from intracellular stores and is rapidly phosphorylated to inositol 1,3,4,5-tetrakisphosphate [IP$_4$], which triggers entry of extracellular calcium through a specialized voltage-independent channel.[6] In the studies presented here, we follow the rapid and early release of intracellular calcium, [Ca^{2+}]$_i$, from internal stores, which we monitor directly for the first time during field exposure in a special cuvette using the fluorescent probe Fura-2, as well as the subsequent influx of extracellular calcium by monitoring transport of the isotope ^{45}Ca^{2+}.

It is important to emphasize that both of these parameters are significantly altered in the activated lymphocyte when mitogen binds to the cell surface during signal transduction. In the absence of mitogen, the lymphocyte is resting and

TABLE 1. Mitogen-activated Signal Transduction in the T-Lymphocyte

Response to Concanavalin A	First Detected
[Ca^{+2}]$_i$, Ca^{+2} influx increase InsP$_3$ release [pH]$_i$ increase PtdInsP$_2$, PtdInsP synthesis	0–5 minutes
c-*fos* mRNA increase c-*myc* mRNA increase Stimulation of glycolysis Increased metabolite uptake (e.g., uridine) Increased inositol incorporation into PtdIns	5–50 minutes
Increase in general RNA synthesis Increase in general DNA synthesis	> 300 minutes

maintains a baseline influx of extracellular calcium and a baseline level of free intracellular calcium. Lymphocyte activation is a normal process in response to extracellular signals that drives the lymphocyte into mitogenesis, followed by clonal expansion or cellular proliferation. As shown in TABLE 1, elevation of free calcium in the T-cell is one of the earliest events of mitogen activation and any field effect on calcium signaling is hypothesized by us to have an effect on subsequent "downstream" events in this pathway such as RNA, DNA, and protein synthesis.[5]

Biological Methodologies

Male Sprague-Dawley rats between 100 and 550 grams were employed in these studies as a source of thymic T-lymphocytes. Thymocytes were harvested and maintained in assay buffer consisting of 145 mM NaCl, 1 mM CaCl$_2$, 5 mM glucose, and 10 mM Na-HEPES at pH 7.4 (37 °C), 1.68 S/m, and 285 mOsm. Human peripheral blood lymphocytes were isolated by density gradient centrifugation using Ficoll-Hypaque; erythrocyte contamination was 5–7%. Cell viabilities as determined by nigrosine dye exclusion before and after field exposures were typically $\geq 95\%$.

Calcium transport across the lymphocyte membrane was monitored by using $^{45}Ca^{+2}$ in an assay in which lymphocytes are rapidly centrifuged through a nonaqueous layer of dibutyl phthalate [DBP].[8] This is a rapid one-step procedure that has the advantage of stripping away loosely bound cell-surface calcium as the cells pellet through the DBP; cell pellets are dispersed into liquid scintillation media and are counted. Early studies involved using a centrifugation assay that required cell manipulation and three cycles of washing the cell pellet before liquid scintillation spectroscopy.[9]

Intracellular calcium was monitored by loading thymocytes with Fura-2/AM. This involved incubation of cells at 1×10^7/mL in the presence of 2 μM Fura-2/AM for 60 minutes at 35 °C with gentle shaking. To determine if thymocytes were adequately loaded and still retained biological activity, washed thymocytes were characterized for their response to the mitogen Concanavalia einsfomis [Concanavalin A, Con-A], which results in an increase in $[Ca^{2+}]_i$, and to the ionophore Ionomycin, as well as $MnCl_2$, which establishes a maximum dynamic range for the probes' response to the influx of extracellular calcium.[10]

Con-A was employed at a mitogenic dose of 1 μg/mL, unless otherwise indicated. All assays were performed at 37.0 ± 0.05 °C.

60-Hz Sinusoidal Magnetic Field Exposures

The solenoidal exposure device used in these studies was fabricated by the Magnet Winding Group at Lawrence Berkeley Laboratory and is shown in FIGURE 2. The coil ($N = 400$ turns, $R = 2.3\Omega$, $L = 20$ mH) was energized with a 60-Hz line current and was operated while immersed in a water-cooled, cylindrical sleeve. Special features of this device are that (1) the solenoid is thermally isolated from the bore of the coil, (2) an internal water bath tank is situated inside the bore and is fed by another water bath to thermoregulate the annular plate holding the cells, and (3) the internal water bath tank is physically isolated from the solenoid so that vibrations are not transmitted to the annular plate housing the cells.

The temperature of the water circulating around the solenoidal coil, the internal water bath tank, and the temperature of the thymocyte cell suspension were monitored using thermistor-type microprobes calibrated against a platinum resistance temperature standard traceable to the National Institute of Technology and Standards (NITS). Temperature stability of the cell suspensions in the annular plate wells was maintained to 37.0 ± 0.05 °C during all experiments.

The time-varying, sinusoidal 60-Hz magnetic field in the bore of the solenoid was mapped using an axial Hall-effect probe and a Bell Model 620 gauss meter (F. W. Bell, Incorporated; Orlando, Florida). This probe and meter were calibrated by the Magnet Field Measurements Group at Lawrence Berkeley Laboratory using a precision Helmholtz coil device. The magnetic field flux density in the active exposure volumes corresponding to each annular plate well was measured to ±3%. With the solenoid unenergized, the local geomagnetic field was mapped using a Model 428B flux-gate meter from Hewlett Packard. The static (DC) magnetic flux

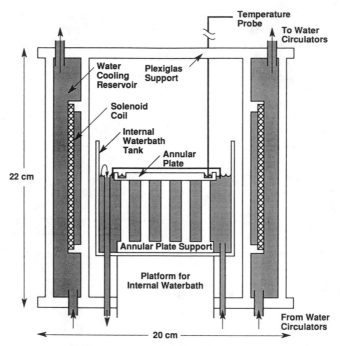

FIGURE 2. Solenoid cell culture exposure system: Special features include a water sleeve to control the temperature of the solenoid coil ($N = 400$, $R = 2.3\Omega$, $L = 20$ mH), an isolated internal water bath system for the bore of the solenoid to hold an annular cell culture plate, and a temperature monitoring probe. Temperature is controlled to ± 0.05 °C.

density was 0.330 gauss in the direction parallel to the solenoid long-axis in the annular plate wells with the plate positioned in the center volume of the bore. With the solenoid unenergized, the ambient 60-Hz magnetic field was mapped along two orthogonal axes, which were themselves orthogonal to the long-axis of the bore. Using a Model 42B-1 AC milligauss meter by Monitor Industries (Boulder, Colorado), we detected a 60-Hz N-S oriented flux density of 8 mG and an E-W oriented flux density of 8 mG.

A critically important feature of these experiments is a specially designed, multiring, acrylic plate for exposing thymocytes (FIGURE 3). Because exposure to the time-varying magnetic field flux density is identical for each well, the consequence of each well having a different radius (r) is that the induced electric field, and thus the induced current in the cell suspension, will vary in direct proportion to r. This is shown in FIGURE 4, where Faraday's law depicts the relationship between the induced electric field and the induced current for a simple circular geometry such as our annular well track. The annular well tracks shown in FIGURE 3 have the following radii (average): 0.75 cm, 2.25 cm, and 3.75 cm. The current density scaling factors are therefore 1, 3, and 5, respectively. Based on an incident 60-Hz magnetic field flux density of 22 mT (rms) and the measured conductivity (σ) of the cell suspension of 1.68 S/m (Yellow Springs Model 35, Yellow Springs, Ohio), the computed induced current in the middle well of the annular plate is 16 μA/cm^2. The calculated power induced in the sample due to joule heating is approximately 130 nW and the temperature excursion expected over a 60-minute period in a nonthermostated sample is computed to be less than 10^{-6} °C.

Note that the right-hand plate in FIGURE 3 is shown with an acrylic plug or dam in each well. This important modification was made for the control plates so that there would be no large circular current loop pathway; this modification has the effect of reducing induced current to negligible values in the annular wells. We calculated this value after first measuring the ambient 60-Hz magnetic field flux density experienced by the control plate, which we positioned in a double-walled Styrofoam bath chamber that was physically remote from laboratory electrical devices and completely shielded with Co-Netic AA Foil (0.254 mm, Magnetic Shielding Corporation, Bensenville, Illinois). This bath was filled with water that was circulated through a thermoregulating water bath so that the temperature in the wells of the annular plates positioned in the bath chamber was isothermal at 37.0 ± 0.05 °C. The ambient 60-Hz magnetic flux density incident upon the plane of the plate was 5 mG; values of 0.6 and 9.0 mG were obtained in the N-S and E-W directions, respectively. Based on the 5-mG value incident to the plane of the plate, we computed that the induced current density experienced by the control thymocytes would be 3.64 × 10^{-3} μA/cm^2, but only if an acrylic plug was absent from the well. Although this value for induced current is reduced by a factor of 4.4 × 10^{-3} compared to that for exposed cells, the actual value for induced current is effectively zero because an acrylic plug was employed in all control wells.

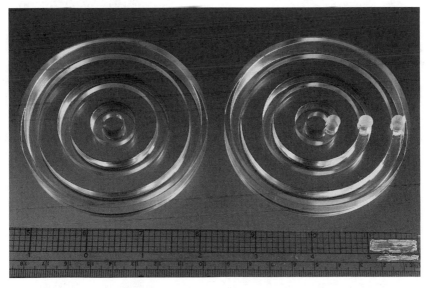

FIGURE 3. Multiwell annular cell culture plates: Annular plates were constructed from optical quality acrylic with three annular tracks having average radii of 0.75 cm, 2.25 cm, and 3.75 cm (1:3:5). Acrylic plugs are positioned in the wells of one plate to block electric field induction around the annular ring. Such plates are used in sham control exposures in a magnetic field–shielded box to ensure that no electric field is induced in these samples.

60-Hz Sinusoidal Electric Field Exposures

Experiments employing the annular ring cell culture dish and a sinusoidal 60-Hz magnetic field, described later, indicate that the induced electric field, in contradistinction to the magnetic field itself, was responsible for the field effect. Therefore, exposures to a spatially uniform 60-Hz sinusoidal electric field were performed using two platinum electrodes (each embedded in an ultrapure agarose diffusion barrier), which were placed at opposing sides of a fluorescence cuvette (FIGURE 5). A signal generator was employed to drive the current through a variable resistor in series with the cuvette; frequency, voltage, and waveform were monitored. By using this

Faraday's Law of Induction

$$V_{peak} = \left| \frac{d(\vec{B} \cdot \vec{S})}{dt} \right| = \pi r^2 \frac{dB}{dt}$$

$$|\vec{E}_{peak}| = \frac{V_{peak}}{2\pi r} = \frac{r}{2} \frac{dB}{dt} = \pi f r B_0$$

$$|\vec{J}_{peak}| = |\vec{E}_{peak}| \cdot \sigma$$

$$|\vec{J}_{peak}| = \frac{\sigma r}{2} \frac{dB}{dt} = \sigma \pi f r B_0$$

V = Potential (Volts)
B = Magnetic Field (Tesla) = $B_0 \sin(2\pi ft)$
S = Area $\perp$ to B (m^2)
E = Electrical Field (V/m)
J = Induced Current Density (A/m^2)
σ = Conductivity of medium (S/m)

Annular Cell Culture Plate

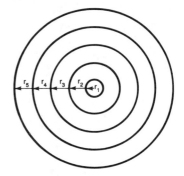

Spatially Uniform B field
$\perp$ to Plane of Culture Dish

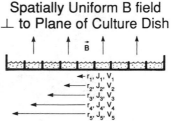

FIGURE 4. Induced electric field in the annular cell culture plate: Faraday's law of induction defines the induced electric field in each annular track. For a uniform incident magnetic field B, the induced electric field E varies directly as the radii of the annular rings.

exposure system and by placing an optical slit in one electrode, it was possible to make fluorescence measurements for the first time to monitor [Ca^{2+}]$_i$ in real time during field exposure.

High-Field NMR Exposures

A Bruker high-field 2.35-T imaging system as shown in FIGURE 6 was used for NMR exposures. This NMR physical environment is a combination of a 2.35-T ultra high static magnetic field, an RF field, and ELF field components associated with the time-varying gradient magnetic field. We employed NMR fields typical of multislice,

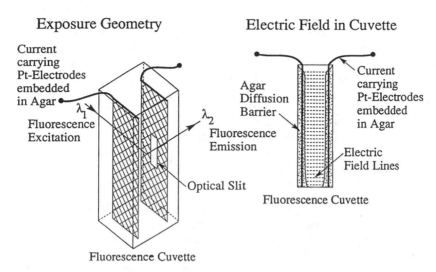

FIGURE 5. Fluorescence cuvette for 60-Hz sinusoidal electric field exposures: Opposing platinum electrodes are embedded in ultrapure agarose (agar). The optical slit enables the direct application of a spatially uniform sinusoidal 60-Hz electric field while simultaneously monitoring sample fluorescence.

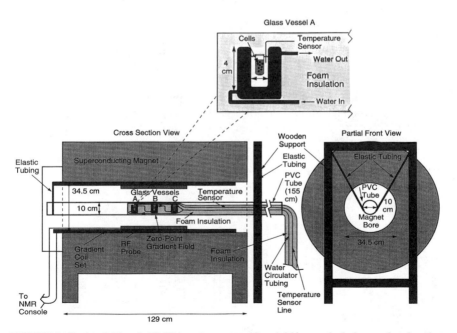

FIGURE 6. Bruker 2.35-tesla NMR imaging system: Special features include sample tubes that are thermostated and that are mechanically isolated from the bore of the magnet via a suspended plastic conduit that is coaxial with the magnet bore. Glass vessels A, B, and C are situated so that A and C are at identical gradient field intensities, whereas the middle vessel, B, is located at the null or zero gradient crossover point.

multiecho imaging sequences (switched gradient, $dB/dz = 10$ mT/m; RF, pulsed 64 μT, 100 MHz carrier). A train of 1 100-μs pulse, α_1, followed by 16 200-μs pulses, α_2, was repeated every 1.2 seconds. The RF pulse and gradient amplitude were calibrated by employing a sphere containing water that was placed at the position occupied by the cellular sample. The RF pulse amplitude was set to produce spin echoes of the greatest amplitude, corresponding to $\alpha_1 = \pi/2$ and $\alpha_2 = \pi$. The RF field amplitude was calibrated using the relationship, $\alpha = \Gamma B \tau$, where Γ is the gyromagnetic ratio of the proton, B is the magnetic flux density, and τ is the pulse duration. The gradient field was calculated from the location of the sphere in a one-dimensional projection image with the spectrometer reference frequency set at resonance in the absence of the gradient: $G = \Delta w / \Gamma \Delta x$, where G is the field gradient, Δw is the frequency of the peak echo spectrum, and Δx is the displacement of the sphere from the isocenter of the magnet.

Rat thymic T-lymphocytes were exposed for 60 minutes in a vibration-isolated, isothermal glass exposure vessel that was positioned on the z-axis at $z = +/-10$ cm ($dB/dt = 1$ T/s, 1 mT B_{peak}). The NMR exposure vessel was thermoregulated at 37.0 ± 0.05 °C and a similar isothermal control vessel was used to simultaneously treat cells 6.5 meters from the NMR system (0.3 mT static, no RF or switched fields). The exposure design enables three glass vessels containing thymocytes to be simultaneously exposed at z equal to -10 cm, 0 cm, and 10 cm. This corresponds to the maximum dB/dt (1 T/s) and to the null or zero gradient crossover point where $dB/dt = 0$. The NMR-exposed thymocytes were isolated from structural vibrations by placing the glass vessel in a hanging plastic tube (155 cm long, 6.6 kg) colinear with the center of the magnet bore suspended from the NMR frame using elastic tubing. The measured spring-mass resonance frequency was 1.7 Hz.

An important link between NMR exposures and ELF fields is identified in this study, we believe, for the first time: the switched magnetic field employed in NMR imaging contains ELF components. We demonstrate this in FIGURES 7 and 8. The NMR gradient magnetic field in FIGURE 7 has 1 pulse followed by 16 pulses. The 16-pulse train components are each on for 30 ms and off for 20 ms, with a cycle time of 50 ms. This corresponds to a fundamental frequency of 20 Hz. To illustrate this, the frequency distribution of the gradient waveform was computed via Fourier analysis (FIGURE 8). The power spectrum corresponds to the square of the amplitude coefficients shown on the y-axis and significant power is associated with 20-, 40-, and 60-Hz components.

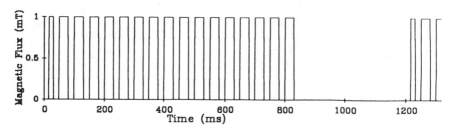

FIGURE 7. NMR switched gradient magnetic field: The pulse train has a series of 16 square-wave pulses with an on-time of 30 milliseconds and an off-time of 20 milliseconds. This 50-millisecond cycle corresponds to a fundamental frequency of 20 Hz (see FIGURE 8).

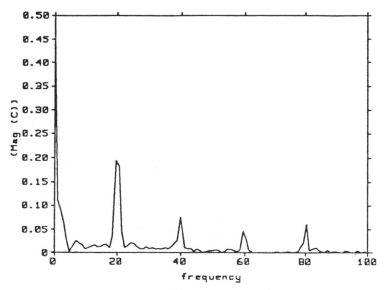

FIGURE 8. Frequency dependence of the NMR switched gradient field: Frequency distribution of the gradient waveform was computed via Fourier analysis. The power spectrum corresponds to the square of the amplitude coefficients shown on the y-axis. The fundamental frequency is at 20 Hz, corresponding to a 50-millisecond cycle time (see FIGURE 7). ELF components are prominent at 20, 40, and 60 Hz.

RESULTS

60-Hz Magnetic Fields: Calcium Influx Is Altered during Mitogen Activation

In these experiments, thymocytes were assessed for calcium uptake using $^{45}Ca^{2+}$ with cells exposed to 60-Hz fields in the absence or presence of the mitogen, Con-A. Field exposures were at 1.0 mV/cm induced electric field using an annular ring average radius of 2.25 cm, 16 $\mu A/cm^2$ induced current density, 220 gauss$_{rms}$, 37.0 ± 0.05 °C, and 60 minutes.

Representative data from a series of experiments employing different animals are shown in FIGURE 9 (Con-A, 20 $\mu g/mL$).[9] Spontaneous or background calcium uptake is shown in the open bars and values are seen to vary for different thymocyte preparations. In the presence of Con-A, calcium uptake is enhanced, but it also varies across animals (hatched bars); the percent Con-A activation is computed as the percent increase due to the addition of Con-A relative to that for background uptake. During 60-Hz field exposure, calcium influx in Con-A-activated thymocytes is further enhanced (solid bars) and this field response also varies across animals. The percent increase in Con-A-activated calcium influx due to the 60-Hz field is computed by first subtracting the background uptake and then comparing Con-A to 60-Hz Con-A uptake. In our studies, 60-Hz fields were found to have no influence on the background calcium uptake. Thus, mitogen activation is critical in eliciting this biological response.

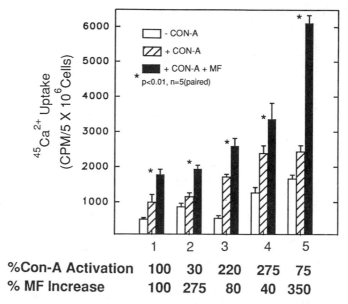

%Con-A Activation   100   30   220   275   75
% MF Increase   100   275   80   40   350

FIGURE 9. Calcium influx in thymocytes exposed to 60-Hz magnetic fields: Calcium influx was monitored by following $^{45}Ca^{+2}$ uptake in thymocytes in the absence of mitogen (−Con-A), in the presence of mitogen (+Con-A), and in the presence of mitogen and the 60-Hz magnetic field (+Con-A, +MF). Data are shown from five experiments employing different animals. Note that the %Con-A activation and the %MF increase vary for thymocyte preparations. Animal age is revealed as a predictor for the level of mitogen activation and response to the MF (see FIGURE 10). Exposures are at 1.0 mV/cm (22 mT), 16 μA/cm², 37 ± 0.05 °C, and 60 minutes.

60-Hz Magnetic Fields: Animal Age Is Correlated with Mitogen Activation and Field-induced Alterations in Calcium Influx

To develop a relationship between the level of mitogen activation observed in thymocytes and the increase in Con-A-stimulated calcium uptake due to 60-Hz fields, experiments were performed employing animals having a wide range in age (weight).[5] A plot was constructed using these two parameters, with animal age shown for each experimental group, and FIGURE 10 clearly shows an age dependence for data from eight different animal experiments. This graph indicates several important findings: (1) animal age is a predictor of Con-A activation and thymocytes from relatively younger animals display the greatest increase in calcium uptake due to Con-A; (2) the 60-Hz field effect is most prominent for thymocytes obtained from relatively old donors, indicating that calcium uptake is increased the greatest during 60-Hz exposures of suboptimally activated cells; and (3) as Con-A activation levels increase for thymocytes from young animals, a diminishingly small response to 60-Hz fields is observed and this suggests that the maximal dynamic response of the cell, once achieved, cannot be further exceeded by exposure to 60-Hz fields. The finding that a decline in Con-A-activated calcium uptake in unexposed thymocytes is correlated with an increase in animal age is consistent with previous reports in the literature.[11]

60-Hz Magnetic Fields: Induced Electric Field Dependence of Mitogen-activated Calcium Influx

Experiments were performed to answer the following question: does the induced electric field, and thus the induced current density in the cell suspension, or the magnetic field itself play a determining role in the 60-Hz effect illustrated in FIGURE 10? To do this, we employed the specially constructed multiring annular cell culture plates fabricated in our laboratory (FIGURE 3) and loaded cells into the outer ring and the inner ring. This resulted in a fivefold reduction in induced current density, from 27 to 5.3 $\mu A/cm^2$ (induced electric field levels of 1.7 and 0.33 mV/cm, respectively), while exposing cells in both wells to the same 220-gauss$_{rms}$ spatially uniform magnetic field. Results are shown in FIGURE 11, which represents data pooled from a series of experiments (*n* represents the number of raw data samples). The addition of Con-A (1–3 $\mu g/mL$) to resting thymocytes resulted in an increase in calcium uptake of approximately 35%. The 1.7-mV/cm 60-Hz field resulted in a further increase over that observed for Con-A alone; this increase corresponds to an approximate doubling of the calcium uptake associated with Con-A activation alone (Con-A uptake minus background). This increase is consistent with the increases shown in FIGURE 9. However, at the induced electric field of 0.33 mV/cm (5.3

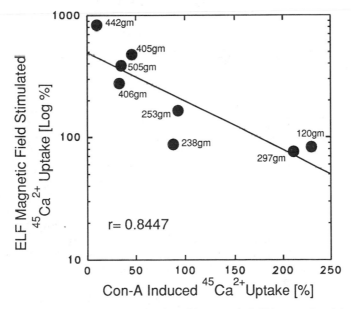

FIGURE 10. Correlation of mitogen activation with magnetic field increase in calcium uptake: An inverse relationship is observed between animal age (weight in grams) and the level of mitogen activation displayed by thymocytes (x-axis)—thymocytes from older animals exhibit suboptimal mitogen activation. The magnetic field increase in Con-A-triggered calcium influx (y-axis) is correlated with this level of mitogen activation (*r*, correlation coefficient): suboptimal mitogen activation is associated with a vigorous response to 60-Hz magnetic fields. Thymocytes from older animals display minimal activation and maximal increases in calcium influx due to exposure to the magnetic field.

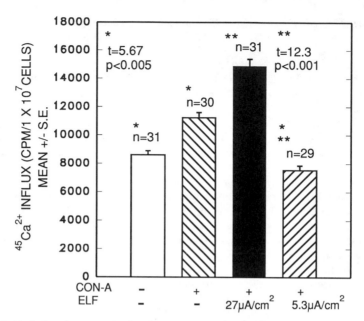

FIGURE 11. Induced current dependence of mitogen-activated calcium influx in rat thymocytes: A uniform 60-Hz magnetic field (220 gauss$_{rms}$) was incident upon a multiring annular cell culture plate (FIGURE 3), resulting in an induced electric field of 1.7 and 0.33 mV/cm and an induced current density of 27 and 5.3 $\mu A/cm^2$, respectively, in the outer and inner annular rings. Exposures are at 37 ± 0.05 °C and 60 minutes.

$\mu A/cm^2$), we detected an inhibition of Con-A-activated calcium uptake and this inhibition was a reduction to levels of background uptake.

These results are significant for several reasons. First, they indicate that, at a relatively low induced electric field of 0.33 mV/cm, the 60-Hz field inhibits (rather than enhances) calcium uptake during mitogen stimulation. This suggests a nonlinear response to the applied field. Second, the field metric of interest in these experiments is clearly the induced electric field because the cellular response was altered by changing the induced electric field while holding the magnetic field flux density constant. Third, the inhibition at low induced current is biologically interesting because this reduction was to background levels seen in the absence of Con-A. This raises the question of whether Con-A binding in itself is altered by the 60-Hz field because inhibition of Con-A binding would result in the background values of spontaneous uptake we observed.

60-Hz Electric Fields: Intracellular Calcium Is Altered in Mitogen-activated Thymocytes

The aforementioned studies assess calcium influx during mitogen-activated signal transduction and report on steady-state calcium influx at 60 minutes. According to TABLE 1, $[Ca^{2+}]_i$ should increase within the first 5 minutes along with calcium influx during signal transduction. To obtain the first real-time assessment of the free intracellular calcium in cells exposed to 60-Hz fields, we have performed studies using the fluorescent probe Fura-2. This approach enables thymocytes to be monitored while Con-A is added and a 60-Hz field is applied to determine instantaneous, real-time changes in $[Ca^{2+}]_i$. Because the studies mentioned earlier established that the induced electric field is responsible for the effect, a special exposure chamber was employed in these studies to apply a spatially uniform 60-Hz sinusoidal electric field. The fluorescence cuvette illustrated in FIGURE 5 with two agar-embedded platinum electrodes was injected with 60-Hz current to achieve a spatially uniform current density of 6 μA/cm^2.

FIGURE 12 shows the real-time monitoring of $[Ca^{2+}]_i$ for thymocytes during Con-A activation in the presence or absence of a 60-Hz electric field. In these experiments, thymocytes were loaded with Fura-2/AM and were followed to determine a baseline value for $[Ca^{2+}]_i$ over several minutes. Traces A, B, C, and D are shown offset in the y-axis direction to identify overlapping traces for times of 0–300 seconds. Subsequently, a 60-Hz field was applied at 6 μA/cm^2 and then Con-A was added (traces C and D), or Con-A was added in the absence of the electric field (traces A and B). It was found that resting thymocytes display a relatively constant level of $[Ca^{2+}]_i$ until Con-A is added (1 μg/mL) at 300 seconds; thereafter, a rapid rise in $[Ca^{2+}]_i$ is observed, which is referred to as the early phase of calcium signaling.

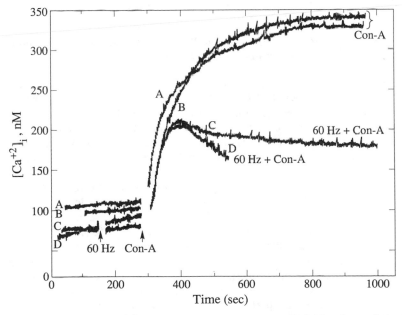

FIGURE 12. Effect of a spatially uniform sinusoidal 60-Hz electric field on intracellular free calcium in thymocytes: Real-time monitoring of intracellular free calcium, $[Ca^{2+}]_i$, in Fura-2-loaded thymocytes (1 × 10^7/mL); (A & B) continual time course before and after the addition of mitogen, Con-A; (C & D) continual time course before and after application of 60-Hz electric fields and after addition of Con-A. Following the first 100 seconds of mitogen-activated calcium release, 60-Hz exposed cells exhibit a reduction in $[Ca^{2+}]_i$. Exposures are at 6 μA/cm^2, 0.38 mV/cm, 1 μg/mL Con-A, and 37 ± 0.05 °C.

Thereafter, $[Ca^{2+}]_i$ stabilizes at approximately threefold above the original baseline level to reach a steady-state plateau phase that is due to influx of extracellular calcium. Traces C and D correspond to the treatment of thymocytes first with 60-Hz fields followed by Con-A and no influence of 60-Hz fields is detected at 300 seconds before Con-A is added. After Con-A is added, $[Ca^{2+}]_i$ is seen to increase in a manner nearly identical to that seen in traces A and B over the next 100 seconds. Thus, thymocytes appear to respond normally to Con-A during exposure to the 60-Hz electric field during the early phase of signal transduction. However, this response is significantly blunted after 100 seconds and a further rise in $[Ca^{2+}]_i$ is not observed.

This inhibition of $[Ca^{2+}]_i$ at 6 $\mu A/cm^2$ is interesting in light of the calcium influx data presented in FIGURE 11, where a similar induced current level leads to inhibition of calcium influx at 60 minutes. Although both parameters change in the same direction, the early rise in $[Ca^{2+}]_i$ reflects the rapid release of intracellular calcium from internal stores in structures such as the mitochondria and ER, whereas the subsequent plateau phase of $[Ca^{2+}]_i$ as well as calcium uptake at 60 minutes reflect a steady-state level of calcium exchange with extracellular calcium through a plasma membrane calcium channel. These results suggest that the outer plasma membrane calcium channel is a site of field interaction. Both the early increase in $[Ca^{2+}]_i$ and a sustained increase in calcium influx are important for effective signal transduction that leads to mitogenesis and cellular proliferation.[10]

NMR Studies: Mitogen Activation Is Correlated with NMR-induced Alterations in Mitogen-activated Calcium Influx

A similar approach to that for the 60-Hz fields was employed in assessing the possible effect of high-field NMR on calcium uptake in thymocytes. Because animal age plays an important role in mitogen activation, we used two groups of animals that represented relatively young and old thymocyte donors. The question we addressed was whether high-field NMR alters calcium uptake in mitogen-activated thymocytes and, moreover, whether a response would correlate with age and thus with the level of mitogen activation.

Relatively young rats (200 g) were assessed for mitogen-activated calcium uptake and FIGURE 13 depicts the results from four treatment groups in which high-field NMR treatments were conducted on thymocytes in the absence or presence of Con-A. The left-hand-side data indicate that high-field NMR has no influence on background calcium uptake in resting thymocytes. In the presence of Con-A alone, an approximately 400% increase in calcium uptake is observed (open bars); this is typical for thymocytes from young animals. For these thymocytes, no influence of high-field NMR was detected during mitogen activation (right-hand-side data).

When similar tests were performed in which thymocytes from relatively old rats (450 g) were employed, we detected a high-field NMR response, but only for mitogen-activated cells. FIGURE 14 indicates (1) that these thymocytes are nonresponsive to mitogen (open bars), (2) that high-field NMR does not influence baseline uptake of calcium in resting thymocytes (left-hand-side data), and (3) that an approximately 22% increase in calcium uptake is detected during high-field NMR for mitogen-stimulated cells. These findings are consistent with results obtained with

60-Hz fields in which thymocytes from older animals, displaying suboptimal mitogen activation, respond to the field (FIGURE 10).

To determine whether human peripheral blood lymphocytes, which represent a mixture of mature T- and B-lymphocytes, respond to high-field NMR, three separate experiments were performed on different dates (FIGURE 15). The responses observed are similar to those shown in FIGURE 14 for suboptimally activated thymic lymphocytes: in the absence of mitogen, no influence of high-field NMR was detected on calcium uptake; however, an approximately 30% increase in calcium uptake was detected in suboptimally mitogen-activated human lymphocytes during high-field NMR.

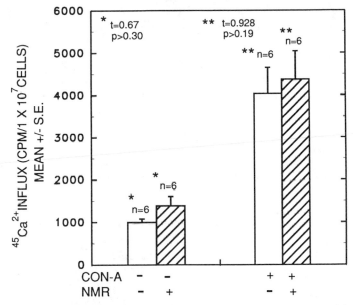

FIGURE 13. Effect of 2.35-T NMR imaging fields on mitogen-activated calcium influx: adolescent rats (200 g). An approximately 400% increase in calcium influx is observed in the presence of Con-A (1 μg/mL). No effect of NMR is detected in resting or mitogen-activated thymocytes. NMR exposure conditions are given in the text; thymocytes are at 37 ± 0.05 °C.

DISCUSSION

It is important that experimental studies in the interdisciplinary field of bioelectromagnetics be equally balanced with regard to excellent biology and engineering. The research presented here pays special attention to engineering and technical approaches to aid in hypothesis testing. For example, the design of our multiring annular cell culture plate based on Faraday's law to test whether the applied magnetic field itself or the induced electric field is the metric of interest proved invaluable in identifying the electric field as the biologically relevant metric. Also, the use of a special cuvette exposure chamber for the direct application of a spatially

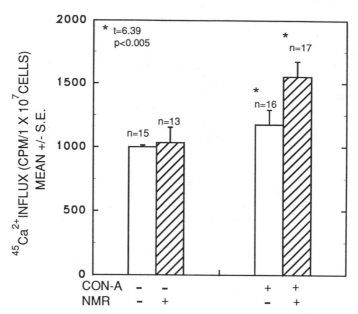

FIGURE 14. Effect of 2.35-T NMR imaging fields on mitogen-activated calcium influx: mature rats (450 g). Minimal to no increase in calcium influx is observed in the presence of Con-A (1 μg/mL). No effect of NMR is observed for resting thymocytes, whereas a 22% increase is observed in mitogen-activated thymocytes. NMR exposure conditions are given in the text; thymocytes are at 37 ± 0.05 °C.

uniform 60-Hz electric field, once the induced electric field was identified as the appropriate metric, enabled the first real-time monitoring of $[Ca^{2+}]_i$ during field exposure. In both the 60-Hz and the NMR studies, special attention was given to the exposure system design to minimize or eliminate confounding factors such as temperature differences and acoustic vibrations.

In bioelectromagnetic studies, it is critical to employ a well-characterized and appropriately relevant biological system. In these studies, we used normal thymic lymphocytes harvested directly from animals and we investigated two physiologically important cellular responses, calcium influx and $[Ca^{+2}]_i$, both critical to lymphocyte signal transduction. Cell signaling and lymphocyte activation have direct *in vivo* relevance to lymphocyte function.[5–7]

An important finding based on these studies is that specific biological constraints operate to restrict the response of lymphocytes to electromagnetic fields. This underscores the need to identify and understand such biological constraints in assessing the possibility of potential health effects. As an example, animal age was shown to be an important factor in defining the level of mitogen activation for a lymphocyte population. In these studies, thymic lymphocytes from relatively young rats displayed maximal mitogen activation with no detectable response to either 60-Hz fields or high-field NMR. This is most likely due to the cells exhibiting a maximal level of activation by Con-A without having further dynamic range to respond to the fields. Thymocytes from older donors, in contrast, showed suboptimal or reduced mitogen activation and were found to respond to both 60-Hz and high-field NMR. Biologically, this is an important constraint and we interpret this finding as evidence that the fields act as a comitogen because synergy is observed between the field and the mitogen; however, this is only for suboptimally activated cells. These studies also emphasize the importance of immune system senescence in defining the biological status of the organism and its potential response to time-varying magnetic fields. In this regard, it would be of interest to assess the field response of human peripheral blood lymphocytes obtained from very young and very old donors.

The biological relevance and focus of the model system employed in these studies is signal transduction in normal lymphocytes. The T-cell activation is well character-ized and cell signaling is known to be initiated by mitogen binding to the T-cell receptor complex at the cell surface. Both of the parameters we monitored, calcium influx and $[Ca^{2+}]_i$, are not altered by fields when the thymocytes are in a resting state: mitogen-triggered signal transduction is critical for a field interaction. Calcium influx and $[Ca^{2+}]_i$ should exhibit parallel changes during the plateau phase of calcium signaling and, in the 60-Hz studies at an induced current density of $\leq 6 \ \mu A/cm^2$, we detected a reduced response for both of these parameters (FIGURES 11 and 12). The changes presented here for $[Ca^{2+}]_i$ are significant in that they represent the first

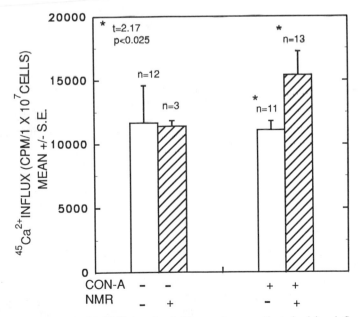

FIGURE 15. Effect of 2.35-T NMR imaging fields on mitogen-activated calcium influx: human lymphocytes. Minimal to no increase in calcium influx is observed in the presence of Con-A (1 μg/mL). No effect of NMR is observed for resting peripheral blood lymphocytes, whereas a 30% increase is observed in mitogen-activated lymphocytes. NMR exposure conditions are given in the text; thymocytes are at 37 ± 0.05 °C.

real-time observations of signal transduction events inside cells during 60-Hz ELF exposures.

What biological significance is associated with such alterations in signal transduction and specifically T-cell activation? Cell signaling is a natural process directly triggered by a molecular event at the cell surface critical to a number of important cellular functions such as protein, RNA, and DNA synthesis. The T-lymphocyte activation *in vivo* is known to result in the modulation of DNA, RNA, and protein synthesis in cellular proliferation that is critical for effectively mounting activities such as T-cell cytotoxicity, which is necessary for immune surveillance. At the molecular level, nuclear events, such as DNA, RNA, and protein synthesis, which are triggered by signal transduction at the cell surface, have been reported to be altered by exposure to sinusoidal and pulsed magnetic fields (see references 12–14 and the sources cited in reference 9). Given the important role that calcium plays in signal transduction and in subsequent gene expression, as well as from the findings presented here, a likely candidate for a common pathway or site of interaction for electromagnetic fields and cellular systems is through modulation of calcium influx and $[Ca^{+2}]_i$. Further studies should help define this interaction pathway. For example, the first event in cell signaling involves ligand binding to a cell surface receptor and an alteration of ligand-receptor binding could explain either up- or down-regulation of calcium signaling. Results presented here could be explained, perhaps most simply, by an inhibition or enhancement of Con-A binding due to these fields and this hypothesis is currently being tested. The Jurkat human T-cell leukemia is a good candidate for such ligand-binding studies because a subclone is available that is T-cell-receptor negative.[15] Alternatively, an alteration in calcium influx and steady-state $[Ca^{+2}]_i$ could be modulated through up- or down-regulation of IP_3-mediated calcium channel activity, as depicted in FIGURE 1. Such an interaction pathway could involve a direct effect of the field on one or more plasma cell membrane components. Whatever the precise molecular interaction pathway, up- or down-regulation of immune function by electromagnetic fields offers the potential for modulating the immune system *in vivo* and for developing applications for treatment of immune system disorders.

A critical finding relating to dosimetry issues addressed by these studies is that the induced electric field is the metric of biological interest for 60-Hz sinusoidal magnetic fields. Use of the multiring cell culture plate clearly shows that mitogen-activated calcium influx scales with the induced electric field and thus with the induced current density experienced by the sample. This has important implications for understanding cellular responses to time-varying magnetic fields. First, an incident uniform magnetic field penetrating a tissue target will be associated with a variety of resultant induced electric field values defined by multiple current loop pathways (see FIGURE 4). For example, at the anatomical level, current loops around the waist and chest are larger than current loops around the head and wrist. At the cellular level, special multicellular aggregates that are in electrical contact with each other may form larger conductive loop pathways in tissue. Epithelial cells, fibroblasts, or neural cells in electrical contact in large extended arrays will form conducting pathways with a large effective radius.[16] This underscores the role that conductive pathways can play in magnetic field interactions that are mediated through induced electric fields.

One similarity between 60-Hz sinusoidal ELF fields and the NMR environment is the presence of ELF components associated with the switched magnetic field, as demonstrated here in FIGURES 7 and 8. This relationship requires further exploration because it raises the important question of whether the time-varying magnetic field in NMR is the operative field component responsible for the cellular responses delineated here. Future studies are under way to test this hypothesis by performing split field exposures in which the switched magnetic, static, or RF field is used separately during exposures. A desirable approach in such studies is to perform instantaneous real-time measurement of $[Ca^{+2}]_i$ (as we have presented here for 60-Hz fields) because, during cell signaling, the $[Ca^{+2}]_i$ transient occurs within the initial 10-minute period following ligand binding. An exposure coil system, or set of DC magnets, can be fitted to a fluorescence spectrometer into which a sample cuvette is placed. We note for our NMR exposures that the computed maximum induced current according to Faraday's law (FIGURE 4) that is associated with a $dB/dt = 1$ T/s for an exposure geometry in which thymocytes are placed in an Eppendorf-type 1.5-mL tube (FIGURE 6) is 0.53 $\mu A/cm^2$. This is an order of magnitude less than we employed in the 60-Hz exposures where we directly monitored $[Ca^{+2}]_i$ (FIGURE 12). An interesting experiment using an acute myeloid leukemia–derived cell line, HL-60,[17] recently suggested that NMR fields and the dB/dt component may elevate baseline intracellular calcium in this leukemic cell after a 23-minute NMR exposure.[18] Such an increase is consistent with the calcium influx data presented here; however, exposure conditions were different and an immortalized leukemic cell line was used that was different than normal primary explanted thymocytes. Other differences were that HL-60 cells were exposed at room temperature (±2 °C) and induced current loops were present in the sample along all three axes, making dosimetry complex.

In summary, the research presented here indicates that cellular responses to time-varying magnetic fields are observed in normal lymphocytes and, importantly, that there are biological constraints that operate to mediate these interactions. One important constraint is that resting lymphocytes do not respond to magnetic fields. We find that lymphocytes activated to undergo signal transduction do respond to time-varying fields, with the additional constraint that suboptimal activation is required, and this depends on animal age. Because these fields operate in synergy with mitogen during signal transduction, the fields act as a comitogen. The special multiring cell culture plate based on Faraday's law of induction was critical in identifying the induced electric field as the biologically relevant metric; this is a significant step forward in understanding how cellular systems respond to time-varying magnetic fields through the induced electric field. The first real-time measurements of $[Ca^{2+}]_i$ during 60-Hz field exposure indicate that the plateau phase of calcium signaling is altered and this implicates the calcium channel in the outer plasma membrane as an interaction site. Additional study will be required to characterize this interaction at the molecular level involving specific signal transduction steps. NMR fields are linked to ELF fields through the switched gradient field component, as shown here, and it will be important to identify which NMR field component or components operate to influence lymphocyte signal transduction.

ACKNOWLEDGMENTS

Assistance in different aspects of these studies from the Bioelectromagnetics Research Group, the NMR Research Group, and the Research Medicine Group at Lawrence Berkeley Laboratory is most gratefully acknowledged.

REFERENCES

1. POLK, C. & E. POSTOW, Eds. 1988. Handbook of Biological Effects of Electromagnetic Fields. CRC Press. Boca Raton, Florida.
2. BUDINGER, T. F. 1979. Thresholds for physiological effects due to RF and magnetic fields used in NMR imaging. IEEE Trans. Nucl. Sci. **26:** 2821–2825.
3. PERSSON, B. R. R. & F. STAHLBERG, Eds. 1989. Health and Safety of Clinical NMR Examinations. CRC Press. Boca Raton, Florida.
4. BEERS, G. J. 1989. Biological effects of weak electromagnetic fields from 0 Hz to 200 MHz: a survey of the literature with special emphasis on possible magnetic resonance effects. Magn. Reson. Imag. **7:** 309–331.
5. LIBURDY, R. P. 1992. ELF fields and the immune system: signal transduction, calcium metabolism, and mitogenesis in lymphocytes with relevance to carcinogenesis. *In* Resonance and Other Interactions of Electromagnetic Fields with Living Systems. C. Ramal & B. Norden, Eds. Oxford University Press. London/New York. In press.
6. ALTMAN, A., T. MUSTELIN & K. M. COGGESHALL. 1990. T lymphocyte activation: a biological model of signal transduction. Crit. Rev. Immunol. **10:** 347–391.
7. METCALF, J. C., G. A. SMITH, J. P. MOORE & R. HESKETH. 1987. The early mitogenic pathway in mouse thymocytes: an analysis of the dual signal hypothesis. *In* International Conference on Lymphocyte Activation and Immune Regulations. S. Gupta, Ed.: 29–44. Plenum. New York.
8. MOHR, F. C. & C. FEWTRELL. 1987. Depolarization of rat basophilic leukemia cells inhibits calcium uptake and exocytosis. J. Cell Biol. **104:** 783–792.
9. WALLECZEK, J. & R. P. LIBURDY. 1990. Nonthermal 60 Hz sinusoidal magnetic field exposure enhances $^{45}Ca^{+2}$ uptake in rat thymocytes: dependence on mitogen activation. FEBS Lett. **271:** 157–160.
10. HESKETH, R., G. A. SMITH, J. P. MOORE & M. V. TAYLOR. 1983. Free cytoplasmic calcium concentration and the mitogenic stimulation of lymphocytes. J. Biol. Chem. **258:** 4876–4882.
11. SEGAL, J. 1986. Studies on the age-related decline in the response of lymphoid cells to mitogen: measurements on Con-A binding and stimulation of calcium and sugar uptake from rats of varying ages. Mech. Ageing Dev. **33:** 295–303.
12. GOODMAN, R., L. X. WEI & A. HENDERSON. 1989. Exposure of human cells to low-frequency electromagnetic fields results in quantitative changes in transcripts. Biophys. Biochem. Acta **1009:** 216–220.
13. GOODMAN, R. & A. HENDERSON. 1988. Exposure of salivary gland cells to low-frequency electromagnetic fields alters polypeptide synthesis. Proc. Natl. Acad. Sci. U.S.A. **85:** 3928–3932.
14. LIBOFF, A., T. WILLIAMS, D. STRONG & R. WISTER. 1984. Time-varying magnetic fields: effect on DNA synthesis. Science **223:** 818–820.
15. YOST, M. G. & R. P. LIBURDY. 1992. Time-varying and static magnetic fields act in combination to alter calcium signal transduction in the lymphocyte. FEBS Lett. In press.

16. POLK, C. 1992. Dosimetric extrapolations across biological systems: dosimetry of ELF magnetic fields. Bioelectromagnetics. In press.
17. LUBBERT, M., F. HERRMAN & H. P. KOEFFLER. 1991. Expression and regulation of myeloid-specific genes in normal and leukemic myeloid cells. Blood **77:** 909–924.
18. CARSON, J. J. L., F. S. PRATO, D. J. DROST, L. D. DIESBOURG & S. J. DIXON. 1990. Time-varying magnetic fields increase cytosolic free calcium in HL-60 cells. Am. J. Physiol. **259:** C687–C692.
19. GUILLAND, L. K., A. GROSSMAN, P. S. RABINOVITCH & J. A. LEDBETTER. 1990. Composite signal transduction in T-cell activation: enhancement, inhibition, and desensitization. *In* Ligands, Receptors, and Signal Transduction in Regulation of Lymphocyte Function, p. 321–357. Amer. Soc. Microbiol. Washington, District of Columbia.

Principles of Nerve and Heart Excitation by Time-varying Magnetic Fields

J. PATRICK REILLY

Applied Physics Laboratory
The Johns Hopkins University
Laurel, Maryland 20723

INTRODUCTION

A time-varying magnetic field has the potential for inducing circulating electrical currents (so-called "eddy" currents) within conducting objects, including the human body. In the case of the magnetic resonance imaging (MRI) procedures, the induced current is a by-product of the pulsed gradient field rather than a requirement of the imaging process. The level of magnetically induced current that can be caused by existing MR imagers is well below levels needed to stimulate excitable tissue. However, recent developments in fast imaging techniques are pressing technology towards rapidly switched gradient fields of such an intensity that nerve or heart excitation may be possible. Consequently, the design of future MRI devices may need to include certain constraints if one wishes to avoid excitatory responses in the exposed subject. The purpose of this article is to review the biological and physical principles through which these responses may be understood.

MAGNETIC INDUCTION PRINCIPLES

Magnetic field strength is characterized in terms of magnetic flux density B, having units of tesla (T). The magnetic field produces electrical forces when the flux density varies with time or when charged particles move within a static field. In accordance with Faraday's law, the induced electric field E is related to the time rate of change of flux density by

$$\int \mathbf{E} \cdot d\mathbf{l} = -\frac{\partial}{\partial t} \int\int \mathbf{B} \cdot d\mathbf{s}, \tag{1}$$

where $d\mathbf{l}$ is an element of length along a closed path and $d\mathbf{s}$ is the element of area normal to the direction of **B**. Boldface terms imply vector quantities; standard fonts indicate scalar quantities. The simplest application of equation 1 is for a closed circular path that encloses a uniform magnetic field, in which case

$$E = -\frac{r}{2}\frac{d\mathrm{B}}{dt}, \tag{2}$$

where the direction of E is along the circumference of the circle and B is the flux

96

density in a direction normal to the loop. When the field varies sinusoidally as $B = B_o \sin 2\pi ft$, the induced field is

$$E = [r\pi f B_o]\cos 2\pi ft, \tag{3}$$

where the term in brackets is the peak induced field during the sinusoidal cycle. It is customary to express only the magnitude of the sinusoidal variation and to omit the cosine term in equation 3. FIGURE 1 illustrates several examples of B and dB/dt waveforms.

The induced electric field causes current to flow within the biological medium. The current density J is related to E through the conductivity σ of the medium in accordance with

$$J = \sigma E. \tag{4}$$

Current density has often been cited as a parameter that characterizes magnetic

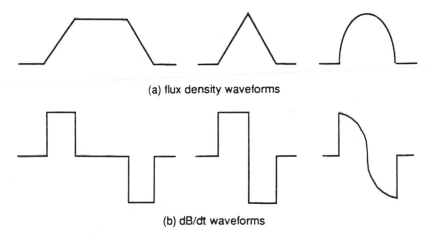

(a) flux density waveforms

(b) dB/dt waveforms

FIGURE 1. Example of flux density and dB/dt waveforms.

induction. Nevertheless, the electric field within the biological medium is a more fundamental parameter when considering electrical stimulation.

A simple model for calculating magnetically induced forces within a volume conductor, such as the human body, treats the volume as if it were made up of concentric rings normal to the direction of the field. According to equation 2, the outermost rings would have the greatest E-field strength. A better model for the human body is a homogeneous prolate spheroid as shown in FIGURE 2. A long wavelength solution for the spheroid model has been developed by Durney and colleagues[1] and has been expressed in applied form by Spiegel.[2] The long wavelength assumption is that the field wavelength is much greater than the dimensions of the biological subject. The induced E-field for three orthogonal orientations of a

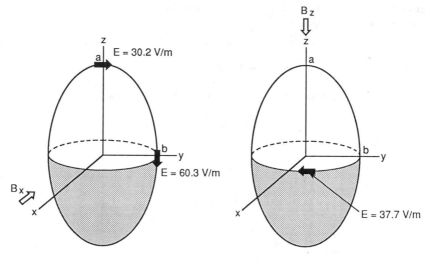

(a) Field perpendicular to long axis   (b) Field parallel to long axis

FIGURE 2. Prolate spheroid model of uniform magnetic field induction. Bold arrows indicate the direction of the induced electric field at the outer boundaries of the spheroid. Indicated values apply to a 60-Hz magnetic field of 1-T strength for semimajor axis $a = 0.4$ m and semiminor axis $b = 0.2$ m.

sinusoidal magnetic field is given by

$$E_1 = \frac{-j2\pi f B_x (a^2 y a_z - b^2 z a_y)}{(a^2 + b^2)}, \tag{5}$$

$$E_2 = \frac{j2\pi f B_y (a^2 x a_z - b^2 z a_x)}{(a^2 + b^2)}, \tag{6}$$

$$E_3 = j\pi f B_z (y a_x - x a_y), \tag{7}$$

where j is the complex operator, indicating a 90° phase shift. The following expression for a pulsed field can be derived from equations 5–7 using arguments of Fourier synthesis:

$$E = -\frac{dB}{dt} \left(\frac{a^2 u a_v - b^2 v a_u}{a^2 + b^2} \right), \tag{8}$$

where a_u and a_v are unit vectors along the minor and major axes, respectively; (u, v) is a location within the ellipse; and B is the component of magnetic flux density in a direction perpendicular to the elliptical cross section. For a circular area, $a = b = r$ and equation 8 is equivalent to equation 2 on the perimeter of the circle.

FIGURE 3 illustrates the variation of the induced E-field for an example ellipse with $a = 0.4$ m and $b = 0.2$ m (representing a frontal cross section of the torso of a large person) and with $dB/dt = 1$ T/s. The induced E-field increases as the measurement point moves from the center of the body to its periphery and is especially great on the minor axis at the perimeter of the ellipse.

Equations 5–8 apply to an idealized body shape of uniform conductivity. In reality, the shape of the body departs from this simple model and the conductivity of the medium is not uniform. These departures from idealized conditions can result in regions within the body where the actual E-field may be enhanced or diminished in comparison with the simple model.

More accurate methods exist for computing the internal E-field. Gandhi and colleagues, for instance, modeled a two-dimensional cross section of the body as a grid of rectangular loops, with each loop incorporating the complex impedance appropriate to the tissue in a particular location of the body.[3] Such methods can represent the body as a two-dimensional object with nonhomogeneous and anisotropic properties. A three-dimensional finite element model might provide even more accuracy, although the computational requirements for implementing one might be rather formidable.

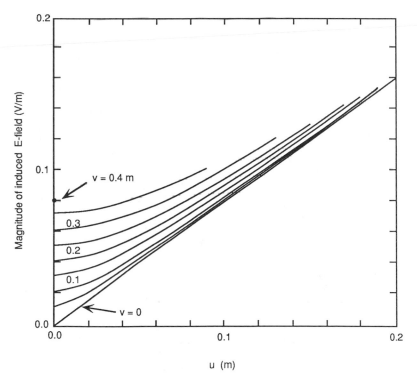

FIGURE 3. Induced E-field with $dB/dt = 1$ T/s in an elliptically shaped conductive medium; semimajor axis $a = 0.4$ m, semiminor axis $b = 0.2$ m.

EXCITATION PRINCIPLES

Nerve Excitation

To understand the properties of a stimulus that determine its excitation potential, it is beneficial to use computational models of electrical stimulation. The model

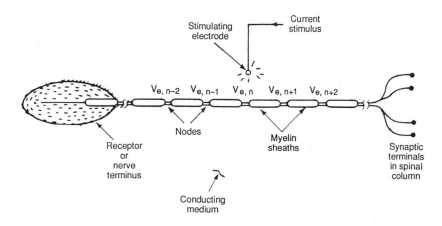

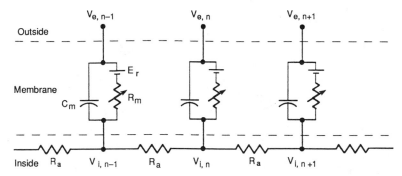

FIGURE 4. Representation of electrical stimulation of myelinated nerve; current flow in the conductive medium results in voltage disturbances V_e at the individual nodes. Upper panel: physical representation of afferent nerve; lower panel: electrical representation.

used here is a representation of a myelinated nerve. Myelinated nerves have much faster conduction times and lower electrical thresholds than unmyelinated nerves. Because of the latter property, the myelinated nerve is the appropriate one to model for electrical excitation studies.

FIGURE 4 illustrates a model for electrical stimulation of a myelinated nerve fiber. As shown in the upper figure, a pattern of voltage disturbances is created within the biological medium by virtue of the electrical stimulus. One can analyze the ability of these disturbances to excite the fiber using the electrical model developed by McNeal[4] (shown in the lower figure). In this model, the fiber is treated as being perfectly insulated by the myelin sheath, except for the nodes of Ranvier. The lower part of the figure represents the nodes as consisting of membrane capacitance C_m and membrane conductance G_m and interconnected by internal axonal resistance R_a. Electrochemical potential sources (not shown) also exist because of differences in ionic concentrations on either side of the membrane.

For subthreshold stimulation, the membrane conductance is approximately constant and linear circuit analysis can be used to evaluate the response of the model. However, the nonlinear electrodynamics of the excitable membrane must be included if one wishes to study threshold responses. The electrodynamics of the myelinated nerve membrane, characterized by Frankenhaeuser and Huxley,[5] are used in the model described herein.

Referring to the lower panel of FIGURE 4, one can write the equations governing the electrical response of the nerve model as

$$\frac{dV_n}{dt} = \frac{1}{C_m} [G_a(V_{n-1} - 2V_n + V_{n+1} + V_{e,n-1} - 2V_{e,n} + V_{e,n+1}) - I_{i,n}], \qquad (9)$$

where $V_n = V_{i,n} - V_{e,n}$ is the voltage difference across the membrane, $V_{e,n}$ is the voltage at the exterior of node n, $V_{i,n}$ is the voltage at the interior of node n, and $G_a = 1/R_a$. The ionic current can be expressed for either a linear or a nonlinear membrane:

$$I_{i,n} = \begin{cases} G_m V_n & \text{linear} & \text{(10a)} \\ \pi d W(J_{Na} + J_K + J_L + J_P) & \text{nonlinear} & \text{(10b)} \end{cases}$$

where W is the internodal gap width, d is the axon diameter, and the J terms are ionic current densities. Equation 10a is a statement of Ohm's law for a linear conductor, whereas equation 10b applies to nonlinear ionic current flow expressed by the Frankenhaeuser-Huxley[5] equations.

Equation 9 is equivalent to the so-called "electrical cable" equation that was developed over 100 years ago by Thompson and Heaviside in connection with the analysis of the first trans-Atlantic telegraph cable. The $V_{e,n}$ values are specified from knowledge about the distribution of the electric field in the biological medium; the V_n values are unknowns for which solutions must be found. The most accurate representation would use a long array, where all nodes of which are described by the nonlinear term in equation 10b. One can save computing time by appropriately selecting a subset of the nodes as being described more simply by equation 10a. The electrical model simulates the real nerve by responding to weak electrical stimuli as would a linear circuit. If, however, the degree of membrane voltage change is adequate, the model represents a stereotypical action potential that propagates from node to node. It is possible to define an electrical threshold as the stimulus intensity that is just adequate to elicit a propagating action potential. A fuller description of excitation models and their properties is given in reference 6.

In order for excitation to occur, a second spatial derivative[a] of the external potentials must exist along the long axis of the nerve fiber or, equivalently, a first derivative of the electric field must exist. If the electric field were uniform and the fiber were infinitely long in both directions, there would in theory be zero net current transfer at every node. Nevertheless, excitation can occur in a locally uniform field if the fiber orientation changes abruptly or if it is terminated (as with receptors, free nerve endings, or motor neuron junctions at muscle fibers). The orientation change or termination creates the equivalent of a spatial derivative of the applied field.

The magnetic field generated by MR imagers induces an E-field that varies only slightly over dimensions equivalent to the axon's internodal spacing. The theoretical calculations presented in this review apply to terminated fibers in a uniform field. This approach leads to theoretical thresholds that correspond reasonably well to many aspects of experimental observations.[7,8]

Strength-Duration and Strength-Frequency Relationships

The so-called Strength-Duration (S-D) function describes the stimulus threshold as a function of the duration of a monophasic current pulse. Ordinarily, an S-D function is described in terms of stimulus current or current density. However, because induced current density is directly proportional to dB/dt (equations 2 and 4), the same functional form applies to the dB/dt waveform. The following equation provides a mathematical curve fit to the S-D curves obtained with the myelinated nerve model and also with data from a wide variety of experiments:[6]

$$\frac{\dot{B}_T}{\dot{B}_o} = \frac{1}{1 - e^{-t/\tau_e}}, \tag{11}$$

where $\dot{B} = dB/dt$, $\dot{B}_T$ is the threshold value, $\dot{B}_o$ is the minimum threshold applying to long pulses, and τ_e is an experimentally determined time constant. Equation 11 is analogous to the more familiar S-D relationship for stimulus current.

Equation 11 can be expressed in terms of the B-field by observing that $B = \dot{B}t$ if $\dot{B}$ is a square wave. The threshold B-field attains a minimum for short duration pulses. As $t \to 0$, $B_T \to B_o = \dot{B}/\tau_e$. The S-D relationship for the normalized B-field is easily shown to be

$$\frac{B_T}{B_o} = \frac{t/\tau_e}{1 - e^{-t/\tau_e}}, \tag{12}$$

where B_T is the threshold B-field and B_o is the minimum threshold for long duration stimuli. Equation 12 is analogous to the more common S-D expression in terms of stimulus charge.

Equations 11 and 12 are shown in FIGURE 5; the threshold value of dB/dt attains a minimum for long stimulus durations and B is a minimum for short duration stimuli. The relationships depicted in FIGURE 5 are for monophasic square-wave pulses (i.e., stimulus current in one direction). Strictly speaking, the dB/dt waveform

---

[a] A second difference calculated as $(V_{e,n-1} - V_{e,n}) - (V_{e,n} - V_{e,n+1}) = V_{e,n-1} - 2V_{e,n} + V_{e,n+1}$ is a discrete version of a second spatial derivative, where $V_{e,n}$ is the external potential at node n.

is always biphasic such that the area under the dB/dt curve is zero. This follows from the fact that B begins and ends at the same (usually zero) value. Nevertheless, the dB/dt waveform can be treated as monophasic from the point of view of excitation if the polarity reversal is sufficiently delayed relative to the tissue time constant, as is often the case with MRI gradient waveforms. In those cases where the biphasic waveform is brief, the thresholds would be elevated above the monophasic value.[7]

The sinusoidal function is a special case of a biphasic waveform. The threshold relation for sinusoidal stimulation describes a Strength-Frequency (S-F) function. Experimental and theoretical data alike follow a U-shaped S-F curve with a minimum threshold at midfrequencies and an upturn at both low and high frequen-

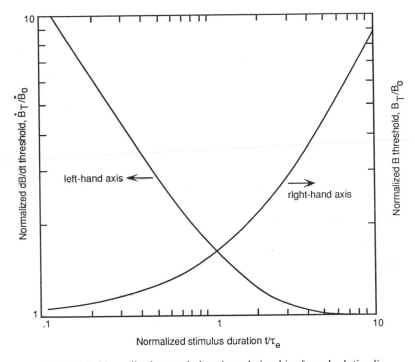

FIGURE 5. Normalized strength-duration relationships for pulsed stimuli.

cies. An empirical fit to the myelinated nerve model as well as to experimental data provides the following S-F expression:[6]

$$\dot{B}_T = \dot{B}_o(1 - e^{-f_e/f})^{-p}(1 - e^{-f/f_o})^{-q}. \tag{13}$$

Here, the first parenthetic expression accounts for the high-frequency upturn in thresholds; the second term accounts for the low-frequency upturn (describing the so-called property of "accommodation"); f_e, f_o, p, and q are experimentally determined parameters. A curve fit to S-F data from the myelinated nerve model provides the values of $p = 0.9$ for continuous sinusoidal stimulation and $p = 1.35$ for single-cycle sinusoidal stimulation; $q = 0.8$ in either case.[6] The frequency parameters will be discussed in the succeeding section.

Equation 13 may be more simply expressed in terms of the asymptotic approximations:

$$\dot{B}_T = \dot{B}_o(f/f_e)^p \quad \text{for} \quad f \gg f_e \tag{14a}$$

$$\dot{B}_T = \dot{B}_o(f_o/f)^q \quad \text{for} \quad f \ll f_o. \tag{14b}$$

The threshold flux density may be determined from equations 13 and 14 using the relationship of $B_T = \dot{B}_T/(2\pi f)$.

Excitation Parameters

Electrical thresholds for nerve stimulation are inversely related to fiber diameter, with the largest myelinated fibers having the lowest thresholds. TABLE 1 lists theoretical thresholds[7] from the myelinated nerve model for fibers of diameters of 5, 10, and 20 μm. This range effectively brackets the diameter distribution of myelinated nerve fibers to be found among skeletal muscle motor neurons and peripheral sensory neurons. The upper row of data in part (a) expresses minimum E-field thresholds applicable to long duration ($t > 1$ ms) pulses. The second row in part (a) expresses minimum thresholds for short pulses ($t < 10$ μs) in terms of the product of E-field and pulse duration.

Whereas the E-field in the medium is the primary force governing stimulation, current density has been often cited in past literature. Part (b) of TABLE 1 expresses thresholds in terms of current and charge density obtained by multiplying E and Et by the conductivity of the medium, with $\sigma = 0.2$ S/m (the approximate geometric mean of the longitudinal and transverse conductivities of skeletal muscle tissue at low frequencies[9]). Current density is cited here to allow for more convenient comparison with other publications; the selection of σ used here for this comparison is somewhat arbitrary.

Because the 20-μm fiber is one of the larger fibers to be found among peripheral nerves, the corresponding threshold value of 6.2 V/m represents a theoretical value for relatively sensitive fibers stimulated by monophasic square-wave pulses. The

TABLE 1. Theoretical Stimulus Thresholds for Uniform Field Excitation of Myelinated Nerve (Single Monophasic Stimuli)[a]

Criteria	Fiber Diameter (μm)		
	5	10	20
(a) field strength			
E_{min} (V/m)	24.6	12.3	6.2
$(Et)_{min}$ (Vs/m)	2.98×10^{-3}	1.49×10^{-3}	0.75×10^{-3}
(b) current density			
J_{min} (A/m^2)	4.92	2.46	1.23
q_{min} (C/m^2)	6.0×10^{-4}	3.0×10^{-4}	1.5×10^{-4}

[a]E_{min} and J_{min} apply to long pulses ($t \geq 1$ ms); $(Et)_{min}$ and q_{min} apply to short pulses ($t < 10$ μs). Current and charge density are determined for $\sigma = 0.2$ S/m.

TABLE 2. Strength–Duration Time Constants for Neural Excitation[a]

Item	Subject	Stimulus Locus	Electrode	Response	τ_e (μs)	Citation
1.	human	forearm	4 cm^2	perception	138	Alon, 1983
2.	human	*	2 mm dia.	pain	760	Notermans, 1966
3.	human	finger	1.1 mm dia.	perception	200–900	Reilly & Larkin, 1984
4.	human	forearm	0.5 cm^2	perception	480	Rollman, 1978
5.	human	finger	0.4 cm^2	perception	217	Hahn, 1958
6.	human	forehead	0.1 mm^2	perception	189	Girvin et al., 1982
7.	human	ulnar nerve	NA	muscle twitch	275	Heckman, 1972
8.	human	muscle	NA	muscle twitch	30–700	Harris, 1971
9.	human	forearm	3.9 cm^2	muscle twitch	140	Crago, 1974
10.	rats, cats	tibialis ant.	10 mm	muscle twitch	85	Crago, 1974
11.	rabbit	tibial nerve	0.1 mm dia.	action potential	80–100	Reilly et al., 1985
12.	cat	A$_\beta$ fiber	in vitro	action potential	30	Li & Bak, 1976
13.	cat	A$_\delta$ fiber	in vitro	action potential	650	Li & Bak, 1976
21.	toad	mye. nerve	in vitro	action potential	148	Tasaki & Sato, 1951
22.	SENN model	mye. nerve	uniform field	action potential	121	Reilly & Bauer, 1987

[a]Table adapted from reference 6.

theoretical thresholds shown in TABLE 1 effectively bracket experimental thresholds obtained with magnetic stimulation if proper allowances are made for waveform factors.[7] From theoretical studies with the myelinated nerve model,[10] it can be concluded that the minimum threshold for a sine wave stimulus has a peak value that is about 17% greater than the peak square-wave threshold. Consequently, the minimum sine wave threshold will be taken as 7.3 V/m (peak) at the most sensitive frequency.

In order to fully describe the S-D and S-F curves, one must also specify the time constant τ_e (equation 11) and the upper frequency constant f_e (equation 13). Thresholds for uniform field excitation obtained with the myelinated nerve model[7] follow an S-D curve with $\tau_e = 120$ μs; thresholds for sinusoidal stimulation by a point electrode[6,10] follow an S-F curve with $f_e = 5400$ Hz and $f_o \approx 10$ Hz. It would be helpful to compare those values with experimental data applicable to stimulation by dB/dt exposure in MR imaging. Unfortunately, most published S-D or S-F data have been obtained with electrode arrangements that produce internal E-field distributions unlike those induced during MR examinations. For instance, much of the data pertaining to nerve stimulation have been obtained with electrodes placed on the surface of the skin or near a nerve. In the case of cardiac stimulation, the preponderance of available data have been obtained with electrodes directly contacting the heart. TABLE 2 lists data from various neurosensory and neuromuscular experiments using square-wave stimuli. TABLE 3 lists values of f_e from neurosensory or neuromuscular experiments using sine wave stimuli. TABLES 4 and 5 list similar data applying to cardiac responses. A more complete version of these tables, along with explanations and citations, may be found in reference 6.

FIGURE 6 represents the data of TABLES 3–5 as a statistical distribution. Although there is a clear separation between nerve and cardiac responses, there remains a very wide range of reported values within those categories. Some of the spread in experimental data can be accounted for by differences in the spatial distribution of the stimulus current. As a general rule, τ_e increases as the voltage disturbances caused by the stimulus current are distributed in a more gradual fashion along the fiber, such as when going from small to large electrodes or when increasing the distance between a small electrode and the fiber. Correspondingly, the frequency constant f_e is expected to fall as the stimulus current becomes more gradually distributed. These effects can be large for both nerve and cardiac responses.[6] In previous work,[7] theoretical values of τ_e and f_e from the myelinated nerve model were used to develop possible MRI exposure limits. The nerve model predicts a value of τ_e that is within the experimental range shown in FIGURE 6, albeit below the median value. Sensory thresholds measured on humans within an MR exposure system[11] follow an S-D curve with a time constant of 148 ± 39 μs, which is a range of values not far from the model's value of 120 μs. The model also predicts a value of f_e that is

TABLE 3. Strength-Frequency Constants for Neural Excitation[a]

Item	Subject	Stimulus Locus	Electrode	Response	f_e (Hz)	Citation
1.	human	hand	gripped wire	perception	500	Dalziel, 1951
2.	human	arm	0.27 cm²	perception	1000	Anderson & Munion, 1951
3.	human	thorax	1.0 cm²	perception	100	Geddes et al., 1969
4.	human	neck	25 cm²	perception	150	Geddes et al., 1969
5.	human	finger	NA	perception	500	Hawkes & Warms, 1960
6.	human	hand	large area grip	tetanus	600	Dalziel, 1954
7.	frog	sciatic nerve	in vitro	action potential	533–1500	Hill et al., 1936
8.	rat	gast. tib.	subcutaneous	muscle twitch	200	LaCourse et al., 1985
9.	toad	mye. nerve	in vitro	action potential	200	Tasaki & Sato, 1951
10.	frog	mye. nerve	in vitro	action potential	500	Wyss, 1963
11.	SENN model	mye. nerve	point electrode	action potential	5400	Reilly, 1985

[a]Table adapted from reference 6.

above the upper end of the distribution in FIGURE 6. At present, there are no appropriate measurements that would directly provide S-F parameters for sinusoidal magnetic field exposure in MR examinations. In the following discussion, a range of values will be used to illustrate how stimulation thresholds depend on τ_e and f_e.

Cardiac Excitation Threshold

The sensitivity of the heart to externally applied stimulation depends critically on the timing of the stimulus with respect to the cardiac cycle. The heart is most sensitive to fibrillation during the so-called "vulnerable" period of the heart after its contractile phase and while it is still partially refractory. The heart is most sensitive to excitation, though, during the diastolic (depolarized) phase. An excitation during the

TABLE 4. Strength–Duration Time Constants for Cardiac Excitation[a]

Item	Subject	Stimulus Locus	Electrode	Response	τ_e (ms)	Citation
1.	guinea pig	papillary musc.	small	excitation	3.8	Weirich et al., 1985
2.	rabbit	left ventricle	1 cm²	excitation	1.75	Roy et al., 1985
3.	dog	trans-chest	8.1 cm dia.	excitation	2.86	Voorhes et al., 1983
4.	dog	ventricle	small	excitation	2.14	Pearce et al., 1982
5.	turtle	ventricle	small	excitation	7.31	Pearce et al., 1982
6.	NA	NA	NA	excitation	0.7–3.9	Irnich, 1980
7.	dog	myocardium	sutured	excitation	0.21	Jones & Geddes, 1977
8.	human	NA	12 mm²	excitation	1.1	Fozzard & Schoenberg, 1972
9.	dog	ventricle	loop & catheter	excitation	2.1	Thalen et al., 1975
10.	sheep	long Purkinje fiber	point	excitation	3.75	Fozzard & Schoenberg, 1972
11.	sheep	Purkinje fiber	pipette	excitation	2.6	Dominguez et al., 1970
12.	human	NA	0.32 cm²	excitation	2.3	Smyth et al., 1976
13.	human	NA	0.18 cm²	excitation	1.7	Smyth et al., 1976
14.	dog	myocardium	7.9 mm²	excitation	1.5	Mouchawar et al., 1989
15.	guinea pig	whole heart	NA	fibrillation	7.7	Weirich et al., 1985
16.	dog	myocardium	sutured	fibrillation	1.7	Jones & Geddes, 1977
17.	dog	whole heart	uniform field	defibrillation	3.9	Geddes et al., 1985
18.	dog	rt. ventricle	catheter	defibrillation	2.8	Wesale et al., 1980
19.	dog	trans-chest	large	defibrillation	4.0	Bourland et al., 1978
20.	pony	trans-chest	large	defibrillation	3.0	Bourland et al., 1978
21.	dog	ventricle	NA	defibrillation	6.5	Konig et al., 1975

[a]Table adapted from reference 6.

TABLE 5. Strength-Frequency Constants for Cardiac Excitation[a]

Item	Subject	Stimulus Locus	Electrode	Response	f_e (Hz)	Citation
1.	guinea pig	papillary musc.	Ag Ag Cl	excitation	278	Weirich et al., 1985
2.	guinea pig	aorta/apex	Ag Ag Cl	excitation	50	Weirich et al., 1983
3.	guinea pig	whole heart	Ag Ag Cl	fibrillation	250	Weirich et al., 1985
4.	guinea pig	aorta/apex	Ag Ag Cl	fibrillation	72	Weirich et al., 1983
5.	dog	ventricle	3.1 cm²	fibrillation	79	Kugelberg, 1976
6.	human	NA	4 mm dia.	fibrillation	148	Kugelberg, 1976
7.	dog	various	various	fibrillation	100	Geddes et al., 1971
8.	dog	trans-chest	8 × 10 cm	fibrillation	100	Geddes et al., 1971
9.	dog	trans-chest	0.5″ wire	fibrillation	120	Geddes et al., 1971

[a]Table adapted from reference 6.

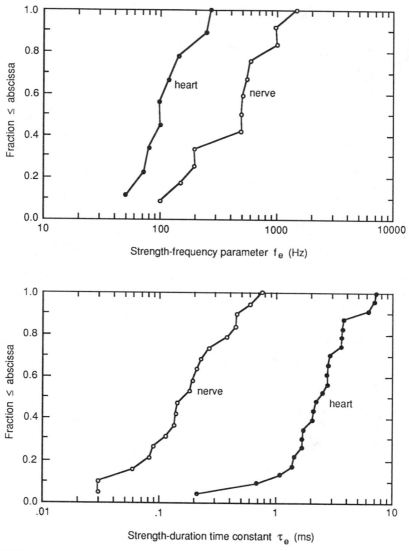

FIGURE 6. Distribution of the measured strength-duration parameter τ_e (lower) and strength-frequency parameter f_e (upper). Data are from various experiments, including different experimental species and procedures.

diastolic period is not necessarily life-threatening, but it will increase the susceptibility of the heart to fibrillation by a subsequent excitatory stimulus. When the stimulus is a series of pulses or a continued sine wave, it can produce a series of extrasystolic excitations. The threshold of fibrillation is reduced with each successive excitation, eventually reaching a value that is only marginally above the excitation threshold.[12,13] In this review, the more sensitive threshold of excitation during the diastolic period will be used as a basis for evaluating magnetic thresholds.

In order to study magnetic stimulation, it is important to establish E-field thresholds for the heart. Unfortunately, there seems to be little experimental data directly establishing E-field or current density thresholds. However, it is possible to estimate current density thresholds from experiments that used large electrodes in contact with the heart by defining current density as the applied current divided by the electrode area. Current density defined this way will correctly give the average value beneath the electrode, but may understate the maximum density because current tends to concentrate at the edges of electrode contact.[14,15]

Roy and colleagues[16] have found that the current density (current ÷ area) required for fibrillation steadily falls with increasing electrode size, eventually reaching an asymptotic minimum of 0.5 mA/cm^2 (average value) with large electrodes. The "minimum" experimental thresholds noted by Roy are about one-half that value, namely, 0.25 mA/cm^2. It is possible to form an estimate of the percentile rank of this so-called "minimum" value. A variety of studies with healthy animal hearts indicate that fibrillation thresholds are log-normally distributed, with a one-percentile value that is about one-half the median.[6] Therefore, one can estimate that Roy's "minimum" thresholds represent approximately the one-percentile rank of a statistical distribution in healthy animal hearts.

Sugimoto et al. found that the excitation threshold for prolonged 60-Hz stimulation is 40% of the fibrillation threshold.[17] If that factor is applied to the "minimum" 60-Hz fibrillation threshold of 0.25 mA/cm^2, the excitation threshold can be estimated to be 0.1 mA/cm^2. That value is close to the theoretical threshold of 0.12 mA/cm^2 mentioned earlier for a 20-μm peripheral nerve fiber. Considering uncertainties in the experimental thresholds and the conductivity of the biological medium, it is reasonable to assume that the minimum E-field thresholds of nerve and heart do not differ greatly. To facilitate the calculation in this review, minimum excitation thresholds for both nerve and heart will be assumed to be equal to the theoretical value for a 20-μm myelinated nerve, namely, 6.2 V/m.

It is worth emphasizing that the assumed threshold criteria are somewhat speculative and they require more thorough experimental investigation. Whether the same excitation threshold would apply to the human heart in a pathological state or under drug treatment also requires examination. Compared with animal data, a much broader distribution of fibrillation thresholds has been reported for patients undergoing open-heart surgery for valve replacement.[18] It is difficult to determine if the greater spread in human open-heart measurements is a consequence of variations in the placement of the cardiac contact electrodes, a reflection of the pathological state of the heart, or the result of some other mechanism. Furthermore, chemical alterations can either enhance or inhibit the electrical activity of the heart.[19] The role of chemical modification on the sensitivity to electrical excitation has not been clearly defined.

MAGNETIC EXCITATION THRESHOLDS

Induced Electric Field

Based on the preceding discussion, it is clear that magnetic excitation thresholds depend on spatial and temporal properties of the field, on the tissue response time

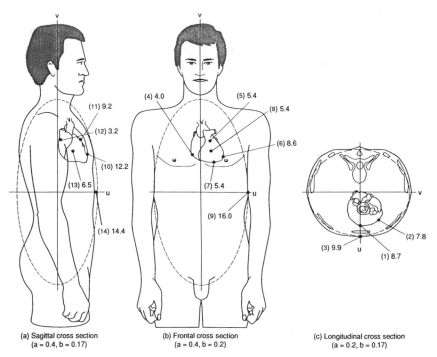

(a) Sagittal cross section
(a = 0.4, b = 0.17)

(b) Frontal cross section
(a = 0.4, b = 0.2)

(c) Longitudinal cross section
(a = 0.2, b = 0.17)

FIGURE 7. Example of the position of the heart within three cross sections of the body; *a* and *b* are semimajor and semiminor axes of equivalent cross-section ellipsoids. Numbered locations are identified with the calculated electric field intensity (V/cm) for magnetic exposure within the ellipse; $d\mathrm{B}/dt = 1$ T/s. Direction of field is perpendicular to the cross section.

constants, and on the location and orientation of the excited organ within the body. To illustrate the relationship among these properties, consider an example with the following assumptions: (a) an ellipsoidal representation of the human torso, (b) uniform conductivity, and (c) uniform magnetic field (amplitude and phase) over the ellipsoidal cross section.

FIGURE 7 illustrates three cross-sectional views of the body, each fitted with an ellipse. The major and minor axis dimensions listed below each view are intended to represent a large person. The diagram includes numbered points and an associated E-field value calculated according to equation 8 with $d\mathrm{B}/dt = 1$ T/s. The induced field on the body periphery is greatest at points 3, 9, and 14 for the longitudinal, frontal, and sagittal cross sections, respectively. Points of maximum induction on the surface of the heart occur at points 1, 6, and 10 on the three cross sections. The heart's outline has been projected on the central cross-sectional plane in each view rather than representing the cross section of the heart in any particular slice. This simplification leads to a somewhat conservative calculation of the E-field as compared with a cross-sectional representation of the heart because the more peripheral points on the heart do not necessarily coincide with the central plane of the body.

Comparison of Nerve and Heart Excitation Thresholds

In accordance with the preceding discussion, a threshold criterion with the value of 6.2 V/m will be used for both nerve and cardiac stimulation by square-wave dB/dt pulses of long duration and the value of 7.3 V/m (peak) will be used for sinusoidal stimuli of moderately low frequency. TABLE 6 lists the dB/dt field necessary to induce 6.2 V/m at the locations in FIGURE 6 where the E-field is greatest on the body periphery (points 3, 9, and 14) or on the heart (points 1, 6, and 10). The tabulated values represent estimated dB/dt thresholds for long duration ($t > 10$ ms) pulsed stimuli. For long duration ($t > 1$ s) sinusoids of low frequency, the listed values should be increased by 17% to indicate the peak sinusoidal threshold. For short pulses or for high frequencies, the listed values should be increased in accordance with S-D or S-F relationships (equations 11 and 13). For closely spaced pulsed trains or short duration biphasic stimuli, other adjustments in the calculated thresholds may be necessary.[7]

In order to apply these relationships, the parameters τ_e and f_e must be specified. FIGURE 8 illustrates S-D curves and FIGURE 9 illustrates S-F curves for nerve and heart with sagittal exposure to the torso by a uniform field. A range of values has been used for τ_e and f_e to represent the spread of experimental data. The curves labeled "nerve" correspond to point 14 in FIGURE 7; the curves labeled "heart" correspond to point 10.

Based on the foregoing analysis and assumptions, thresholds of excitation for peripheral nerves and the heart do not appear to differ greatly if the stimulus is a pulsed waveform of long duration or a sinusoid of low frequency. On the other hand, the use of short duration pulses or of higher frequency sinusoids can provide a wide margin between the nerve and heart excitation thresholds.

Experimental Magnetic Thresholds for Nerve and Heart

Data are available from numerous and diverse experiments involving magnetic stimulation of nerve and heart; several of these (discussed next) involved human subjects with large-area magnetic field exposure.

TABLE 6. Magnetic Field Time Derivative Necessary to Induce a 6.2-V/m E-Field at Selected Body Loci[a]

B-Field Orientation	Ellipse b, a (cm, cm)	Body Locus	dB/dt (T/s)
longitudinal	17, 20	1	71.3
		3	62.6
frontal	20, 40	6	72.1
		9	38.8
sagittal	17, 40	10	50.8
		14	43.1

[a]Points 3, 9, and 14 apply to peripheral nerve; points 1, 6, and 10 apply to the heart.

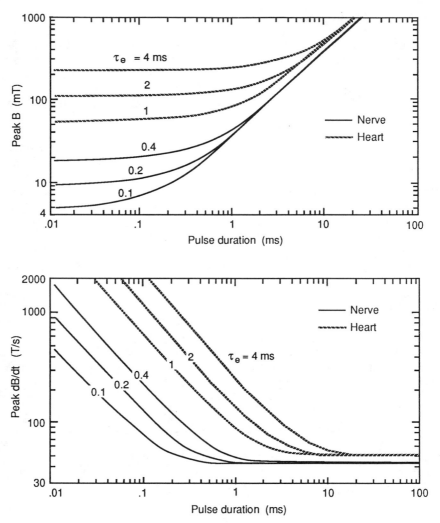

FIGURE 8. Calculated excitation thresholds for sagittal exposure of the torso to a pulsed magnetic field. Curve parameter τ_e applies to the strength–duration time constant of excitable tissue. Upper panel: peak flux density; lower panel: peak dB/dt.

Two subjects tested by Cohen and colleagues[20] reported sensations in the lower back and facial regions when the torso was exposed to pulsed sinusoidal fields of a frequency of 1.4 kHz, a repetition frequency of 14 Hz, and a peak dB/dt of 86 T/s. Simultaneous ECG recordings failed to show any effect of the applied field. From FIGURE 9, it is expected that human peripheral nerves might be excited with a 1.4-kHz field at the cited experimental levels, but that cardiac excitation would require significantly higher fields.

Subjects tested by Budinger and associates[21] reported mild sensations in the lower back when exposed to a longitudinal field of 60 T/s peak. Perception thresholds were found to be proportional to frequency over the tested range of 600 to 2000 Hz. Subjects reported painful stimulation at about twice the perception threshold. The very small dynamic range from perception to pain is consistent with

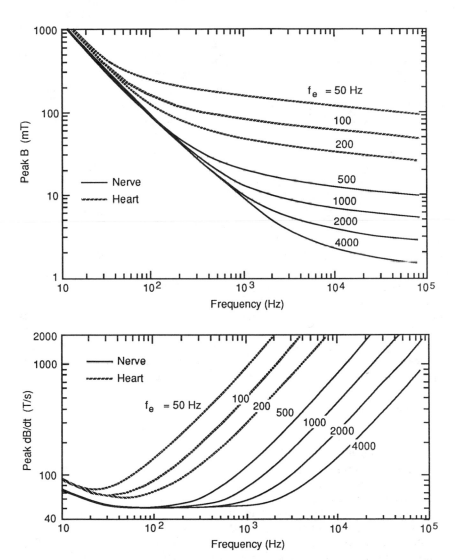

FIGURE 9. Calculated excitation thresholds for sagittal exposure of the torso to a sinusoidal magnetic field. Curve parameter f_e applies to the upper frequency constant of excitable tissue; lower frequency constant $f_o = 10$ Hz. Upper panel: peak flux density; lower panel: peak dB/dt.

cutaneous stimulation by sinusoidal currents[6] and can be attributed to the fact that suprathreshold sinusoidal currents result in rapid neural recruitment and in multiple synchronous action potentials.

Various other experiments with magnetic stimulation have been carried out on laboratory animals, nerve preparations, or limited regions of the human anatomy.[22-29] These experiments have been reviewed previously in the context of MRI exposure.[7,8] When appropriate consideration is given to the stimulus waveform or to its spatial distribution, it is found that experimental thresholds of peripheral nerve excitation fit within the theoretical range given in TABLE 1.

Cardiac excitation by magnetic stimuli has also been examined experimentally. At a pulse duration of 530 μs, the longitudinal magnetic threshold for an ectopic heartbeat in dogs was reported to be a factor of 13.5 ± 3.7 above the threshold of skeletal muscle stimulation.[11] In comparison, the theoretical model for human exposure predicts that the 1-percentile threshold of ectopic stimulation would occur at a factor of 6 above the peripheral nerve stimulation threshold; the 50-percentile cardiac threshold would be a factor of 12 above the nerve threshold (using $\tau_e = 120$ μs for nerve and $\tau_e = 3$ μs for the heart; longitudinal magnetic exposure). A more careful analysis of the relative human and canine anatomy would be required before these data could be confidently used for human exposure applications.

McRobbie and Foster[25] examined the ECG of rats subjected to repetitively pulsed magnetic stimuli having a maximum dB/dt in the range of 3 to 30 T/s. These investigators were unable to produce cardiac abnormalities, even for stimuli that caused violent muscle contractions. The magnetic waveforms used in these experiments were damped sinusoids, with frequencies in the range of 670 to 2000 Hz and with decay time constants of about 1.5 s. For sinusoidal stimulation in the frequency range, one expects cardiac thresholds to be significantly above neuromuscular thresholds (FIGURE 9). Consequently, the lack of cardiac stimulation in these experiments is not surprising.

Silny[29] placed coils around dogs such that the magnetic field was either along or perpendicular to the long axis of the body. With a single 50-Hz stimulus, Silny observed salvos of ectopic beats at applied fields above 2 T. That field is about six times the theoretical 1-percentile cardiac stimulation threshold for continuous sinusoidal exposure in humans; it is about three times greater than the median threshold. In order to compare the calculated human thresholds with the observed canine data, it is necessary to account for the relative sizes of the subjects, the geometric configuration of the body and heart, and the distribution of the magnetic field strength within the exposure areas, that is, information that is lacking in the Silny report. Nevertheless, one can conclude that the observed canine thresholds ought to be greater than human thresholds because (1) the canine subject is smaller than a human and (2) the coil placement in Silny's tests, with the heart roughly in the center of the coil, may not have been optimum for cardiac stimulation.

Willis and Brooks[27] studied rats and guinea pigs under magnetic exposure. These investigators were unable to observe cardiac abnormalities with dB/dt pulses of 2 T/s maintained for about 25 μs. The applied exposure was well below the predicted cardiac threshold (FIGURE 8), especially considering the small size of the animal subjects. Therefore, the lack of observed effect is to be expected.

DISCUSSION

By assuming uniform spatial properties for the magnetic field, rather simple mathematical models can be used for the induction process. In recent years, considerable attention has been given to so-called "focal" stimulation by small coil systems. Studies of focal stimulation include magnetic stimulation of the brain, central nervous system, and peripheral nerves. Potential clinical applications include measurement of central motor conduction time, monitoring of spinal cord function during surgery, evaluation of visual cortex function, and evaluation of nerve function. The principles discussed in this review also apply to focal magnetic stimulation. However, a thorough analysis of focal stimulation in general requires more sophisticated models for calculating the induced field and its spatial gradient.[6]

Published papers that deal with stimulation by large-area magnetic exposure indicate that the predictions with the simple models used here are not inconsistent with currently available experimental data. However, this apparent lack of disagreement is not the same as experimental verification. To confidently predict the thresholds of stimulation for MRI magnetic field exposure would require carefully designed experiments that take into account the stimulus waveform, its spatial distribution, and the anatomical properties of the test subject. The following paragraphs emphasize some of the areas of uncertainty particularly needing theoretical and experimental clarification.

Induction Model: A more realistic induction model should account for the subject's body shape and the nonhomogeneous and anisotropic properties of the various internal tissues and organs. Such a model should include the ability to employ metallic implants.

Tissue Time Constants: Tissue time constants (τ_e, f_e, f_o) determined experimentally vary over a very wide range and have been derived under conditions that differ from the magnetically induced stimulus. These parameters need to be evaluated under conditions appropriate to the magnetic stimulus.

Excitation Thresholds: Minimum excitation thresholds applicable to MRI exposure have not been adequately established. The assumptions used in this article have required some judgment and speculation. The threshold criterion used for the electric field needs further experimental clarification.

Patient Pathology and Drug Treatment: The influence of cardiac pathology on electrical thresholds and the effects of drug treatment have received little attention to date. Some evidence exists to indicate the possibility of heightened sensitivity in patients with cardiac pathology.

It is certain that many outstanding questions will be clarified in future research. In selecting criteria for the acceptability of electrical exposure, however, there will surely remain questions that cannot be answered with scientific objectivity. Frequently, these are policy or judgment issues that are settled on the basis of historical precedent or some other basis. Policy issues may include the population percentile that should be assumed for a threshold reaction or the safety factor that should be applied to theoretical predictions. Although a purely scientific approach cannot define the "correct" criteria of exposure, it is a critical aid to the process of criteria selection.

REFERENCES

1. DURNEY, C. H., C. C. JOHNSON & H. MASSOUDI. 1975. Long wavelength analysis of plane wave irradiation of a prolate spheroid model of a man. IEEE Trans. Microwave Theory Tech. **23**(2): 246–253.
2. SPIEGEL, R. J. 1977. Magnetic coupling to a prolate spheroid model of a man. IEEE Trans. Power Appar. Syst. **96**(1): 208–212.
3. GANDHI, O. P., J. F. DEFORD & H. DANAI. 1984. Impedance method for calculation of power deposition patterns in magnetically induced hyperthermia. IEEE Trans. Biomed. Eng. **31**(10): 644–651.
4. MCNEAL, D. R. 1976. Analysis of a model of excitation of myelinated nerve. IEEE Trans. Biomed. Eng. **23:** 329–337.
5. FRANKENHAEUSER, B. & A. F. HUXLEY. 1964. The action potential in the myelinated nerve fiber of *Xenopus laevis* as computed on the basis of voltage clamp data. J. Physiol. **171:** 302–315.
6. REILLY, J. P. 1992. Electrical Stimulation and Electropathology. Cambridge University Press. London/New York.
7. REILLY, J. P. 1989. Peripheral nerve stimulation by induced electric currents: exposure to time-varying magnetic fields. Med. Biol. Eng. Comput. **27:** 101–110.
8. REILLY, J. P. 1991. Magnetic field excitation of peripheral nerves and the heart: a comparison of thresholds. Med. Biol. Eng. Comput. **29**(6): 571–579.
9. FOSTER, K. R. & H. P. SCHWAN. 1986. Dielectric permittivity and electrical conductivity of biological materials. *In* Handbook of Biological Effects of Electromagnetic Fields. C. Polk & E. Postow, Eds.: 27–96. CRC Press. Boca Raton, Florida.
10. REILLY, J. P., V. T. FREEMAN & W. D. LARKIN. 1985. Sensory effects of transient electrical stimulation—evaluation with a neuroelectric model. IEEE Trans. Biomed. Eng. **32**(12): 1001–1011.
11. BOURLAND, J. D., J. A. NYENHUIS, G. A. MOUCHAWAR, L. A. GEDDES, D. J. SCHAEFER & M. E. RIEHL. 1991. Z-Gradient coil eddy-current stimulation of skeletal muscle and cardiac muscle in the dog. Society of Magnetic Resonance in Medicine, Tenth Annual Meeting, August 10–16, San Francisco.
12. ROY, O. Z., G. C. PARK & J. R. SCOTT. 1977. Intracardiac catheter fibrillation thresholds as a function of the duration of a 60 Hz current and electrode area. IEEE Trans. Biomed. Eng. **24**(5): 430–435.
13. ANTONI, H. 1985. Pathophysiological basis of ventricular fibrillation. *In* Electrical Shock Safety Criteria. J. F. Bridges, G. L. Ford, I. A. Sherman & M. Vainberg, Eds.: 33–43. Pergamon. Elmsford, New York.
14. CARUSO, P. M., J. A. PEARCE & D. P. DEWITT. 1979. Temperature and current density distributions at electrical surgical dispersive sites. *In* Proceedings of the Seventh New England Bioengineering Conference (Troy, New York, March 22–23), p. 373–376.
15. LANE, J. F. & T. J. ZEBO. 1967. Volume potential fields developed in cats' limbs during the passage of constant current pulses. *In* Digest Seventh Int. Conf. Med. Biol. Eng. (Stockholm, August 14–19), p. 207.
16. ROY, O. Z. 1980. Summary of cardiac fibrillation thresholds for 60 Hz currents and voltages applied directly to the heart. Med. Biol. Eng. Comput. **18:** 657–659.
17. SUGIMOTO, T., S. F. SCHAAL & A. G. WALLACE. 1967. Factors determining vulnerability to ventricular fibrillation induced by 60 cps alternating current. Circ. Res. **21:** 601–608.
18. WATSON, A. B., J. S. WRIGHT & J. LOUGHMAN. 1973. Electrical thresholds for ventricular fibrillation in man. Med. J. Aust. **1:** 1179–1182.
19. ANTONI, H. 1992. Electrical properties of the heart. *In* Electrical Stimulation and Electropathology. Chapter 5. Cambridge University Press. London/New York.
20. COHEN, M. S., R. M. WEISSKOFF, R. R. RZEDZIAN & H. C. KANTOR. 1990. Sensory stimulation by time-varying magnetic fields. Magn. Reson. Med. **14:** 409–414.
21. BUDINGER, T. F., H. FISCHER, D. HENTSCHEL, H. E. REINFELDER & F. SCHMITT. 1990. Neural stimulation dB/dt thresholds for frequency and number of oscillations using sinusoidal magnetic gradient fields. Society of Magnetic Resonance in Medicine, Ninth Annual Meeting, August 18–24, New York.

22. IRWIN, D., S. RUSH, R. EVERMY, E. LEPESCHKIN, D. B. MONTGOMERY & R. J. WEGGEL. 1970. Stimulation of cardiac muscle by a time-varying magnetic field. IEEE Trans. Magn. **MAG-6:** 321–322.

23. POLSON, M. J. R., A. T. BARKER & S. GARDINER. 1982. The effect of rapid rise-time magnetic fields on the ECG of the rat. Clin. Phys. Physiol. Meas. **3:** 231–234.

24. POLSON, M. J. R., A. T. BARKER & I. L. FREESTON. 1982. Stimulation of nerve trunks with time-varying magnetic fields. Med. Biol. Eng. Comput. **20:** 243–244.

25. MCROBBIE, D. & M. A. FOSTER. 1984. Thresholds for biological effects of time-varying magnetic fields. Clin. Phys. Physiol. Meas. **5:** 67–78.

26. UENO, S., K. HARADA & Y. OOMURA. 1984. Magnetic nerve stimulation without interlinkage between nerve and magnetic flux. IEEE Trans. Magn. **20:** 1660–1662.

27. WILLIS, R. J. & W. M. BROOKS. 1984. Potential hazards of NMR imaging: no evidence of the possible effects of static and changing magnetic fields on cardiac function of the rat and guinea pig. Magn. Reson. Imag. **2:** 89–95.

28. MCROBBIE, D. & M. A. FOSTER. 1985. Cardiac response to pulsed magnetic fields with regard to safety in NMR imaging. Phys. Med. Biol. **30**(7): 695–702.

29. SILNY, J. 1986. The influence of threshold of the time-varying magnetic field in the human organism. *In* Biological Effects of Static and Extremely Low Frequency Magnetic Fields. J. H. Bernhardt, Ed.: 105–112. M. M. Verlag. Munich.

Stimulation by Time-varying Magnetic Fields

MICHAEL L. ROHAN AND RICHARD R. RZEDZIAN

Advanced NMR Systems
Wilmington, Massachusetts 01887

INTRODUCTION

In this review, we present work in progress at Advanced NMR Systems on the stimulation of nerves by time-changing magnetic fields ($d\mathrm{B}/dt$).

The $d\mathrm{B}/dt$ effects in MRI are caused by the interaction of the time-changing gradient fields with the nerves and muscles of the human body. The mechanism for these effects is that a changing magnetic flux through a conductive surface causes electric fields or voltages to be induced in that conductor; in MRI, the gradient fields have a changing flux through the body of the patient, which results in voltages that may interact with nerves or muscles and cause stimulation. Thresholds for the occurrence of these effects are under investigation.

Efforts in the assessment of $d\mathrm{B}/dt$ effects in MRI are twofold: calculations have been done to model the system using changing, but spatially uniform magnetic fields using an ellipsoidal and homogeneously conductive model for the body; laboratory efforts are under way to find the stimulation thresholds in canines using scaled-down gradient coil systems.

This review presents a description of the gradient fields used in MRI imaging for better inclusion in predictions of stimulation, introducing a simple parametrized model for those fields. Additionally, statistics on high speed gradient scanning at Advanced NMR Systems over the last six years are presented to add to the existing information.

The analysis methods used to date are based on plane wave magnetic fields such as those produced by transmission lines; the fields used in MRI have several nonzero field components, each of which varies spatially. Furthermore, MRI uses two types of gradient coils (axial and transverse) that have different field distributions and require separate consideration. An additional concern is the geometric considerations that a spatially varying field requires; such a field cannot be characterized by only a peak value, but must be at least scaled by a volumetric form factor.

A model for the $d\mathrm{B}/dt$ situation for a transverse coil is shown in FIGURE 1.

MECHANISMS

The physical mechanism for stimulation is well known: a time-changing magnetic field passing through a conductive area produces an electric field and that electric field stimulates a muscle or nerve. The strength of the electric field depends on the rate of change of the magnetic field, on the area through which the magnetic field passes, and on the angle between the magnetic field and the area. This behavior is

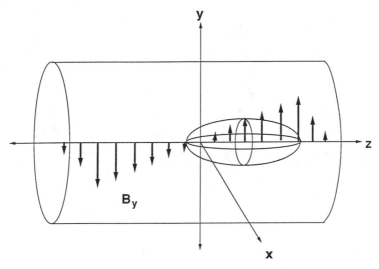

FIGURE 1. Transverse gradient "cross field".

summarized in FIGURE 2 and in the following equation:

$$\oint \vec{E} \cdot d\vec{\ell} = \int \frac{d\vec{B}}{dt} \cdot d\vec{A}$$

or, for the simple case of a circular cross section and a spatially uniform and uniformly changing magnetic field, the tangential electric field at the edge is

$$E = \frac{R}{2} \frac{dB}{dt} \cos(\theta),$$

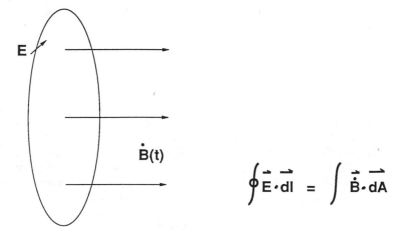

FIGURE 2. Mechanism for induced electric fields.

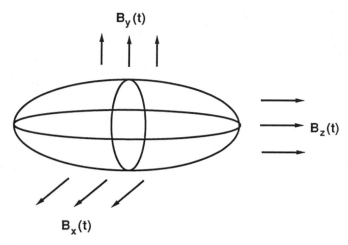

FIGURE 3. Field components and relevant planes for MRI.

where θ is the angle between the magnetic field and the normal to the surface. We can see from this expression that, in predicting the dB/dt effect, we must consider the dB/dt value integrated over the volume within the conducting body (rather than a peak field in the magnet bore). We must be concerned with the existence of all three components of the gradient field (not just the imaging component) and thus the direction of the magnetic field or dominant field component. Finally, we need to consider the cross section of the body normal to the field. This situation is illustrated in FIGURE 3, which shows the cross sections relevant to the three possible field components in MRI using the ellipsoidal model for the body proposed in reference 1.

In the end, it is the induced electric field inside the body and its interaction with the nervous or muscular system that is the threshold to be calculated; any use of the magnetic field to measure such a threshold must consider all the parameters that produce that electric field, voltage, or current.

GRADIENT COIL FIELDS

There are two types of gradient coils used in MRI, namely, the axial coil (Z coil) and the transverse coils (X and Y coils). The fields produced by these two types of coils are different and will produce different induced voltages for the same gradient pulses. To describe these fields, we use stylized linear models that are general enough to apply to all gradient systems. The simplifications made for these models are listed when they are made. For each coil, we list the field component that produces a significant flux and neglect the less significant components; a complete solution would consider all components, but a system open to regulation and publication must be characterizable and comparable to other systems and thus we introduce some simple measurements to characterize the dB/dt of these coils.

Axial Coil

The field of an axial coil is usually expressed for imaging purposes as

$$\vec{B} = Gz\hat{z}.$$

Because of the finite length of a gradient coil, this expression is valid in only a small area about the center of the coil; the field everywhere has an envelope that goes to zero at large z. This envelope function is labeled $f_1(z)$ in FIGURE 4. The axial coil has a radial field component required by Maxwell's $\nabla \cdot \vec{B} = 0$ equation. The "ideal" radial field, $B_r = Gr/2\hat{r}$, also has an envelope in z, labeled $f_2(z)$ in FIGURE 5. The envelope functions are the result of edge effects in the coil and are not derived here. There is no azimuthal field component for the axial coil. The total field of the axial coil can then be written as

$$\vec{B} = Gzf_1(z)\hat{z} + G(r/2)f_2(z)\hat{r},$$

where $f_1(z)$ and $f_2(z)$ are z-dependent envelope functions reflecting the finite length of the coils. The forms of $f_1(z)$ and $f_2(z)$ are shown in a simplified form in FIGURES 4 and 5. The figures use linear functions for the field profiles; the actual fields have curvature towards or away from the axis.

In considering stimulation by an axial coil, we consider the three elements for inducing voltage that were discussed earlier: average flux through an area, the cross-sectional area in question, and the angle between them. The z component of an axial coil is easily characterizable, with a fairly uniform field and a well-defined cross section; its peak location is out some distance along the z axis.

The radial component of the axial coil does not have a cross-sectional area as easily identifiable as the z component does. For a first approximation, this component can be neglected in characterizing an axial coil.

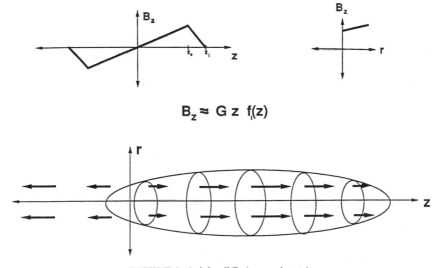

$$B_z \approx G \ z \ f_1(z)$$

FIGURE 4. Axial coil B_z (approximate).

Transverse Coil

The X and Y gradient coils are transverse coils. The X coil is the same as the Y coil, rotated 90°; our discussions of the Y coil will apply to the X coil by substituting x for y. The field of a transverse Y coil is characterized for imaging purposes as

$$\vec{B} = Gy\hat{z}.$$

Again, because of the finite length of a gradient coil, this is true only in a small area about the center and there is a further z dependence elsewhere, which can be included as an envelope function that goes to zero for large z. The transverse coil has a second field component in the direction of the gradient, which is required by

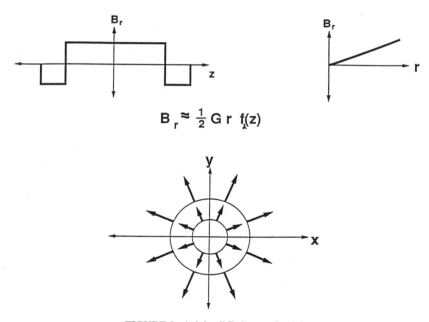

FIGURE 5. Axial coil B_r (approximate).

Maxwell's $\nabla \cdot \vec{B} = 0$ equation. There is no field component in the third direction. The field of a transverse Y coil can be written as

$$\vec{B} = Gyf_2(z)\hat{z} + Gzf_1(z)\hat{y},$$

where $f_1(z)$ and $f_2(z)$ are z-dependent envelope functions reflecting the finite length of the coils. Stylized profiles for $f_1(z)$ and $f_2(z)$ are shown in FIGURES 6 and 7. These transverse envelope functions are similar to those for the axial coils and thus are labeled the same; they arise for the same reasons. As with the axial coil, these straight line drawings do not show the curvature inherent in the fields.

In considering stimulation by a transverse coil, we can see that the total flux through a transverse slice of the body due to B_z is zero; stimulation would occur in

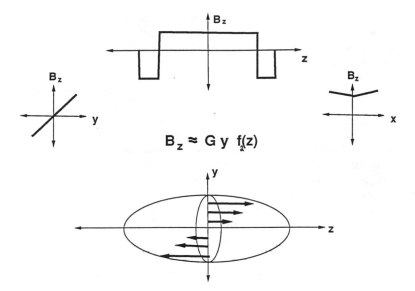

FIGURE 6. Transverse coil B_z (approximate).

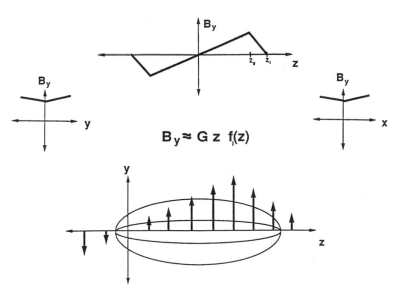

FIGURE 7. Transverse coil B_y (approximate).

smaller cross-sectional areas above and below $y = 0$ caused by nonuniform fields. A stimulation threshold calculated from the peak dB/dt would be much smaller than one considering the actual fields involved because the field is zero in the center and thus both the intersecting areas and fields are significantly less than the use of the peak field and cross section would indicate.

The second field component (B_y) of a transverse coil (shown in FIGURE 7) is more significant. The cross-sectional area for a unipolar flux is larger and the peak field involved will be larger because of the greater extent of the coil along its axis (note that the imaging B_z component and the "cross field" B_y component have the same gradient G); a threshold prediction using the peak field and the cross-sectional area would require a form factor to account for the nonuniform field. This "cross field" dB/dt is the dominant of the two components in the transverse coil and, for a first approximation, it can be used to set the threshold for stimulation. This statement is valid for most coils used in cylindrical MRI systems that use volume transverse coils; it will not be valid for shorter transverse coils.

CHARACTERIZATION

Characterization of the dB/dt in a pulse sequence requires consideration of the field from the gradient coil and of the pulse sequence in use. We can consider these two separately: the field of the gradient coil can be characterized by its field distribution at a standard 1-G/cm operation and the pulse sequence parameters of peak gradient strength and waveform can be determined for each MRI experiment independently. This allows an easier comparison between experiments on different systems.

Our goal is parametrization in a manner that will allow the calculation of voltages induced within the body for comparison with established thresholds.

We characterize dB/dt with the dominant field components for each coil (identified earlier as B_z for axial coils, B_x for transverse x coils, B_y for transverse y coils) and by using the ellipsoidal cross sections introduced by Reilly.[1] The standard ellipse used here has an axis of 80 cm in z and 40 cm in x and y. For calculation of flux through a cross section, we use the linear field models described earlier:

$$-G_z(z + z_1)\hat{z} \quad \text{for} \quad -z_1 < z < -z_0 \quad (1)$$

$$\mathbf{B}_{model} = G_z z\hat{z} \quad \text{for} \quad -z_0 < z < z_0 \quad (2)$$

$$-G_z(z - z_1)\hat{z} \quad \text{for} \quad z_0 < z < z_1 \quad (3)$$

for the axial coil and

$$-G_y(z + z_1)\hat{y} \quad \text{for} \quad -z_1 < z < -z_0 \quad (4)$$

$$\mathbf{B}_{model} = G_y z\hat{y} \quad \text{for} \quad -z_0 < z < z_0 \quad (5)$$

$$-G_y(z - z_1)\hat{y} \quad \text{for} \quad z_0 < z < z_1 \quad (6)$$

for the transverse coils. We use these to find an average flux for comparison (integrating over the ellipse). For example, a transverse coil whose field peaks at the center of the standard ellipse ($z = 40$ cm) will have an averaged flux density equal to 57% of its peak.

The dB/dt for an axial coil can be characterized by measurement of two field strengths and two distances. We measure the maximum B_z value found along the z axis and the distance of this point from $z = 0$; we then measure the B_z value at the same z location, but at a specified radius (corresponding to the edge of a standard ellipse). The two field measurements are averaged to provide a peak B_z number. A corresponding peak field could be found with a computer model of the coil by averaging the B_z field inside a specified cross section at the peak location in z. Last, we measure the distance at which the B_z becomes zero again on the z axis. The axial characterization is shown in FIGURE 8.

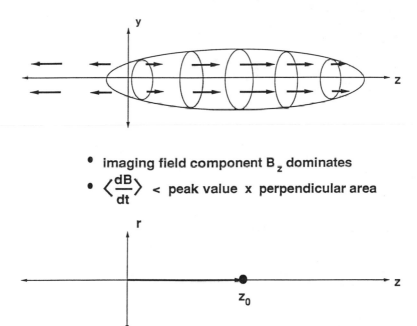

FIGURE 8. Axial dB/dt characterization.

The dB/dt for a transverse coil can be characterized by a similar method. In the laboratory, we measure the B_y field along the z axis and record the value and position of its peak. We also measure the B_y strength at the same z location and at a specified y position corresponding to the edge of a standard ellipse; these two field numbers are averaged to provide a peak field at the peak z location. The position along the z axis where the B_y field returns to zero is also recorded. The flux through planes perpendicular to y can be calculated using a linear model with these numbers (numerically, the average flux through ellipses perpendicular to y can also be calculated). The transverse characterization is shown in FIGURE 9.

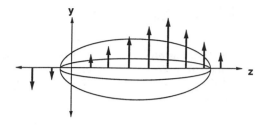

- "cross" field component B_y dominates
- $\left\langle \dfrac{dB}{dt} \right\rangle$ < peak value x perpendicular area

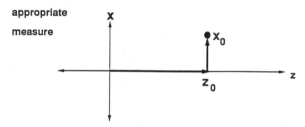

FIGURE 9. Transverse dB/dt characterization.

The field distributions above can be done for any gradient coil at a nominal 1-G/cm operation. Evaluation of particular pulse sequences then involves only multiplication by the imaging waveform of interest, in units of G/cm. The dB/dt values quoted here are calculated in this manner; to evaluate a gradient waveform at 1 kHz and 2.0 G/cm, we multiply our field distribution in gauss at 1 G/cm by a factor of $2\pi \cdot 1000 \cdot 2.0$.

Consideration must be given to the interaction of operation of different gradient coils at the same time; in some of the echo planar results quoted later, the pulse sequence consists of a resonant gradient pulse train at 1 kHz with a smaller gradient pulse of 7 kHz applied at the zero-crossings of the first. Threshold calculations and determination for this multicoil, multifrequency situation are not addressed here.

CLINICAL SCANNING

We present data from six years of clinical scanning at Advanced NMR Systems (ANMR) along with data from two studies at the Massachusetts General Hospital (MGH) using an ANMR retrofitted scanner. The data are inconclusive for any attempt to confirm stimulation at these gradient strengths; a dB/dt study at higher gradients is needed for this. The data presented in TABLE 1 are from clinical trials and research using the Instascan pulse sequence, which uses a high strength resonant read gradient and simultaneous high frequency phase gradient pulses. We note that the $d\text{B}/dt$ figures presented here are not the same as those from a previous work on the ANMR system;[2] numbers in this paper have been recalculated using the methods above and with peak rather than rms values.

The data listed here (with the exception of the 1.4-kHz data) were not produced in $d\text{B}/dt$ studies, but rather in the course of routine clinical research. Events were reported by volunteers who were asked to note unusual sensations; if they did, the study was stopped with no attempt at repeating or confirming the sensations or at identifying the source (acoustic stimulation was not tested). All events listed were reported by researchers participating in the studies who were aware of the possibility of such events, although the studies included significant numbers of both researchers and patients. The data at 1.4 kHz are from a $d\text{B}/dt$ study previously published[2] that attempted to locate and confirm gradient stimulation. Data from canine work are not included; we note that reference 2 reports an attempt at canine cardiac stimulation.

The data presented cover four configurations of scanner hardware and several pulse sequences. The 2.0-T system had a shortened gradient system with a longitudinal field extent of 45 cm, whereas the 1.5-T system had a longitudinal extent greater than 60 cm. For each configuration, the $d\text{B}/dt$ figures for both the read gradient and a higher frequency phase gradient are reported; the phase gradient cross field is perpendicular to the read cross field (one is B_x and the other is B_y). Both read and phase gradient fields were supplied by transverse coils. The read gradients are continuous sinusoidal trains of 32 to 64 cycles; the phase gradients are single unipolar half-sine pulses at the zero-crossings of the read gradient. Note that the listing for "double phase" gradients describes an experiment with two unipolar half-sine phase gradient pulses at each read gradient zero-crossing.

Both peak and spatially averaged $d\text{B}/dt$ values are listed for each item to emphasize the differences in peak and average flux values. The low value for the 2.0-T system is a result of the different coil configuration; the short extent of this coil and a reversal of the cross field within the standard ellipse produce a low integrated flux and the imaging component B_z may be the dominant component in this coil.

DISCUSSION

This review has presented a parametrized model of the gradient fields in MRI for use in standardization and in prediction of thresholds for a better understanding and

TABLE 1. Clinical Scanning Data at ANMR and MGH (Transverse $d\text{B}/dt$)

System	Gradient	Peak $d\text{B}/dt$	$\langle d\text{B}/dt\rangle$	Volunteers	Images	Events
2.0 T	1.6 kHz, 8.0 kHz	43 T/s, 18 T/s	~0	60	11,000	0
		48 T/s, 18 T/s	~0	2		1
1.5 T	1.4 kHz, 7.0 kHz	61 T/s, 27 T/s	~31, 15 T/s	2		2
1.5 T	1.0 kHz, 7.0 kHz	36 T/s, 27 T/s	~19, 15 T/s	31	10,000	2
	double phase			4		1
1.5 T/MGH	1.0 kHz, 7.0 kHz			26 head	>6000	0
				62 abd.	>15,000	3

prediction of clinical results. The next step in calculation of a dB/dt threshold is the determination of induced voltages and fields in the MRI experiment using the fields and pulse sequences employed in MRI.

The clinical data presented, summarizing six years of scanning at ANMR and MGH on a resonant gradient system, are inconclusive for the establishment of a repeatable pattern of stimulation because of the small number of potential events (8 out of 40,000 images). The data are qualitatively inconclusive because a head scan should be the most sensitive scan for stimulation, placing the abdomen in the transverse cross field, but this is not reflected in the list of potential events.

Further calculational work involves analysis of these MRI fields in a conducting ellipsoidal model, a look at the conductive paths and impedances in the body for more accurate prediction, and eventually the finite element modeling of the MRI experiment in the body.

REFERENCES

1. REILLY, J. P. 1990. Peripheral nerve and cardiac excitation by time-varying magnetic fields: a comparison of thresholds. FDA Report No. MT90-100.
2. COHEN, M. S., R. M. WEISSKOFF, R. R. RZEDZIAN & H. L. KANTOR. 1990. Magn. Reson. Med. **14:** 409–414.

Session II Summary

STEPHEN R. THOMAS

Department of Radiology
University of Cincinnati
Cincinnati, Ohio 45221

Fundamental to the process of data acquisition in magnetic resonance imaging (MRI) and spectroscopy (MRS) is the rapid switching (on, off, polarity reversal) of magnetic gradient fields. Power transfer to tissues, and hence the potential for biological effects, may occur principally through interaction with the electric fields induced by changing magnetic fields as described by classical electromagnetic relationships. This session was designed to explore the aspects of biological interactions and the potential consequences associated with rapid, time-varying magnetic fields.

A generalized approach to this topic might be developed around the following interrogative outline: (1) What biological effects are important for consideration? Are they reversible? Do they represent a projected health risk? (2) What are the "known" thresholds for stimulation of these effects? What is the degree of variability in the data defining these thresholds? (3) What models are required for predictive calculation of these biological effects? How realistic are the proposed models? What are the calculational uncertainties? (4) Ultimately, what safety precautions and regulatory guidelines are appropriate for implementation? What should be the impact of calculational predictions versus human experimental data/evidence on establishment of these guidelines? What degree of conservatism is prudent?

The authors of the contributions in this session have addressed a number of these questions (although not all) specific to rapidly switched magnetic fields. First, most of the attention by far focuses on excitatory responses, which include such phenomena as visual magnetophosphenes (reversible, considered to have no risk), accelerated bone regrowth/healing, peripheral neuromuscular stimulation, and cardiac excitation/fibrillation (definite associated risk). Another biological response for consideration involves cellular membrane activation processes and the influence of time-varying magnetic fields on intracellular transport (e.g., signal transduction influencing calcium kinetics).

Second, the magnetic field rate of change (dB/dt) threshold levels for biological effects are recognized as being dependent upon a multiplicity of factors including tissue type (bioconstituent composition, normal versus pathologic status), orientation relative to the magnetic field, location within the body, and excitation waveform (fundamental frequency, presence of harmonics, rise/fall times). Threshold values for excitatory response are directly related to the magnitude of the electric field (or current density) induced by dB/dt. Estimates of the threshold for nerve cell stimulation may vary by orders of magnitude (10 mA/m^2 to 1 A/m^2) depending on the cell type and experimental model employed. This wide range underscores the importance of reaching scientific agreement upon (a) protocols for threshold determination and (b) end points of significance for biological effects.

Third, because the primary mode of physical interaction of time-varying magnetic fields with tissue takes place via induction of electric fields (and currents), the use of traditional electromagnetic formalism (Maxwell's equations, Faraday's law of induction) serves as the agreed-upon starting point. A general approach is to calculate the magnitude of the induced electric field (or current density) resulting from a given $d\mathrm{B}/dt$. Elements of the models include the geometric distribution of body tissue (e.g., concentric rings normal to the magnetic field, prolate spheroid) and assumptions concerning electrical properties (conductivity, resistivity), response time, and homogeneous characteristics of the tissues. Experimental verification of the models or investigations to confirm the existence of bioeffects require carefully controlled procedures by which confounding variables are eliminated (e.g., vibration, thermal fluctuation).

Finally, theoretical calculations must be based on practical protocols for clinical MRI and MRS systems both for assessment of potential biological consequences and for establishment of operational guidelines. Although perhaps controversial according to points mentioned earlier, most commonly implemented MRI pulse protocols appear to operate below levels that would stimulate excitable tissue. However, the advent of echo planar techniques employing strong extremely rapidly switched gradients to obtain an image in less than 50 ms may provide $d\mathrm{B}/dt$ values approaching 100 T/s. Initial observations report peripheral nerve stimulation in human subjects under these scan conditions. Current federal guidance would put the upper limit at 20 T/s for pulse widths of 120 ms or greater. (Higher values of the switched gradient field would be permitted for shorter pulse widths.) Thus, developing technologies for MRI systems are extending the upper dynamic range for time-varying magnetic fields. Therefore, an accurate and complete understanding of the consequences of rapidly switched magnetic fields is required. The contributions presented in this session are directed toward this objective.

Absorption and Distribution Patterns of RF Fields

OM P. GANDHI AND JIN-YUAN CHEN

Department of Electrical Engineering
University of Utah
Salt Lake City, Utah 84112

INTRODUCTION

Over the past five to ten years, magnetic resonance imaging (MRI) has become an important tool for medical diagnostic applications. There are several aspects of the intense magnetic fields that require close scrutiny from the point of view of patient safety. These include larger static magnetic fields, large spatial gradients of the magnetic fields, rapidly switched magnetic fields, and higher and higher frequency RF magnetic fields. In this report, we will examine the absorption and distribution patterns of radio-frequency (RF) magnetic fields, which in emerging techniques may be of frequencies as high as 200 MHz. Highly simplified homogeneous spherical, cylindrical, and disk models have in the past been used to obtain power depositions due to RF magnetic fields.[1,2] Because only homogeneous models have been used, these models, naturally, are incapable of providing information on distributions of RF absorption (specific absorption rates or SARs). For RF dosimetry, we have developed an anatomically based model of the human body[3] and a new numerically efficient method called the impedance method that we and our colleagues have used to obtain SAR distributions for frequencies up to 63 MHz.[4-6] In the impedance method, we represent the body or the parts thereof by a three-dimensional network of impedances, each of which represents a certain subregion of the body typically about 1–1.5 cm in length. Durney *et al.*[7] have recently generalized the impedance network formulation using the complete set of Maxwell's equations, which should therefore be usable at any frequency. This generalization involves inclusion of inductances in addition to the resistance-capacitance equivalent impedances that were used previously.[4-6]

THE ANATOMICALLY BASED MODEL

As previously described in references 3 and 4, the inhomogeneous model of the human body is taken from the book, *A Cross-Section Anatomy*, by Eycleshymer and Schoemaker.[8] This book contains cross-sectional diagrams of the human body that were obtained by making cross-sectional cuts at spacings of about 1 inch in human cadavers. The process for creating the data base of the human model was the following: first of all, a 0.25-inch grid was taken for each single cross-sectional diagram and each cell on the grid was assigned a number corresponding to one of the sixteen tissue types (muscle, fat, bone, blood, intestine, cartilage, liver, kidney,

131

TABLE 1. Tissue Properties Used for the Human Model[9,10]

Tissue Type	Mass Density ρ (1000 kg/m³)	64 MHz σ (S/m)	ϵ_r	128 MHz σ (S/m)	ϵ_r	192 MHz σ (S/m)	ϵ_r
air	0.0012	0.0	1.0	0.0	1.0	0.0	1.0
muscle	1.05	0.84	84	1.14	70	1.25	56
fat/bone	1.2	0.06	8.3	0.07	7.0	0.07	7.0
blood	1.0	0.84	79	1.11	72	1.15	65
intestine	1.0	0.38	39	0.56	34	0.60	30
cartilage	1.0	0.06	8.3	0.07	7.0	0.07	7.0
liver	1.03	0.58	87	0.64	70	0.72	56
kidney	1.02	0.91	111	1.02	85	1.08	67
pancreas	1.03	0.81	125	1.02	85	1.08	70
spleen	1.03	0.81	125	0.84	98	0.88	95
lung[a]	0.33	0.26	26	0.31	22	0.21	12
heart	1.03	0.69	97	0.77	72	0.85	59
nerve/brain	1.05	0.48	97	0.55	77	0.60	62
skin	1.0	0.80	66	0.78	64	0.80	57
eye	1.0	0.64	98	1.90	85	1.90	82

[a]We have used 33% lung tissue and 67% air for the conductivity and dielectric constant of the lung.

pancreas, spleen, lung, heart, nerve, brain, skin, eye) or to air. Thus, the data associated with a particular layer consisted of three numbers for each square cell: x and y positions relative to some anatomical reference point in this layer, usually the center of the spinal cord, and an integer indicating which tissue that cell contained. Because the cross-sectional diagrams available in reference 8 are for somewhat variable separations, typically 2.3–2.7 cm, a new set of equispaced layers was defined at 0.25-inch (0.635-cm) intervals by interpolating the data onto these layers. Because the 0.25-inch cell size is too small for the memory space of readily accessible computers, the proportion of each tissue type was calculated next for somewhat larger cells of sizes equal to 0.5 inches (1.27 cm), combining the data for $2 \times 2 \times 2 = 8$ cells of the smaller dimension. Without changes in the anatomy, this process allows some variability in the height and weight of the body. We have taken the final cell size of 1.31 cm (rather than 0.5 inches) to obtain the total height and body weight of 176.85 cm and 70.0 kg, respectively.

The electrical properties of the various tissues used for the human model are given in TABLE 1 for frequencies of 64, 128, and 192 MHz that have been used for SAR calculations. In TABLE 1, σ is the electrical conductivity and ϵ_r is the relative permittivity or the dielectric constant of the respective tissues. Also given in TABLE 1 are the mass densities ρ used for the various tissues for SAR calculations.

THE IMPEDANCE METHOD

For low-frequency dosimetry problems (≤ 40 MHz for the human body) in which quasi-static approximations may be made, the impedance method has been found to be highly efficient as a numerical procedure for calculation of internal current densities, induced electric fields, and SARs. In this method detailed in references 4 and 5, the biological body or the exposed part thereof is represented by a three-dimensional (3-D) network of impedances whose individual values are obtained from the complex conductivities $\sigma + j\omega\epsilon$ for the various locations of the body, where σ is the electrical conductivity, $\omega = 2\pi f$ is the radian frequency, and $\epsilon = \epsilon_r\epsilon_o$ is the electrical permittivity in terms of the dielectric constant ϵ_r and the permittivity ϵ_o of free space ($= 8.85 \times 10^{-12}$ F/m).

The anatomically based model with a cell size of 1.31 cm (nominal 0.5″) consists of 45,024 cells (subvolumes) for which the volume-averaged tissue properties are taken. Each of these cells can then be represented by a network of impedances whose individual values in different directions are given by the following expression:

$$Z_m^{i,j,k} = \frac{\Delta_m}{\Delta_n\Delta_p(\sigma_m^{i,j,k} + j\omega\epsilon_m^{i,j,k})}, \tag{1}$$

where i, j, k indicate the cell index; m is the direction (which can be x, y, or z) for which the impedance is calculated; and $\sigma_m^{i,j,k}$ and $\epsilon_m^{i,j,k}$ are the electrical conductivities and permittivities for the cell i, j, k in the m-th direction. Δ_m is the thickness of the cell in the m-th direction, and Δ_n and Δ_p are the widths of the cell in directions at right angles to the m-th direction. For exposure to time- and space-varying magnetic fields, voltages (electromotive forces or EMFs) are induced for the various loops of the 3-D

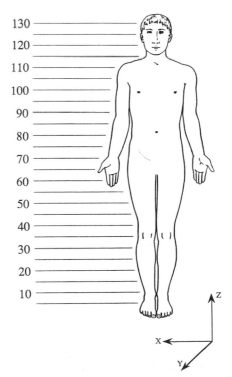

FIGURE 1. The layer-numbering scheme used for the model of the human body. Each layer is 1.31 cm from its neighbors. Layer no. 1 is 0.655 cm above the bottom of the feet and layer no. 135 is 0.655 cm below the top of the head.

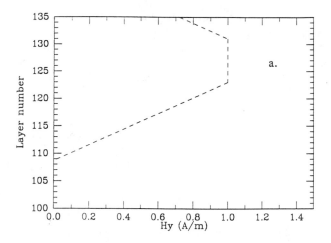

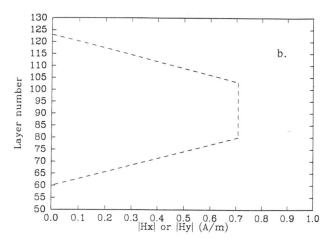

FIGURE 2. (a) Intensity profile for the linearly polarized magnetic field centered at layer no. 127 passing through the eyes of the model; $\mathbf{H} = \mathrm{H}_y\hat{y} = 1$ A/m. (b) Intensity profile for the circularly polarized magnetic field. The magnetic field is polarized in the xy plane; $\mathbf{H} = 0.707(\hat{x} + j\hat{y})$, $|\mathbf{H}| = 1$ A/m.

equivalent impedance network, whose values are given by the following expression:

$$V_m^{i,j,k} = -\frac{d}{dt}\int \mathbf{B}^{i,j,k} \cdot d\mathbf{S} = -\left(\frac{d}{dt}\,\mathrm{B}_m^{i,j,k}\right)\Delta_n\Delta_p, \tag{2}$$

where $\mathrm{B}_m^{i,j,k}$ is the component of the magnetic field for cell i, j, k in the m-th direction and $\Delta_n\Delta_p$ is the area of the loop in the plane at right angles to the m-th direction.

From equation 2, it can be seen that both time- and space-varying magnetic fields can indeed be handled using the impedance method formulation.

From equation 1, the equivalent impedances $Z_m^{i,j,k}$ can be considered to be composed of parallel combinations of resistances and capacitances whose values are given by $\Delta_m/(\sigma_m^{i,j,k}\Delta_n\Delta_p)$ and $(\epsilon_m^{i,j,k}\Delta_n\Delta_p)/\Delta_m$, respectively. A handicap of the impedance method as presently formulated is that, whereas it accounts for Faraday's law of induction $[\oint \mathbf{E} \cdot d\ell = (-d/dt) \int \mathbf{B} \cdot d\mathbf{S}]$ through equation 2, it ignores Ampère's circuital law given by the following equation:

$$\oint \mathbf{H} \cdot d\ell = \int \sigma\mathbf{E} \cdot d\mathbf{S} + \epsilon \int \frac{d\mathbf{E}}{dt} \cdot d\mathbf{S}. \qquad (3)$$

Durney et al.[7] have included equation 3 as well in obtaining the modified equivalent impedance network that should be applicable at any frequency. They have shown that this should result in modifying the equivalent circuit in each of the arms of the impedance network by the addition of a series inductance $L = \mu\Delta/4$, where μ is the permeability ($=\mu_o$) for the tissues and Δ is the cell size assumed to be cubical as for the presently used network. For this generalized formulation, it is possible to calculate $L = 4.1$ nH for the cell size of $\Delta = 1.31$ cm. At the highest frequency of 192 MHz, this series inductance would amount to an impedance of 4.9 ohms as compared to the impedance of the parallel resistance-capacitance (RC) combination of impedance $49.7-j23.8$ ohms for muscle at one extreme and $510-j544$ ohms for fat or bone at the other extreme. Because the added impedance in each of the arms due to this inductance is no more than 10% for muscle even at the highest frequency of interest and is, in fact, considerably smaller for other frequencies and less-conducting tissues,

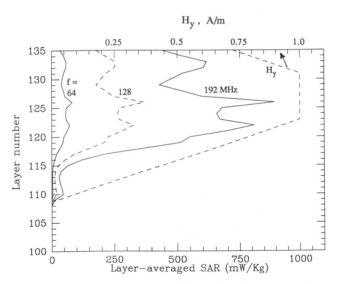

FIGURE 3. Layer-averaged SARs for the model of the human body for the linearly polarized RF magnetic fields of FIGURE 2a. The frequencies taken for the calculations are 64, 128, and 192 MHz.

we have neglected this additional complexity of the equivalent circuit in the first instance and have used the conventional impedance method for the present calculations.

RESULTS

The layer-numbering scheme used for the model of the human body is shown in FIGURE 1. Each layer is 1.31 cm from its neighbors. Layer no. 1 is 0.655 cm above the bottom of the feet and layer no. 135 is 0.655 cm below the top of the head. To

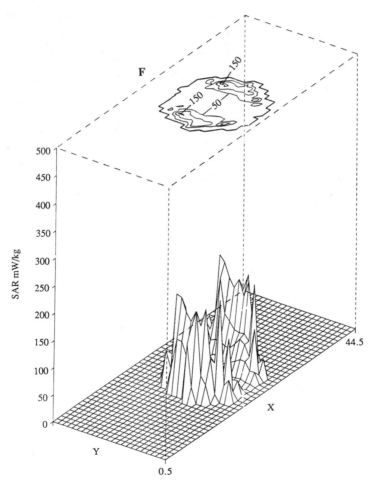

FIGURE 4a. SAR distributions for layer no. 128, which is 1.31 cm above the plane passing through the center of the eyes; $\mathbf{H} = \mathrm{H}, \hat{y} = 1 \, \mathrm{A/m}$. The plots on the top of the parallelopiped are contour plots of the data plotted within the parallelopiped. F denotes the front of the face. In this figure, f = 64 MHz and the separation between contour lines = 50 mW/kg.

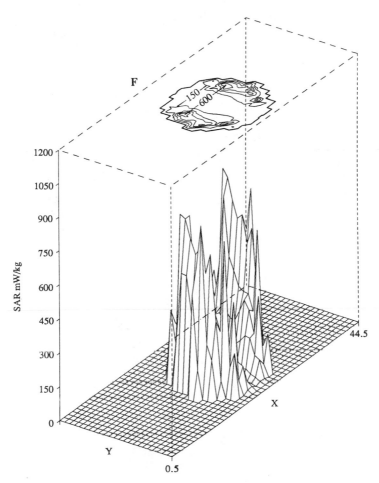

FIGURE 4b. Same as the caption to FIGURE 4a, except that f = 128 MHz and the separation between contour lines = 150 mW/kg.

calculate the induced current densities, we have assumed the following two configurations[a] for the applied RF magnetic fields:

(1) A linearly polarized magnetic field oriented from front to back of the head with an assumed field intensity of 1 A/m that is uniform over a region of ±5.24 cm (four cell widths) on either side of a central plane (layer no. 127) through the eyes of the model. Beyond this region of uniformity, the magnetic field tapers linearly to zero at the rate of 14% for every two cell widths, that is, 2.62 cm (see FIGURE 2a).

[a]These configurations were originally suggested by Daniel J. Schaefer of General Electric Company, Milwaukee, Wisconsin.

(2) A circularly polarized magnetic field centered at layer no. 91 of the model (a section of the torso) having the intensity profile as shown in FIGURE 2b. The field is polarized in the xy plane (see FIGURE 1 for the coordinates) and is constant with x and y; it varies only with z. The field has a constant magnitude of 1 A/m (0.707 A/m for each of the components H_x and H_y that are 90° phase-shifted from each other) for the cross-sectional planes of the body that are 42.6 and 72.7 cm below the top of the head, respectively. The magnitude of the magnetic field tapers linearly to zero both below and above these planes at the rate of 10% for every two cell widths, that is, 2.62 cm.

The fields described in these two configurations can only be thought of as approximations because the tapers of the x and y components of the magnetic fields

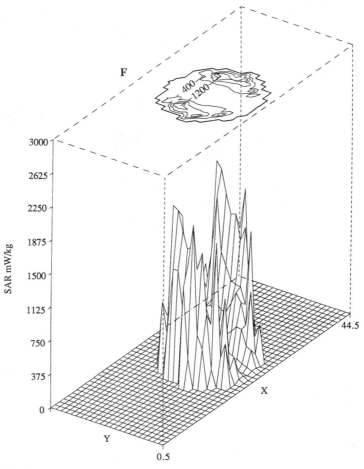

FIGURE 4c. Same as the caption to FIGURE 4a, except that f = 192 MHz and the separation between contour lines = 400 mW/kg.

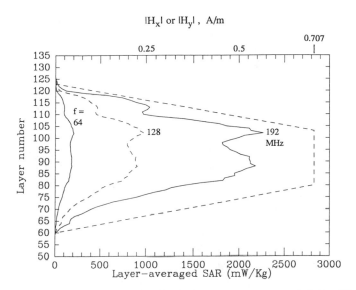

FIGURE 5. Layer-averaged SARs for the circularly polarized RF magnetic fields of FIGURE 2b. For layer nos. 80 to 103, $\mathbf{H} = 0.707(\hat{x} + j\hat{y})$, $|\mathbf{H}| = 1$ A/m.

in the edge regions would cause other nonzero components of the magnetic fields. These additional components will depend on the type of applicator used. Due to the lack of available data on these components, we have neglected them for these initial computations. Also, because of the unavailability of the data, we have neglected phase differences of the applied magnetic fields across the body, which in any case are likely to be fairly small for imaging applications. We have taken frequencies of 64, 128, and 192 MHz for the RF magnetic fields.

From the calculated currents in the various equivalent impedances, it is also possible to calculate the current densities $\mathbf{J}$ and hence the electric field $\mathbf{E}$ for the various cell centers in the body. The SAR for each of these cells can then be calculated from the relationship,

$$\text{SAR} = \frac{\sigma |\mathbf{E}|^2}{\rho}, \tag{4}$$

where ρ is the volume-averaged mass density for the respective cells.

The layer-averaged SARs for the linearly polarized RF magnetic fields of FIGURE 2a are shown in FIGURE 3 for 64, 128, and 192 MHz, respectively. Also shown in this figure is the assumed variation of the applied magnetic field. The SAR distributions for layer no. 128 through the eyes are shown in FIGURES 4a, 4b, and 4c, where the plots on the top of the parallelopipeds are contour plots of the data plotted within the respective parallelopipeds. For each of these figures, F represents the front of the body, that is, the face. Note that, as expected, we get double-peaked distributions (see the plots of the data within the parallelopipeds) because the induced currents are flowing around the applied magnetic field and increasing current densities and hence larger SARs are expected as we get further away from the center along the x axis. Nonuniformity of the SAR distributions is, of course, the result of the anatomically based heterogeneities of the tissues.

For the linearly polarized magnetic fields of FIGURE 2a, the highest local SARs are observed for layer no. 126 through the nose. The highest local SARs calculated at 64, 128, and 192 MHz are 0.64, 2.94, and 7.14 W/kg, respectively.

The layer-averaged SARs for the circularly polarized RF magnetic fields of FIGURE 2b are shown in FIGURE 5, where the assumed variation of the magnetic field is also given. The SAR distributions for a representative torso section (layer no. 91) are shown in FIGURES 6a, 6b, and 6c together with the contour plots at 64, 128, and 192 MHz, respectively. These SAR distributions also show an expected behavior because double-peaked SARs along the x and y axes are expected due to the applied

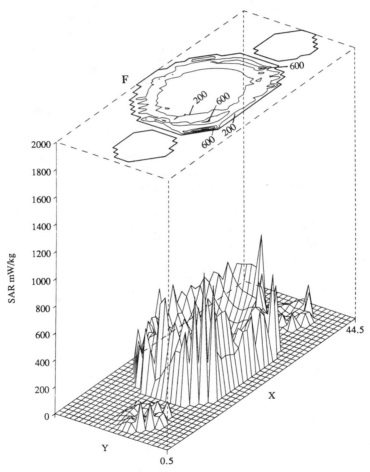

FIGURE 6a. SAR distributions for layer no. 91 corresponding to the central plane of the applied circularly polarized RF magnetic fields of FIGURE 2b. The plots on the top are the contour plots of the data. F denotes the front of the body. In this figure, f = 64 MHz and the separation between contour lines = 200 mW/kg.

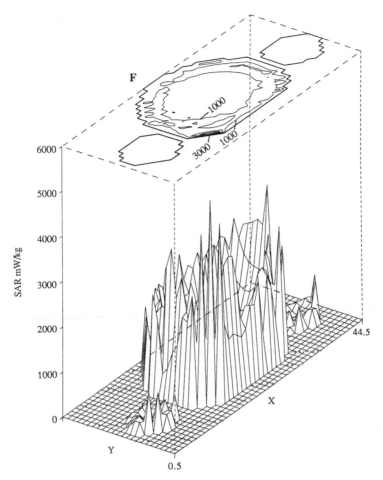

FIGURE 6b. Same as the caption to FIGURE 6a, except that f = 128 MHz and the separation between contour lines = 1000 mW/kg.

H_y and H_x, respectively. A trough-type SAR distribution is consequently obtained for these circularly polarized RF magnetic fields. The highest local SARs are calculated for layer no. 102 just below the armpit, where SARs as high as 1.04, 5.02, and 12.04 W/kg are calculated for 64, 128, and 192 MHz, respectively.

DISCUSSION

The three-dimensional impedance method has been found to be a very versatile and numerically efficient method capable of allowing detailed modeling of the tissue heterogeneities. As seen in equation 2, it is possible to include both the time- and space-varying magnetic fields in this formulation. Even though we have used the sinusoidally varying RF magnetic fields for the SAR calculations given in this discussion, it should also be possible to use the impedance method for calculation of induced current densities and electric fields due to spatially varying, rapidly switched magnetic fields used for MRI. For time-varying magnetic fields, it should be possible to write the various frequency components and solve the problem for the currents

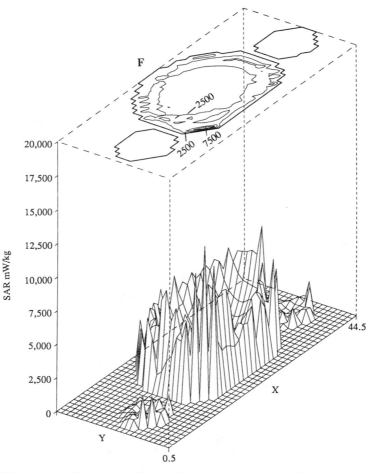

FIGURE 6c. Same as the caption to FIGURE 6a, except that f = 192 MHz and the separation between contour lines = 2500 mW/kg.

induced at the different frequencies, which may then be combined to obtain the time-domain variations of the induced current densities and electric fields at various points of the body. Because the frequencies involved with switched magnetic fields are on the order of a few kHz, it would be necessary to include anisotropy in the conductivity of the skeletal muscle for the formulation of the impedance model. It has been reported that the conductivity of the skeletal muscle is different in different directions, being a factor of 12–15 times higher along muscle fibers than in the transverse directions.[11,12] As seen from equation 1, this anisotropy of the tissue properties is not difficult to include in formulating the impedance method and would result in different impedance values for a given cell in different directions.

As seen from the results shown in FIGURES 3 and 5, there are negligible induced currents (and hence SARs) for parts of the body that are removed a few cell widths from the exposed volumes. It has therefore been possible to use truncated models even though a detailed model of the whole body was indeed available for the calculations. Because of the reduced volumes that need to be modeled, it should be possible to employ smaller cell sizes than the 1.31-cm cubical cells that have been used to date. Utilizing the super-minicomputer Hewlett Packard Model 9000 (32 Mbytes of RAM), we have been able to use impedance models with up to 600,000 cells for run times of few tens of minutes. Using somewhat larger memory workstations (such as APOLLO RGB/DN 10,000; 64 Mbytes of RAM), we expect to be able to go up to 2 million cells, which should allow us cell sizes on the order of a few millimeters. With such resolutions and by recognizing that the cell sizes could be different in different directions (equation 1), it should be possible in the future to locate the nodes of the impedance networks at the interfaces between the various tissues so that the relative lack of conduction through low-conductivity tissues such as fat, bone, etc., may be modeled properly.

REFERENCES

1. BOTTOMLEY, P. A., R. W. REDINGTON, W. A. EDELSTEIN & J. F. SCHENCK. 1985. Estimating radiofrequency power deposition in body NMR imaging. Magn. Reson. Med. 2: 336–349.
2. BUCHLI, R., M. SANER, D. MEIER, E. B. BOSKAMP & P. BOESIGER. 1989. Increased rf power absorption in MR imaging due to rf coupling between body coil and surface coil. Magn. Reson. Med. 9: 105–112.
3. SULLIVAN, D. M., O. P. GANDHI & A. TAFLOVE. 1988. Use of the finite-difference time-domain method in calculating EM absorption in man models. IEEE Trans. Biomed. Eng. 35: 179–186.
4. GANDHI, O. P. & J. F. DEFORD. 1988. Calculation of EM power deposition for operator exposure to RF induction heaters. IEEE Trans. Electromagn. Compat. 30: 63–68.
5. ORCUTT, N. & O. P. GANDHI. 1988. A 3-D impedance method to calculate power deposition in biological bodies subjected to time-varying magnetic fields. IEEE Trans. Biomed. Eng. 35: 577–583.
6. GRANDOLFO, M., P. VECCHIA & O. P. GANDHI. 1990. Magnetic resonance imaging: calculation of rates of energy absorption by a human torso model. Bioelectromagnetics 11: 117–128.
7. DURNEY, C. H., D. A. CHRISTENSEN & P. MCARTHUR. 1990. An equivalent circuit for Maxwell's equations. Paper presented at the Twelfth Annual Meeting of the Bioelectromagnetics Society, San Antonio, Texas (June 14–18).
8. EYCLESHYMER, A. C. & D. M. SCHOEMAKER. 1970. A Cross-Section Anatomy. Appleton–Century–Crofts. New York.
9. JOHNSON, C. C. & A. W. GUY. 1972. Nonionizing electromagnetic wave effects in biological materials and systems. Proc. IEEE 60: 692–718.
10. STUCHLY, M. A. & S. S. STUCHLY. 1980. Dielectric properties of biological substances—tabulated. J. Microwave Power 15: 19–26.
11. EPSTEIN, B. R. & K. R. FOSTER. 1983. Anisotropy in dielectric properties of skeletal muscle. Med. Biol. Eng. Comput. 21: 51–55.
12. ZHENG, E., S. SHAO & J. G. WEBSTER. 1984. Impedance of skeletal muscle from 1 kHz to 1 MHz. IEEE Trans. Biomed. Eng. BME-31: 477–481.

Homogeneous Tissue Model Estimates of RF Power Deposition in Human NMR Studies

Local Elevations Predicted in Surface Coil Decoupling

PAUL A. BOTTOMLEY AND PETER B. ROEMER

General Electric Corporate Research and Development Center
Schenectady, New York 12301

INTRODUCTION

The earliest investigation of the radio-frequency (RF) power deposited in tissue during a whole-body proton (^{1}H) NMR imaging experiment[1] preceded by years the capability of performing such studies at NMR frequencies, ν, above a few MHz,[2-4] where power deposition problems become more acute. This fact bears witness to the serious concerns about the safety of the technology for human applications extant from the outset. The mechanism for RF power deposition in tissue in an NMR experiment is the induction of eddy currents and joule heating by the RF magnetic field, with the tissue having nonzero electrical conductivity at these frequencies.

The aforementioned investigation[1] derived analytic solutions for the spatial distribution of the RF field and power deposited in a semi-infinite plane of homogeneous tissue and in an infinitely long cylinder of homogeneous tissue, both immersed in uniform RF fields. The power deposition, or specific absorption rate (SAR), was computed in cylinders comprising a variety of normal and tumor tissues whose electrical properties were measured over the NMR frequency range of 1–100 MHz. Because the models predicted that the greatest power deposition occurred near the surface,[1] curves relating the surface SAR in torso- and head-sized muscle and brain cylinders to NMR frequency, NMR pulse-width, and pulse sequence duty-cycle were later deduced[5] to assist in interpreting guidelines for RF exposure issued by government regulatory agencies[6-8] in the context of operating parameters commonly used in actual NMR imaging studies.

The two main quantities of concern when considering the risks of RF heating in tissue are the total RF power absorbed by the body per unit body mass, which measures the total heat load with which the body must cope, and the local peak levels of power deposited in tissue, which, if excessive, could cause local tissue damage. United States regulatory guidelines for the local peak SAR in any gram of tissue and the SAR averaged over the whole body, as well as alternate guidelines based on temperature changes measured *in vivo*, are summarized in TABLE 1.[7,8]

To test experimentally the predictions of the simple homogeneous tissue models, the average power and the maximum power deposited in homogeneous tissue spheres, truncated tissue cylinders, and tissue cylinders with transverse RF fields, all immersed in uniform NMR excitation fields, were then estimated and compared with measurements of the total power deposited in nine adults during a 63-MHz NMR

144

imaging exam.[9] Happily, reasonable agreement between experiment and theory was found for the average values in some of the cylindrical model geometries. However, the theoretical estimates for the maximum SAR at the surface significantly overestimated the experimental values derived by measuring the incremental power increase with increasing torso size in the subjects studied. The latter observation was linked to the presence of a peripheral adipose layer of variable thickness and low conductivity, which does not substantially increase surface power deposition with increasing torso radius.[9]

Now, NMR imaging and *in vivo* spectroscopy experiments are being performed in the presence of an RF irradiation that is applied in addition to the usual imaging and spectroscopy excitation sequences—and usually at the ^{1}H NMR frequency—for extended, if not continuous, periods during the course of an NMR exam.[10–13] This

TABLE 1. Regulatory Guidelines for RF Power Deposition in Clinical Studies

Reference	Quantity	Limit[a]
6 (UK)	body temperature increase	1 °C
	local temperature increase	
	in any 1 g of tissue	1 °C
	or	
	body average SAR	0.4 watts/kg
	peak SAR in any 1 g of tissue	4 watts/kg
7 (USA)	body average SAR	0.4 watts/kg
	or	
	core body temperature increase	1 °C
	local temperature	no explicit limits
8 (USA)	body average SAR	0.4 watts/kg
	peak SAR in any 1 g of tissue	8 watts/kg
	head average SAR	3.2 watts/kg
	or	
	core body temperature increase	1 °C
	local temperature, head	38 °C
	local temperature, trunk	39 °C
	local temperature, extremities	40 °C

[a]This refers to the limit below which heating is of no concern.

additional irradiation can advantageously alter the contrast in ^{1}H NMR images.[10] It can improve the signal-to-noise ratio and resolution in NMR spectroscopy[11–13] by collapsing multiplet resonances, providing nuclear Overhauser enhancement, and generally sharpening resonance lines, as exemplified in FIGURE 1.[13] The additional, decoupling RF magnetic field irradiation is typically applied at power levels of several watts with small NMR surface coils rather than volume coils in order to provide maximum enhancement per unit current input and to minimize the total RF power deposition. However, the field produced by a surface transmitter coil is very nonuniform over a volume comparable to the coil size. Thus, models that assume a homogeneous applied RF field are inappropriate. In fact, the RF power is almost entirely deposited in the tissue adjacent to the surface coil, so there is potential for significant, if not hazardous, local RF heating.[13]

Here, we review the predictions of the homogeneous tissue models in which the RF magnetic field is applied both with NMR coils that produce substantially uniform RF fields across the coil volumes (when the sample is absent) and by surface decoupling NMR coils that generate nonuniform RF fields. The spatial distribution of the power deposited in surface coil decoupling experiments depends on coil geometry, but only circular-shaped[12] and figure-eight-shaped[13] configurations have thus far been deployed. Calculations of the spatial distribution of the SAR in a semi-infinite plane of homogeneous tissue produced during decoupling with these

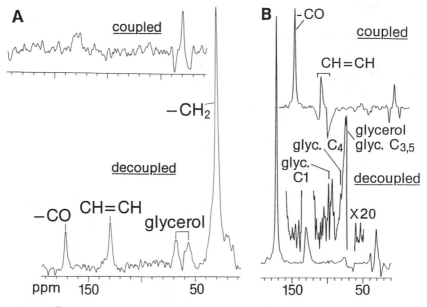

FIGURE 1. [13]C surface coil spectra obtained in 1 s from the human leg with (bottom) and without (top) ^{1}H irradiation at 63 MHz with an input of $W = 3$ watts provided by an 8×13–cm figure-eight-shaped coil (A). The sequence repetition period, T, was 0.5 s and the spectrometer gain was kept constant.[13] Panel B shows cardiac-gated ^{13}C DRESS spectra from 2-cm-thick slices in the heart with (bottom) and without (top) ^{1}H decoupling at $W = 3$ watts from the same coil. Enhancements of up to fivefold in the leg and heart muscle ^{13}C spectra produced by the ^{1}H decoupling irradiation are evident.

surface coils are presented and compared with United States guidelines.[7,8] The theoretical analyses assume that the power deposited from electric fields emanating directly from the coils is rendered negligible relative to that induced by the coil's magnetic fields, for example, by interposing a Faraday screen between the coil and the tissue or by using NMR coils with distributed tuning capacitance.[14]

TISSUE CYLINDERS AND SPHERES IN UNIFORM RF FIELDS

The eddy current loops induced in a tissue sphere and cylinder immersed in a uniform axial RF magnetic field, $B_1 \sin(2\pi vt)$, and in a tissue cylinder with transversely oriented field are sketched in FIGURE 2.[9] An important consequence is that the eddy currents themselves generate an RF magnetic field that opposes and partially cancels the applied field within the sample, thereby rendering the field nonuniform, reducing the flux linking each loop, and reducing the power deposition relative to what would occur if the field were kept uniform within the sample as well as outside of it.[1] Nevertheless, the calculation assuming that the field is uniform inside the sample is simple and instructive and will be used later to gauge the importance of the cancellation effect by comparison with results obtained without the assumption. We include it presently.

Uniform RF Field inside the Sample

The induced electric fields, E, in the loops of radius r in FIGURES 2A and 2B with B_1 fields axial (superscript a) and linearly polarized are given by Faraday's law to be $|E| = \pi r \nu B_1 \cos(2\pi\nu t)$. The value of B_1 in the NMR experiment is fixed by the flip-angle θ, the pulse duration τ, and the nuclear gyromagnetic ratio γ at $B_1 = 2\theta/\gamma\tau$ for square excitation pulses.[5] The SAR is

$$P = |E|^2/2\rho s, \qquad (1)$$

where ρ is the tissue conductivity and s is its specific gravity. Therefore, for ^{1}H NMR with an RF pulse repetition period of T,

$$P_{c,s}^a(r) = 4C(r\nu\theta)^2/(\pi^2\rho\tau Ts) \qquad (2)$$

for both cylinder and sphere (subscripts c and s) in mks units, where $C = 6.81 \times 10^{-19}$. Thus, the SAR varies quadratically with NMR frequency and radius, with maximum values of $P(R)$ at the surface ($r = R$) and with values decreasing rapidly to zero at the sample center. The average SAR is obtained by integrating equation 2 over the respective volumes:[9]

$$\overline{P}_c^a = P_{c,s}^a(R)/2 \quad \text{and} \quad \overline{P}_s^a = 2P_{c,s}^a(R)/5. \qquad (3)$$

When the RF field is transverse (superscript t) to the cylinder (FIGURE 2C), the induced electric field components perpendicular to the axis cancel if the cylinder is infinite in extent, yielding

$$P_c^t(r, \phi) = 4P_{c,s}^a(r) \cos^2\phi, \qquad (4)$$

with a higher average at $\overline{P}_c^t = P_{c,s}^a(R)$ and a much higher maximum SAR value at $4P_{c,s}^a(R)$ than occur in the axial B_1 cylindrical and spherical configurations.

However, the perpendicular components do not cancel for truncated cylinders. If the length of cylinder exposed to the transverse field is $\sim 2R$, peak power again reduces to about $P_{c,s}^a(R)$ because the eddy current loops are no longer infinite in extent. The average value for the truncated cylinder with transverse field will then be around $P_{c,s}^a(R)/2$, as in the axial field case.

Nonuniform RF Field within the Sample

The exact solutions (superscript e) for the power deposition in infinitely long homogeneous tissue cylinders with the boundary condition that the field be uniform

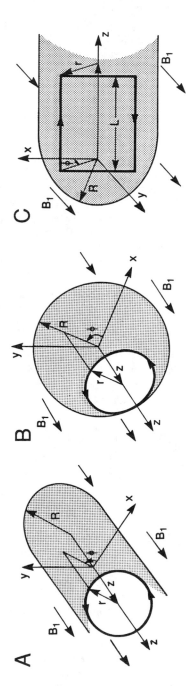

FIGURE 2. Geometry and coordinate systems for cylindrical (A, C) and spherical (B) homogeneous tissue models.[9] The RF magnetic field, $B_1 \sin 2\pi\nu t$, is along the cylindrical axis in part A and is transverse to it in part C. Induced eddy current loops are drawn bold in each model.

outside the sample are deduced by solving the cylindrical wave equation for the RF fields in the tissue[1,9,15] and by then invoking equation 1. For the infinite cylinder models, the transverse and axial solutions are mutually related in the same way as equations 2 and 4:[9]

$$P_c^{a,e}(r) = 4P_{c,s}^{a}(r)|I_1(Kr)|^2|KrI_0(KR)|^{-2}, \qquad (5)$$

$$P_c^{t,e}(r, \phi) = 4P_c^{a,e}(r)\cos^2\phi. \qquad (6)$$

Here,

$$K = \omega\{\tfrac{1}{2}\epsilon\mu([1 + (\rho\epsilon\omega)^{-2}]^{1/2} - 1)\}^{1/2} + j\omega\{\tfrac{1}{2}\epsilon\mu([1 + (\rho\epsilon\omega)^{-2}]^{1/2} + 1)\}^{1/2} \qquad (7)$$

is the complex ($j = \sqrt{-1}$) wave number, $\omega = 2\pi\nu$, ρ and ϵ are the tissue resistivity and permittivity, μ is the permeability (assumed to be that of free space), and I_n are modified n-th order Bessel functions of the first kind. The first term in the series expansion of the quotient of quadratic terms in equation 5 is 0.25, so equations 2 and 4 are identical to the first-order expansion of equations 5 and 6. FIGURE 3 plots equation 5 for head- and torso-sized cylinders; the curves for the transverse model are obtained by scaling FIGURE 3 by $4\cos^2\phi$.

Comparison with Experiment

We now compare the theoretical estimates for the surface and average SAR with values derived experimentally. The power applied to an $L = 0.5$ m whole-body NMR coil during 0.7-ms $\theta = \pi$ NMR pulses in a 63-MHz body NMR imaging experiment with T = 0.2 s using a GE 1.5-T imaging/spectroscopy system was measured with an RF wattmeter on nine normal adult volunteers weighing $M = 65$–102 kg. The proportion of this power that is deposited in the body depends on how much power is lost in the cable connecting the meter to the NMR coil and on how much is lost in the coil itself. The latter can be determined by measuring how much the body loads the coil. The total time-averaged power, W, deposited in the body by the pulses is given by

$$W = \left(\frac{\tau}{T}\right) W_i\left[1 - \frac{Q(\text{loaded})}{Q(\text{empty})}\right], \qquad (8)$$

where W_i is the power input to the coil during the pulses with the loss in the cable connecting the meter to the coil subtracted and where Q(loaded) and Q(empty) are the coil quantity factors measured with and without the coil on the subject.[9,15]

The total body-averaged SAR as defined by the regulatory agencies (superscript R) is just $\overline{P}^R = W/M$. However, because all of the body is not exposed to the RF field, we define $\overline{P} = W/m$ for a fairer comparison with the theoretical estimates, where m is the mass of the 0.5-m section of the body assumedly exposed to the RF.

The SAR at the surface can be estimated by observing how W varies with the radius of the subject:[9]

$$P(R) = \delta R \cdot \partial W/\partial R = (10^{-3}/2\pi RLs)\partial W/\partial R, \qquad (9)$$

where δR is the increase in radius resulting in a 1-g increase in torso mass. This calculation should be interpreted cautiously because it assumes that incrementing δR does not result in any nonlinear redistribution of the SAR elsewhere within the torso. FIGURE 4 plots the relationship between W and R for the nine subjects with the B_1 field directed horizontally and transversely from left to right across the subject,

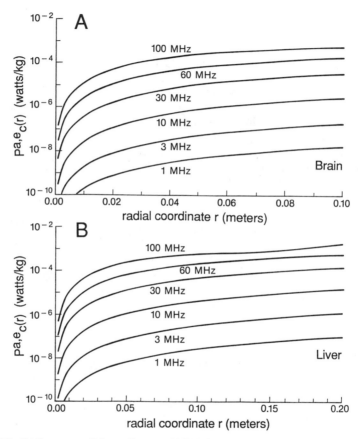

FIGURE 3. SAR versus radial coordinate and NMR frequency in a 10-cm-radius homogeneous brain tissue cylinder (A) and in a 20-cm-radius liver cylinder (B), with $\tau T = 10^{-1}$ s^2 and $\theta = \pi$. Curves were computed from equations 5 and 7 with published brain and liver resistivity and permittivity dispersions.[1,9] The curves are valid for the transverse model if scaled by a factor of $4\cos^2\phi$, as per equation 6 with ϕ being the polar angle.

yielding $\partial W/\partial R = 127 \pm 25$ watts/meter.[9] With the field directed in the orthogonal transverse direction (anterior/posterior), power deposition increased 1.5- to 2-fold, indicating a significant effect of the body's asymmetry on power deposition.

TABLE 2 compares the experimental and theoretical estimates. As expected, the discounting of the effect of the eddy currents in reducing the field inside the body in the uniform field approximations results in significant overestimation of the SAR

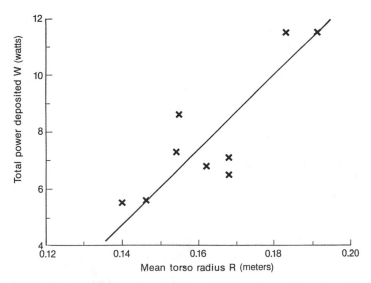

FIGURE 4. Total power W deposited in the body at 63 MHz with $\tau = 0.7$ ms, T $= 0.2$ s, and $\theta = \pi$, with a 50-cm-long NMR coil, as a function of the average torso radius (circumference/2π) for nine adult male volunteers.[9] The line is a least-squares fit giving $\partial W/\partial R = 127 \pm 25$ watts/meter, which is used in equation 9 to estimate surface power deposition.

levels compared with the exact and measured values. The exact cylindrical model estimates of the average SAR agree reasonably well with experiment, but most models overestimate the SAR, especially at the surface. Torso images show that a large fraction of the surface tissue of the torso is typically made up of adipose, whose

TABLE 2. Comparison of Theoretical and Experimental Estimates of the SAR

Method	Average SAR $\underline{P}$ (watts/kg)	Surface SAR $P(R)$ (watts/kg)
Measured		
total body,[a] field horizontal	0.096 ± 0.012	
field horizontal[b]	0.19 ± 0.03	0.25 ± 0.06
field vertical[b]	0.33 ± 0.05	0.4 ± 0.1
Cylindrical model, axial field		
field uniform within, $R = 16$ cm	0.66	1.3
exact solution, $R = 16$ cm	0.26^c	0.52
exact solution, $R = 20$ cm	0.24^c	0.48
Cylindrical model, transverse field		
field uniform within, $R = 16$ cm	1.3	5.3
truncated, uniform field	0.66^c	1.3
exact solution, infinite cylinder	0.48^c	1.9
Spherical model		
field uniform within	0.52	1.3

[a]W/M, as defined by regulatory guidelines.
[b]W/m, where m is the approximate torso mass lying in the coil. Surface SAR values are from equation 9.
[c]Calculated from surface values assuming equations 2–4.

resistivity is about 10-fold that of muscle or liver.[1] Therefore, from equation 1, the SAR in adipose is expected to be some 10-fold lower than in muscle or liver. The experimental estimates of the surface SAR should thus be lower than the model estimates by an amount proportional to the fraction of adipose tissue in the increment δR, which goes some way in explaining the difference between the experimental and theoretical surface SAR estimates. This implies that peak power deposition in humans occurs at levels deeper than the surface adipose, for example, in underlying muscle or liver.

Note also that the surface SAR in the exact models does not increase much from R equal to 0.16 to 0.2 meters (TABLE 2). This is attributable to the fact that the increase in flux resulting from the increased area of the eddy current loops in the larger cylinder is partially offset by greater attenuation or phase-cancellation of the RF field at its center, which is another mitigating factor affecting the comparison of surface SAR estimates.

Power Deposited by Nonsquare RF Pulses

Many RF pulses used for NMR imaging are not square, but are amplitude-modulated to excite a tailored NMR frequency response. The Gaussian-modulated and sinc $(\sin[t]/t)$–modulated pulses used for selective excitation are common examples. The different rms power contents of such pulses relative to the square pulse can be accommodated by adjusting the value of τ in equation 2 and its dependents. By integrating a Gaussian function of full-width–half-maximum τ_g and a sinc function whose central lobe width is τ_z and by comparing them to a square function, we can obtain[9]

$$P(\text{Gaussian pulse}) = 0.669P(\tau_g) \quad \text{and} \quad P(\text{sinc pulse}) = 2P(\tau_z), \qquad (10)$$

where τ_g and τ_z replace τ in equation 2 for P.

SURFACE COIL DECOUPLING IN SEMI-INFINITE TISSUE PLANES

Unlike the RF pulses used in NMR sequences, the RF power levels in decoupling experiments are traditionally measured, monitored, and applied directly in watts, continuous, rather than via flip-angle, B_1, or NMR timing parameter adjustment. This simplifies our present purpose. Again, it is very important for the proper estimation of tissue losses to exclude all of the other power losses that occur between the wattmeter measurement and the tissue. Even for an efficient surface coil, these losses will typically account for nearly half of the power output from the decoupler amplifier and, if the RF is applied continuously for extended periods, the fraction deposited in the coil may be sufficient to cause thermal damage to the coil.[13] From equation 8, $W = W_i[1 - Q(\text{loaded})/Q(\text{empty})]$ watts of the time-averaged input W_i to the coil is deposited in the tissue, whereas $(W_i - W)$ watts heats up the coil.

The average power deposited in an M-kg subject from a W-watt decoupling field is just $\overline{P}^R = W/M$ watts/kg. This works out to 14 milliwatts/kg for a 70-kg subject and a 1-watt input. Thus, the 0.4 watts/kg FDA guideline limit for average SAR (TABLE

1) would be of no concern for decoupler levels of up to $W = 29$ watts, a figure above most present decoupling needs. However, the peak power deposited locally by the coil is of concern.

To determine the spatial distribution of the power deposited in tissue, $P(r)$, we again assume that the coil design minimizes direct electric field losses from the coil to the sample. In this case, because the applied RF field is no longer uniform and because it depends on coil geometry, we calculate the SAR numerically from the vector potential $\mathbf{A}$ and Faraday's law, assuming that the sample appears to the surface coil as a semi-infinite plane of tissue of uniform conductivity and dielectric constant. Because decoupling surface coils are much smaller than body coils, we shall also assume that the sample does not significantly perturb the field.[13] The induced electric field at a location $\mathbf{r}$ in the sample is

$$\mathbf{E}(\mathbf{r}) = \frac{d\mathbf{A}}{dt} = \frac{\omega\mu}{4\pi} \int \frac{\mathbf{I} \cdot dl}{|\mathbf{r} - \mathbf{r}'|}, \tag{11}$$

where the line integral is evaluated around the length l of the coil carrying current $\mathbf{I}$ and $|\mathbf{r} - \mathbf{r}'|$ is the vector distance between a point $\mathbf{r}'$ on the coil and the point in the sample $\mathbf{r}$. $P(\mathbf{r})$ is then obtained upon substitution of equation 11 in equation 1.

The total power input to the tissue is related to $P(\mathbf{r})$ via

$$W = \int P(\mathbf{r})d\mathbf{V} = \int \frac{|\mathbf{E}(\mathbf{r})|^2}{2\rho s} d\mathbf{V} \tag{12}$$

integrated over the entire sample volume or, in practice, numerically over 4 m³ of the sample. Computation of

$$q = P(\mathbf{r})/\int P(\mathbf{r})d\mathbf{V} \quad [\text{kg}^{-1}] \tag{13}$$

then relates $P(\mathbf{r})$ to W via

$$P(\mathbf{r}) = qW \quad [\text{watts/kg}], \tag{14}$$

which, incidentally, is independent of ρ (the assumption that the sample does not perturb the field notwithstanding).

Coil Geometry

Local power deposition depends on the coil geometry via equation 11. $P(\mathbf{r})$ was computed numerically for two geometries: a 6.5-cm circular surface coil and an 8 × 13–cm figure-eight-shaped surface coil.[13] These coils are comparable in that they have optimum sensitivities at about the same depth of ~ 7 cm (i.e., the ratio $B_1/\sqrt{Z}$, where Z is the total sample noise resistance and B_1 is the field produced for a given coil current, is maximum at about 7 cm for each coil[16]). This coil size is a reasonable choice for human studies.[4,13] FIGURE 5 shows an NMR surface coil probe built with a figure-eight decoupler coil and a 6.5-cm spiral detection coil. The advantage of the figure-eight coil is that it is inherently electrically orthogonal to the circular coil.[13] Mutual interactions between the coils during decoupling and simultaneous detection are therefore minimized.[13]

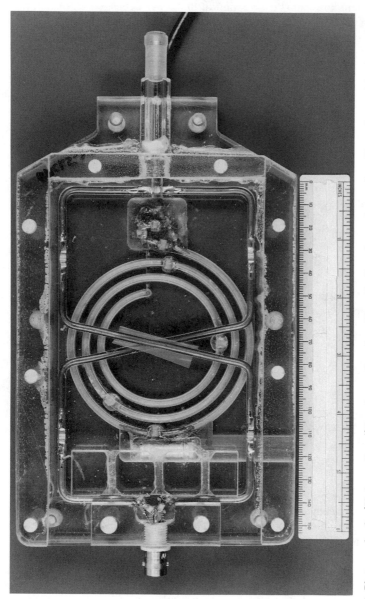

FIGURE 5. Photograph of a ¹H decoupling, ¹³C surface coil probe with a distributed capacitance, 8 × 13-cm figure-eight decoupling coil on top, accessed via the connector at right.[13] The coil former is made of Plexiglas, which forms an air-cooling chamber around the figure-eight coil with air input at left. The circular three-turn spiral ¹³C coil has windings with diameters of 5, 6.5, and 8 cm. (Note that the measuring ruler has been intentionally placed upside down.)

Contour plots of the transverse magnetic fields responsible for NMR produced by these coils are shown in FIGURES 6 and 7. As expected, the field of the figure-eight coil is twice or more extensive along its long axis. Given that the deposited power is derived from the eddy currents generated by this more extensive field, it is unsurprising that the figure-eight coil results in 2.5-fold more power, W, deposited in the tissue for the same transverse (NMR) RF field strength as the circular coil.

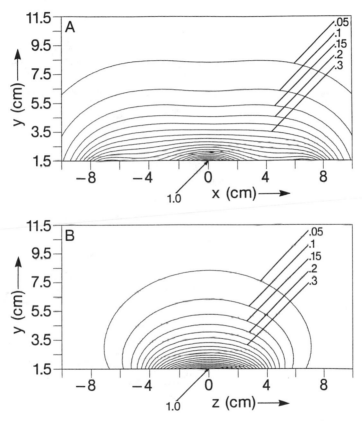

FIGURE 6. Computer contour plots of the magnitude of the transverse RF field produced by the 8 × 13–cm figure-eight decoupling surface coil (FIGURE 5) in the xy (A) and yz (B) planes. The coil is oriented with the zx plane with its long axis in the x direction. The contour interval is 0.05 units normalized to 1 at (0, 1.5, 0), where the top of the probe is located at $y = 1.5$ cm.

Spatial Distribution of the SAR

Contour plots of the SAR induced by all of the components of the RF magnetic field produced by the two surface coils in the xy and yz planes, as computed from equations 1 and 11, are shown in FIGURES 8 and 9. The coils are offset from the sample by 1.5 cm to allow space for a separate detection coil (e.g., as in FIGURE 5), foam padding, etc. The contour plots scale linearly with coil dimension.

For both coils, some 90% of the power is deposited within 2 cm of the surface, with maximum power deposition occurring closest to the wires. The q values relating numbers on the contours to the total power deposited (equations 13 and 14) are tabulated in TABLE 3. Peak values on the contours are therefore 11.9 watts/kg for $W = 1$ watt into the sample with the figure-eight coil and 4.7 watts/kg for the circular coil. However, because the power is so highly localized, the peak averaged over any 1 g of tissue as defined by the United States regulatory guidelines (TABLE 1) is reduced

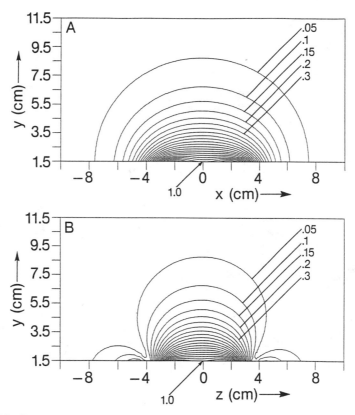

FIGURE 7. Computer contour plots of the transverse RF field produced by the circular 6.5-cm coil in the xy (A) and yz (B) planes. The contour interval is 0.05 units normalized to 1 at (0, 1.5, 0), where the top of the probe is located at $y = 1.5$ cm.

to about 60% of these values, or 7 watts/kg and 3 watts/kg for the two coils per watt W input, respectively. Thus, with average decoupling power levels of 1–10 watts continuous, United States regulatory guidelines for local power deposition (TABLE 1) can easily be exceeded.

Note that q, and therefore peak power deposition, decreases 30–50% if the sample is moved to 2.5 cm from that coil. However, W must now be increased a

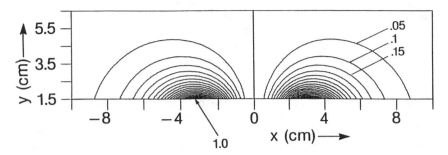

FIGURE 8. Contour plot of local RF power deposition in the *xy* plane of the circular surface coil. The contour interval is 0.05 units normalized to 1 at (0, 1.5, 0), where the top of the probe is at *y* = 1.5 cm, and uniform biological tissue fills the half-space *y* ≥ 1.5 cm. For *W* = 1 watt input to the tissue, peak power deposition is 4.7 watts/kg. The plot is cylindrically symmetric about the coil axis.

corresponding amount to maintain the same transverse RF field (as per FIGURES 6 and 7) and the corresponding decoupling/Overhauser enhancements.

DISCUSSION

We have investigated theoretically models describing the RF power deposited in tissue in NMR experiments assuming the body is a cylinder or sphere of homoge-

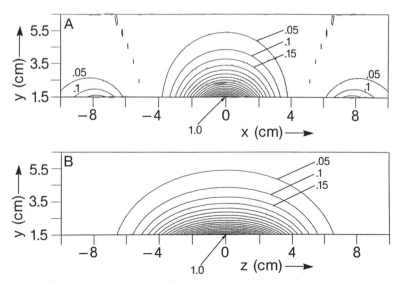

FIGURE 9. Local RF power deposition in the *xy* (A) and *yz* (B) planes produced by the figure-eight coil. The contour interval is 0.05 units normalized to 1 at (0, 1.5, 0), where the top of the probe is at *y* = 1.5 cm, and uniform biological tissue fills the half-space *y* ≥ 1.5 cm. For W_s = 1 watt input to the tissue, power deposition at (0, 1.5, 0) is 11.9 watts/kg.

neous tissue and have demonstrated that these models can yield reasonable estimates of the average RF power deposited in actual body NMR imaging experiments.[1,5,9] However, the models overestimate the surface power deposition in comparison to values obtained by measuring the incremental power required as the radii of the subjects increase. This is likely due to tissue heterogeneity. The difficulty in reliably predicting the local peak SAR levels in real heterogeneous bodies is the principal shortcoming of homogeneous tissue models. For many NMR experiments, even at 63 MHz, average SAR levels should not exceed United States regulatory guidelines and potential problems can be overcome by increasing τ or T.

With *in vivo* decoupling NMR experiments at average power levels of several watts or more, our calculations show that United States regulatory guidelines for the peak SAR can be exceeded and may pose a problem for human studies.[13] Again, however, the peak calculations may be mitigated in practice by tissue heterogeneity. Because the surface of 5–10 mm or more is usually adipose, whose conductivity is about a tenth of that of muscle, the coil separation is effectively increased by this distance for a fixed W. Also, the use of gated decoupling or various pulse decoupling sequences will reduce power deposition by the fraction of the pulse duty-cycle (increases in the field amplitude during the pulses notwithstanding). Even so, the

TABLE 3. q Values for Scaling Surface Coil Contour Plots of the SAR

Separation of Sample from Coil (cm)	q (1/kg)	
	Figure-eight-shaped Coil	Circular Coil
1.5	11.9	4.7
2.0	9.95	3.7
2.5	8.52	2.3

levels involved are sufficiently high to warrant careful monitoring of the power levels in each individual case. Our calculations also show that the body average power deposition in surface coil decoupling studies at power levels of several watts is well below the regulatory guidelines and should not be a problem.

Although no direct heating effects have been reported and peak power deposition is still below values typically used for shortwave diathermy, we emphasize the need for proceeding with considerable caution in regard to surface heating and potential local tissue damage, particularly in the head near the eyes and in the testes, when using surface coil decoupling at input power levels of the order of 1 watt or more. Also, because power deposition increases approximately as the square of the NMR frequency to produce the same NMR effect, excessive peak power deposition could preclude ^{1}H nuclear Overhauser enhancement and perhaps some forms of ^{1}H decoupling in humans at main magnetic field strengths of 4 tesla or more. For some ^{1}H applications, the sensitivity advantage of, for example, 4 tesla over lower fields might thus be negated.

ACKNOWLEDGMENTS

We are grateful for the important contributions and support from E. R. Andrew, W. A. Edelstein, R. W. Redington, and J. F. Schenck over the 15-year course of this work.

REFERENCES

1. BOTTOMLEY, P. A. & E. R. ANDREW. 1978. Phys. Med. Biol. **23:** 630–643.
2. HOLLAND, G. N., R. C. HAWKES & W. S. MOORE. 1980. J. Comput. Assist. Tomogr. **4:** 429–433.
3. EDELSTEIN, W. A., J. M. S. HUTCHISON, G. JOHNSON & T. REDPATH. 1980. Phys. Med. Biol. **25:** 751–756.
4. BOTTOMLEY, P. A., H. R. HART, W. A. EDELSTEIN, J. F. SCHENCK, L. S. SMITH, W. M. LEUE, O. M. MUELLER & R. W. REDINGTON. 1983. Lancet **ii:** 273–274.
5. BOTTOMLEY, P. A. & W. A. EDELSTEIN. 1981. Med. Phys. **8:** 510–512.
6. NRPB (National Radiological Protection Board ad hoc Advisory Group on Nuclear Magnetic Resonance Clinical Imaging). 1983. Br. J. Radiol. **56:** 974–977.
7. YOUNG, F. E. (United States Food and Drug Administration). 1988 (March 9). Fed. Regist. **53:** 7575–7579.
8. UNITED STATES FOOD AND DRUG ADMINISTRATION (FDA). 1988 (August 2). Guidance for Content and Review of a Magnetic Resonance Diagnostic Device 510(k) Application: Communication to Manufacturers. FDA. Rockville, Maryland.
9. BOTTOMLEY, P. A., R. W. REDINGTON, W. A. EDELSTEIN & J. F. SCHENCK. 1985. Magn. Reson. Med. **2:** 336–349.
10. WOLF, S. D. & R. S. BALABAN. 1989. Magn. Reson. Med. **10:** 135–144.
11. LUYTEN, P. R., G. BRUNTINK, F. M. SLOFF, J. W. A. H. VERMEULEN, J. I. VAN DER HEIJDEN, J. A. DEN HOLLANDER & A. HEERSCHAP. 1989. NMR Biomed. **1:** 177–183.
12. SHULMAN, G. I., D. L. RUTHMAN, T. JUE, P. STEIN, R. A. DE FRONZO & R. G. SHULMAN. 1990. N. Engl. J. Med. **322:** 223–228.
13. BOTTOMLEY, P. A., C. J. HARDY, P. B. ROEMER & O. M. MUELLER. 1989. Magn. Reson. Med. **12:** 348–363.
14. SCHENCK, J. F., H. R. HART, T. H. FOSTER, W. A. EDELSTEIN & M. A. HUSSAIN. 1986. *In* Magnetic Resonance Annual. H. Kressel, Ed.: 123–160. Raven Press. New York.
15. MANSFIELD, P. & P. G. MORRIS. 1982. NMR Imaging in Biomedicine, pp. 184–191 and 312–314. Academic Press. New York.
16. BOTTOMLEY, P. A., H. C. CHARLES, P. B. ROEMER, D. FLAMIG, H. ENGESETH, W. A. EDELSTEIN & O. M. MUELLER. 1988. Magn. Reson. Med. **7:** 319–336.

Increased Radio-Frequency Power Absorption in Human Tissue due to Coupling between Body Coil and Surface Coil

PETER BOESIGER, RETO BUCHLI, MARTIN SANER, AND
DIETER MEIER

Institute of Biomedical Engineering and Medical Informatics
University of Zurich
and
Swiss Federal Institute of Technology
CH-8044 Zurich, Switzerland

INTRODUCTION

In magnetic resonance imaging or spectroscopy with surface coils, the danger may arise that excessive tissue heating could occur if the surface coil, acting as a receiver-only coil, strongly couples to the transmitter coil during the transmitting phase. These heating effects are caused by the induction of a strong current in the receiver coil and the subsequently occurring superposition of the radio-frequency (rf) field of the receiver coil to the field of the transmitting coil in the tissue.[1]

In clinical magnetic resonance imaging examinations, extreme coupling usually is avoided by the geometrical arrangement of the two coils or by electronic decoupling circuits, which detune and short-circuit the receiver coil during the transmitting phase. In receiver coil circuits that are equipped with fixed or mechanical tuning capacitors, a short-circuiting may be achieved in a passive way by a pair of antiparallel clipping diodes that restrict the maximum voltage over the tuning capacity. Varicap-equipped receiver coils usually are protected by PIN or VARACTOR diodes, which are actively switched during the transmitter phase and which short-circuit the tuning capacitors.

However, in both cases, the decoupling circuits may fail. Thus, worst-case scenarios may occur, for example, if the following factors coincide:

(1) the surface coil is placed with its axis parallel to the (linearly polarized) transmitter rf field so that the rf magnetic flux through the surface coil and thus the induced voltage in the surface coil are maximum;

(2a) mechanical tuning and matching capacitors or fixed capacitors are used in the surface coil and the protecting clipping diodes fail;

or

(2b) the electronic rf decoupling circuit (PIN or VARACTOR diode circuit) of the varicap-equipped resonance circuit of the surface coil breaks down;

(3) the failure occurs after the rf power optimization has been performed and the transmitting body coil as well as the receiving surface coil still remain tuned after the decoupling breakdown.

To analyze the problem, a disk-shaped phantom filled with saline solution with an electrical conductivity similar to that of human tissue ($\sigma = 1.5$ S/m) was built (FIGURE 1). The circular surface coil is placed concentrically on the face of the phantom in such a way that the coil center and the phantom center coincide. For easy

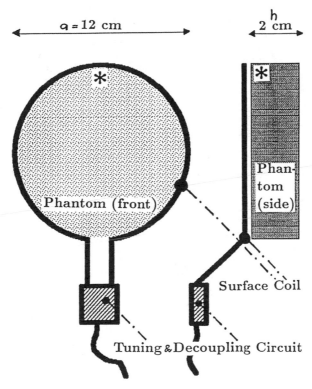

FIGURE 1. Disk-shaped phantom and receiver-only surface coil in front view (left) and from the side (right). The circular surface coil is placed concentrically on the face of the phantom. An asterisk (*) indicates the area at which the total rf field amplitude B_{tot} and the temperature rise ΔT were determined.

calculations, the radius of the coil has been chosen to be equal to that of the phantom. Because it is well known that the field strength of the surface coil and therefore the temperature rises near the wires and thus at the rim of the phantom are highest,[2,3] a sponge was immersed into the phantom. Hence, fluid motions inside the phantom, which might smear out any occurring local temperature rises and temperature gradients, are avoided.

THEORETICAL CONSIDERATIONS

The local temperature rise ΔT of the saline solution, which is produced by the local power loss P of the radio-frequency field per volume element V, is calculated to be

$$\Delta T = \frac{Dt}{C} \frac{P}{V}, \tag{1}$$

where

D = duty cycle of the pulse sequence,

t = total MRI examination time,

C = specific heat capacity of the phantom.

The specific local power loss of the electric field in the saline solution is

$$\frac{P}{V} = (\tfrac{1}{2})\sigma E^2,$$

where E stands for the electric rf field amplitude and σ stands for the conductivity of the saline solution. Assuming a harmonically oscillating magnetic rf field, E may be calculated by the solution of the Faraday equation, $\mathbf{E} = -d\mathbf{B}/dt$, where $\mathbf{B}$ denotes the magnetic rf field. Applying Stokes theorem through integration over a concentrical circular plane of radius r within the disk-shaped phantom, we obtain E = $-(d\mathrm{B}/dt)r/2$, with E and B being the amplitudes of $\mathbf{E}$ and $\mathbf{B}$, respectively. The time derivative of the harmonically time-dependent sinusoidal rf field is $d\mathrm{B}/dt = i\omega\mathrm{B}$, where ω stands for the resonance frequency of the protons at 1.5 teslas in our case. Thus, the electric field becomes E = $-i\omega\mathrm{B}r/2$ and, finally, the local time average rf power deposition per unit volume is given by

$$\frac{P}{V} = (\tfrac{1}{8})\sigma\omega^2 \mathrm{B}^2 s r^2, \tag{2}$$

where s is a correction factor, introduced because the rf shows a limited penetration depth into the interior of the phantom and into the human tissue.

The amplitude of the total rf magnetic field $\mathbf{B}$ in the worst-case scenario is given as B = $|\mathbf{B}_1 + \mathbf{B}_2|$, with $\mathbf{B}_1$ as the field of the transmitting body coil and $\mathbf{B}_2$ as the field that occurs due to the current I_2 induced in the surface coil by the coupling of the two coils. B can be calculated to be

$$B = |\mathbf{B}_1 + \mathbf{B}_2| = |\mathbf{B}_1 + m\mathrm{I}_2|, \tag{3}$$

where I_2 denotes the current induced in the surface coil during the rf pulses and m denotes the magnetic field–per–current ratio. Putting equations 2 and 3 into equation 1, we obtain a temperature rise of

$$\Delta T = \left(\frac{Dt}{8C}\right)\sigma\omega^2 a^2 s |\mathbf{B}_1 + m\mathrm{I}_2|^2. \tag{4}$$

I_2 can be calculated by straightforward calculations applying the electrical equivalent circuits of the two coupled resonance circuits. However, because many parameters going into such calculations are difficult to obtain, another approach is taken: namely, because (in case of resonance) the rf voltage U_2, which is induced in the surface coil, and I_2 are in phase, the time average rf power P_2 delivered to the surface coil is $P_2 = U_2 I_2 / 2$. Therefore, the induced current is $I_2 = 2P_2 / U_2$. According to Faraday's law, the rf voltage induced in the circular surface coil of radius a is

$$U_2 = i\omega B_1 \pi a^2. \tag{5}$$

Nearly all the rf power P_2 delivered to the surface coil by its coupling to the transmitter coil is absorbed by the saline solution of the phantom. Thus, the total power loss P_2 can be calculated through integration of the local power loss (equation 2) over the whole volume of the phantom:

$$P_2 = \int_0^a \int_0^h \int_0^{2\pi} \left(\frac{P}{V}\right) dV = \int_0^a \left(\frac{P}{V}\right) 2\pi r h \, dr = \left(\frac{\pi}{16}\right) \sigma \omega^2 a^4 h s m^2 I_2^2, \tag{6}$$

where h stands for the thickness of the disk-shaped phantom and the symbol a stands for its radius, which is identical with the radius of the surface coil. The induced current I_2 is now calculated with equations 5 and 6 and with $I_2 = 2P_2 / U_2$, which leads to

$$I_2 = \frac{8iB_1}{\sigma \omega a^2 h s m}. \tag{7}$$

Because the B_2 field at resonance has a phase shift of 90° with respect to the B_1 field, we end up with the following local temperature rise near the wires of the surface coil:

$$\Delta T = \left(\frac{Dt}{C}\right) \left[(1/8)\sigma \omega^2 a^2 s B_1^2 + \left(\frac{8B_1^2}{\sigma \omega a^2 h^2 s m^2}\right) \right]. \tag{8}$$

The first part of equation 8 stands for the heating effect of the transmitting B_1 field of the body coil, whereas the second part describes the additional heating of the field B_2, which is caused by the induced current I_2 in the surface coil. The retrospective effect of the field B_2 on the body coil is neglected. Tedious calculations show that the omission of these reflections leads to minimal errors as long as the conductivity σ is of the order of that of human tissue.

RESULTS

Theoretical calculations and experiments on a commercial whole-body MRI scanner with 1.5-tesla field strength have been performed for a single-slice multispin echo sequence with a repetition time of $T_R = 500$ ms and with six echoes with echo times between 50 and 300 ms. Because eight measurements were performed, this leads to a total examination time of 15 minutes with a duty cycle of $D = 0.026$. The remaining parameters are summarized in TABLE 1. Similar results can be expected

TABLE 1. Parameters of the Experimental Setup

D	duty cycle of the pulse sequence	0.026
σ	electric conductivity of the phantom solution	1.5 S/m
ω	frequency of the oscillating magnetic field	$2\pi \times 64$ MHz
a	radius of the surface coil (one-turn coil)	6 cm
s	correction factor	0.7
B_1	transmitting radio-frequency field amplitude	11.7 μT
h	phantom height	2 cm
m	magnetic field–per–current ratio	28 μT/A
T_R	repetition time	500 ms
T_E	echo time (6 echoes)	50–300 ms
nav	number of averages (measurements)	8
t	total MRI examination time	15 min

from multislice spin echo examinations. The mean magnetic field–per–current ratio, m, is calculated according to references 4 and 5.

With these parameters, the local temperature rises were calculated for the two cases of a phantom without a surface coil and a phantom with a surface coil, which was equipped with mechanical tuning and matching capacitors. The results are summarized in TABLE 2. Due to the unpredictable behavior of the varicaps in the experiment with varicap tuned surface coils, no calculations were done for this setup.

Using a linearly polarizing transmitter coil, the B_1 field that is needed to produce a π-pulse within 2 ms is 11.7 μT. At a frequency of 64 MHz, the skin depth is 5.2 cm for the phantom solution with a conductivity of 1.5 S/m. The reduction of the rf power deposition due to the skin effect can be calculated by integration of an exponential function over the phantom thickness, from which a correction factor of s = 0.7 is derived for the phantom thickness of h = 2 cm. For the experimental setup applied here, m is 28 μT/A. The induced current I_2 is calculated according to equation 7 to be 4 A; the corresponding induced magnetic B_2 field is 112 μT.

Finally, the local temperature rises and the local specific power absorption rates (SAR) are calculated. The heat capacity C of the saline solution is almost equal to the heat capacity of water (4.2×10^6 W/°C · m³) and is slightly higher than that of tissue. The transmitting B_1 field produces a local temperature rise ΔT of 0.06 °C and a local SAR of 0.3 W/kg; the induced B_2 field leads to a local temperature rise ΔT of 5.2 °C and a local SAR of 24 W/kg.

The experiments were performed on a Philips Gyroscan S15 whole-body imager with 1.5-tesla field strength. The amplitude of the total magnetic rf field **B** was

TABLE 2. Calculated and Measured Values of the Total Magnetic rf Fields **B** and the Local Temperature Rises ΔT of the Phantom Solution for the Three Experiments

	Magnetic Field		Temperature Rise	
Type of Experiment	B_{calc}	B_{meas}	ΔT_{calc}	ΔT_{meas}
Without surface coil	12 μT	14 μT	0.06 °C	0.1 °C
Surface coil with mech. tun. cap.	112 μT	94 μT	5.20 °C	4.7 °C
Surface coil with varicaps	—	6 μT	—	0.1 °C

measured with a calibrated cylindrical one-turn search coil of 1.5-cm radius[6] located at the same position inside the surface coil where the temperature rises were determined. Measurements were done for all three cases; the results are summarized in TABLE 2. The measured magnetic fields were 14 μT for the case without surface coil, 6 μT with varicap tuned surface receiver circuits, and 94 μT for circuits equipped with mechanical tuning capacitors. Each measurement was repeated at least five times. Possible calibration and positioning errors of the measuring coil might amount to experimental errors of about 20%. Corresponding temperature rises of 0.1 ± 0.1 °C, 0.1 ± 0.1 °C, and 4.7 ± 0.6 °C, respectively, were measured.

CONCLUSIONS

The experimental results are in good agreement with those of the corresponding calculations. They indicate that an SAR = 0.3 W/kg is achieved without a surface coil. A considerable temperature rise due to coupling effects may be observed if mechanical or fixed tuning capacitors are used in the surface coil circuit. The corresponding SAR can locally exceed several watts/kg body weight, so dangerous temperature rises may occur.

By using varicap-equipped undecoupled surface coils in such a way that maximum coupling is achieved, the power absorption does not rise. Obviously, the varicaps used to tune and match the surface coil do not work accurately when the coupling effects become too strong and the voltage amplitude exceeds a certain limit. This breakthrough of the varicaps, which could be experimentally verified, leads to a detuning of the receiver circuit. Therefore, the current induced in the surface coil is substantially reduced.

REFERENCES

1. BUCHLI, R., M. SANER, E. B. BOSKAMP & P. BOESIGER. 1989. Magn. Reson. Med. **9**: 105.
2. GADIAN, D. G. & F. ROBINSON. 1979. J. Magn. Reson. **34**: 449.
3. GOTTSCHALK, S. C., R. C. GAUSS, G. X. KAMBIC, E. SOLEM & A. A. STEIN. 1986. Fifth Annu. Meet. Soc. Magn. Reson. Med. (Montreal, Canada).
4. DURAND, E. 1968. Magnetostatique. Masson. Paris.
5. HOFMANN, H. 1976. Das Elektromagnetische Feld. Springer-Verlag. Berlin/New York.
6. HUTCHISON, J. M. S. 1986. Eur. Econ. Community Eurospin **6**.

Effects of RF Power Absorption in Mammalian Cells[a]

STEPHEN F. CLEARY, LI-MING LIU, AND
GUANGHUI CAO

Department of Physiology and Biophysics
Medical College of Virginia
Richmond, Virginia 23298

INTRODUCTION

Optimization of the safety, fidelity, and efficacy of *in vivo* nuclear magnetic resonance imaging (NMRI) and nuclear magnetic resonance spectroscopy (NMRS) requires detailed knowledge of the interactions and effects of radio-frequency (RF) electromagnetic radiation and static and time-varying gradient magnetic fields. In contrast to recent concern about putative deleterious magnetic field effects, *in vivo* and *in vitro* studies of RF radiation effects conducted for over three decades have documented a number of effects of human exposure. This communication summarizes the effects of RF radiation on mammalian cells as they may pertain to NMRI and NMRS. In this context, it should be noted that few studies of cellular effects of RF fields, as employed in NMRI and NMRS, have been reported. Thus, whereas the RF bioeffects data base provides general insight regarding safety aspects, specific questions about RF field-induced cell physiologic perturbations induced by NMRI or NMRS fields remain unanswered. It has been suggested, for example, that exposure of mammalian cells to RF radiation simulating NMRS, but without the dc magnetic field component, may detectably affect cellular energy metabolism and proliferation.[1-3]

Recent results document RF-induced direct cell physiological alterations without the intervention of heating. Consequently, the safety and fidelity of NMRI and NMRS applications must involve consideration of direct as well as indirect thermal effects of RF absorption. Because effects of cell heating per se are relatively well understood, attention will focus on emerging information on the direct or nonthermal effects of RF radiation on mammalian cells. So far, mechanisms explaining direct RF cellular effects are lacking. It should be noted, though, that this situation is not unique to RF electromagnetic frequencies. There is increasing evidence that electric and/or magnetic fields at frequencies varying from static or extremely low frequency (ELF) to high frequency millimeter wavelength microwaves induce physiological alterations of unknown causation.[1] There is an obvious need for further insight regarding electromagnetic field effects on living systems for NMRI and NMRS safety assessments.

[a]This research was supported by Grant No. NIH 1 R01 OH 02148 from the National Institute for Occupational Safety and Health.

CELLULAR EFFECTS

Whereas a variety of cellular effects of RF exposure were reported, distinguishing direct effects from indirect thermal effects proved difficult because, in many instances, RF-induced heating was not controlled or adequately quantitated. Unambiguous evidence of direct RF cellular interactions was provided by studies of (a) cation binding and fluxes, (b) energy metabolism, and (c) proliferation.

Cation Fluxes and Binding

Studies of the effects of RF radiation on erythrocyte cation permeability identified the plasma membrane as an interaction site. Both passive and active membrane transport of potassium (K^+), its tracer analogue rubidium (Rb^+), and sodium (Na^+) were altered by exposure to 1-kHz,[4] 2450-MHz,[5] and 8.3-GHz[6] RF radiation, respectively. RF radiation affected cation transport only in specific temperature ranges (e.g., near 20 °C). This led to the conclusion that the effect involved RF interaction with a temperature-dependent membrane phase transition.[6] Cation permeability alterations that depended upon the composition of the cell suspension medium[6] also involved the shedding of erythrocyte membrane protein.[5] The inhibitory effect of RF radiation on erythrocyte active K^+ transport was attributed to a direct frequency and electric field strength–dependent interaction with membrane Na^+/K^+ ATPase.[7]

An effect of RF radiation in the NMR frequency range was reported in reference 8. Rabbit erythrocytes exposed in whole blood suspensions, for 2 h at 22.5 °C, were hemolyzed by 50- or 100-MHz continuous wave (CW) RF fields at field strengths of 400 V/m or greater. Hemolysis due to exposure to 10-MHz RF radiation required a field strength of at least 900 V/m. The apparent frequency dependence of erythrocyte hemolysis was further indicated by the lack of an effect following exposure to comparable intensities of 2.45- or 8.3-GHz RF radiation.[1] The specific mechanism(s) for RF radiation-induced hemolysis was not determined. The effect was attributed to an irreversible alteration of the membrane permeability of a sensitive cell subpopulation (e.g., aged cells) resulting in osmotic lysis.[8]

The relevance of such *in vitro* studies to NMRI and NMRS safety and fidelity is uncertain. These data provided evidence of direct RF intensity- and frequency-dependent cell physiological alterations, but the RF-enhanced membrane cation permeability was associated with a membrane phase change at temperatures near 20 °C, well below the normal body temperature of 37 °C. Because phase changes in the range of 10 to 40 °C were reported in erythrocyte and other cell membranes, the possibility of RF effects on membrane cation permeability *in vivo* could not be excluded. Effects of RF on membrane cation permeability *in vitro* that occurred near 20 °C generally involved specific absorption rates (SARs) somewhat in excess of 4 W/kg.

In addition to direct RF field effects on cell membrane cation fluxes, extremely low frequency (ELF)–modulated RF fields altered Ca^{+2} binding on chick brain and neuroblastoma plasmalemma surfaces. Altered binding, induced by low intensity (5–50 V/m) RF fields, was characterized by multiple biphasic modulation and intensity responses, referred to as modulation and intensity "windows", respectively.

Such responses deviate from classical dose or dose-rate responses characterized by well-defined unique thresholds.

Bawin et al.[9,10] reported modulation windows for Ca^{+2} efflux from chick brain exposed to 147-MHz radio-frequency (RF) electromagnetic radiation, amplitude-modulated (AM) at specific frequencies between 6 and 20 Hz. Blackman and co-workers[11,12] detected intensity (power-density) windows for this phenomenon and subsequently found similar responses using modulated 50-MHz RF radiation.[13] Sheppard et al.[14] also observed a Ca^{+2} efflux intensity window in response to modulated RF radiation. Dutta et al.[15,16] reported multiple intensity windows for Ca^{+2} efflux from neuroblastoma cells in culture exposed to 915- or 147-MHz RF radiation amplitude-modulated at 16 Hz. The dependence of this phenomenon on modulation frequency per se was documented by studies of the effects of ELF sinusoidal electric or magnetic fields.[17] As in the case of RF modulation, intensity and modulation windows were detected for enhanced Ca^{+2} efflux from chick brain tissue in vitro.[17] Also of potential significance with respect to NMRI or NMRS was the fact that the location of the Ca^{+2} efflux modulation windows depended upon the magnitude and orientation of the local static magnetic field.[18]

The physiological significance of the modulated RF-induced alteration in brain cell Ca^{+2} binding is not well understood. However, the central role of this cation in neuronal signaling and other cell processes indicates a potential involvement of this phenomenon in central or peripheral nervous system alterations in vivo. Evidence of behavioral alterations in monkeys exposed to ELF-modulated fields was reported,[19] as was RF-induced Ca^{+2} release from cat brain tissue in vivo.[20]

Cell Energy Metabolism

RF radiation effects on cell energy metabolism provided additional evidence of direct frequency-dependent alterations.[21] A 2-min exposure to 200- or 591-MHz RF radiation induced dose-dependent increases in nicotinamide adenine dinucleotide (NADH) fluorescence at SARs of less than 1 W/kg, whereas exposure to 2450 MHz was ineffective. Brain cell levels of adenosine triphosphate (ATP) decreased following exposure at 200 or 591 MHz, but not at 2450 MHz. The only RF frequency that affected brain cell creatine phosphate (CP) levels was 591 MHz. Rat brain energy metabolism was also altered by amplitude- and pulse-modulated 591-MHz RF radiation under nonthermal exposure conditions.[22] Altered cell energy metabolism, as reflected in ATP concentrations, has also been detected in erythrocytes exposed to 27-MHz CW RF radiation under isothermal conditions.[23] These results are of potential significance with respect to the fidelity of in vitro studies of tissue energy metabolism via NMRS. They suggest that RF radiation at frequencies and intensities used in this procedure may affect the assay end point, namely, cell energy metabolism.

Cell Proliferation

Cell proliferation, due to its role in growth, development, immune responses, and neoplasia, is of obvious physiological significance. Whereas direct effects of RF radiation on cell proliferation, such as with lymphocytes, were suggested by results of *in vivo* studies, the involvement of indirect effects of radiation-induced temperature elevations could not be ruled out.[24] However, *in vitro* studies, conducted under isothermal conditions at 37 °C, provided evidence of direct dose or dose-rate effects of RF radiation on cell proliferation.[2,3,24] *In vitro* cellular studies of the effects of ELF electric or magnetic fields, as well as clinical applications of ELF magnetic fields for tissue repair, provide additional evidence of direct effects of nonthermalizing electromagnetic fields on cell proliferation.[25,26] Taken as a whole, these results indicate an unexpected, and as yet unexplained, effect of electromagnetic fields over a wide frequency range on cell proliferation, a conclusion that is not inconsistent with respect to field effects on other physiological end points. Although mechanisms are unknown, the cell plasma membrane appears to be a likely interaction site.

Lymphocytes

Fresh whole human blood, obtained from healthy donors, was exposed or sham-exposed *in vitro* for 2 h to 27- or 2450-MHz CW RF radiation under isothermal conditions at normal body temperature (i.e., 37 ± 0.2 °C). After exposure, mononuclear cells were removed and cultured at 37 °C with or without stimulation by the mitogen phytohemagglutinin (PHA). Proliferation was assayed by pulse labeling with ^{3}H-thymidine (^{3}H-TdR) at 3 days after RF exposure. Exposure to either RF frequency at SARs of 50 W/kg or more resulted in statistically significant suppression of ^{3}H-TdR incorporation. Exposure in the range of 25 to 50 W/kg caused statistically significant increased ^{3}H-TdR incorporation in both PHA-activated and unactivated lymphocytes. The biphasic dose-dependent response, the isothermal exposure conditions, and the PHA-dependence led to the conclusion that RF radiation directly affects lymphocyte proliferation, independent of cell heating.[3] Dose-fractionation (i.e., two 1-h exposures 24 h apart) caused similar lymphocyte responses, indicating a possible cumulative RF exposure effect.[24]

The effects of RF pulse modulation on lymphocyte proliferation were investigated by exposure to 27-MHz RF radiation at 37 ± 0.2 °C. Modulation consisted of a 2-s RF pulse every 5.3 s (duty cycle, 0.38). Lymphocytes were activated with PHA (0.1 μg/μL). A 2-h exposure to 27-MHz CW radiation at an SAR of 25 W/kg resulted in a statistically significant 38% mean increase in ^{3}H-TdR uptake (ANOVA *p*-value, 0.0001). Pulse-modulated (PM) 27-MHz exposure, at the same time-averaged SAR (peak SAR, 66.3 W/kg), caused a similar (24%) statistically significant mean increase in ^{3}H-TdR incorporation (ANOVA *p*-value, 0.026). Evidence of dose-dependent differences in the effects of CW versus PM 27-MHz radiation was detected at an SAR of 50 W/kg. Whereas there was a statistically significant 25% decrease in uptake following CW exposure (ANOVA *p*-value, 0.0008), PM exposure (maximum SAR, 132.5 W/kg) induced a highly statistically significant 79% increase in ^{3}H-TdR incorporation (ANOVA *p*-value, 0.0001). Exposure to 27-MHz PM RF radiation at an SAR of 100 W/kg resulted in a statistically significant (ANOVA *p*-value, 0.008) 57% reduction in ^{3}H-TdR incorporation, which was consistent with the suppressive effect of 27-MHz CW radiation at SARs of 50 W/kg or higher. The results of these studies indicate that exposure to high SAR RF radiation, such as may

TABLE 1. ^{3}H-TdR Incorporation in PHA (0.1 μg/μL)–stimulated Human Peripheral Lymphocytes at 3 Days after a 2-h Isothermal (37 ± 0.2 °C) Exposure to CW or PM 2450-MHz RF Radiation at SARs of 5 W/kg (46 V/m) or 0.5 W/kg (14.5 V/m)

SAR (W/kg)		^{3}H-TdR Ratio	ANOVA
Average	Maximum	Exposed/Sham	p-Value
5 (CW)	5	0.95	0.22[a]
5 (PM)	14.9×10^3	0.81	0.0001
0.5 (CW)	0.5	0.90	0.43
0.5 (PM)	1.49×10^3	0.82	0.002

[a]The p-value for logarithmic transformed data = 0.05.

be encountered due to nonuniform or partial-body occupational exposure, may alter cell proliferation *in vivo*.

The results of *in vitro* studies of the effects of RF radiation on human lymphocytes in relation to NMRI or NMRS exposures are summarized in TABLES 1 and 2. These data, obtained under the same isothermal (37 ± 0.2 °C) exposure conditions used in experiments at higher SARs, but at SARs of 0.5 or 5 W/kg, indicate that, at these RF intensities, a 2-h exposure to either 27- or 2450-MHz CW or PM RF radiation affects cell proliferation.

A 2-h exposure of human lymphocytes to 2450-MHz CW or PM RF radiation at 0.5 or 5 W/kg resulted in a consistent 13% mean suppression of proliferation after 3 days of culture in the presence of 0.1 μg/μL PHA. As indicated in TABLE 1, the suppression was statistically significant (ANOVA p-value of untransformed or logarithmic transformed data, <0.05), except in the case of the 10% reduction that occurred following exposure to CW RF radiation at 0.5 W/kg.

Isothermal exposure of PHA-stimulated (0.1 μg/μL) human lymphocytes for 2 h to 27-MHz CW or PM RF radiation at a time-averaged SAR of 5 W/kg resulted in a 13% reduction in ^{3}H-TdR incorporation at 3 days after exposure, as indicated in TABLE 2. The effect of CW RF exposure was statistically significant (ANOVA p-value, 0.003). Whereas suppression of ^{3}H-TdR uptake following 27-MHz PM exposure was not statistically significant, the p-value for the two-tailed unbalanced randomized block ANOVA for logarithmic transformed data was marginally significant (p = 0.08). The 18% reduction in ^{3}H-TdR uptake following CW exposure at 0.5

TABLE 2. ^{3}H-TdR Incorporation in PHA (0.1 μg/μL)–stimulated Human Peripheral Lymphocytes at 3 Days after a 2-h Isothermal (37 ± 0.2 °C) Exposure to CW or PM 27-MHz RF Radiation at SARs of 5 W/kg (65.8 V/m) or 0.5 W/kg (20.8 V/m)

SAR (W/kg)		^{3}H-TdR Ratio	ANOVA
Average	Maximum	Exposed/Sham	p-Value
5 (CW)	5	0.87	0.0003
5 (PM)	13.3	0.87	0.189[a]
0.5 (CW)	0.5	0.82	0.05
0.5 (PM)	1.33	1.24	0.0002

[a]The p-value for logarithmic transformed data = 0.08.

W/kg was statistically significant ($p = 0.05$). Unexpectedly, exposure to PM 27-MHz RF at this same time-averaged SAR caused a statistically significant 24% increased uptake, in contrast to other data at SARs of 0.5 or 5 W/kg for either RF frequency. Whereas this may indicate a frequency- and modulation-dependent effect, a statistical artifact cannot be ruled out. Additional studies are being conducted to determine the effects of exposure of lymphocytes to 27-MHz CW and PM RF radiation at an SAR of 0.5 W/kg.

Glioma

To test the generality of the effects of isothermal RF radiation exposure on cell proliferation, parallel *in vitro* studies were conducted using glioma [human (LN71) or rat (RT2)]. These glioma cell lines afforded an opportunity to investigate the RF effects on transformed cells derived from two mammalian species in comparison with the effects on normal human lymphocytes summarized earlier.

Exposure of glioma cells *in vitro* for 2 h to 27- or 2450-MHz CW RF radiation modulated the rates of DNA and RNA synthesis at 1, 3, or 5 days after exposure. The biphasic glioma dose response, at either frequency, was similar to the lymphocyte dose response over a comparable intensity range. Exposure to SARs of 50 W/kg or less increased the incorporation rates of ^{3}H-TdR and tritiated uridine (^{3}H-UdR), whereas higher intensity RF exposure suppressed DNA and RNA synthesis. Statistically significant time-dependent alterations in cell polynucleotide synthesis were detected for up to 5 days after exposure. The procedures and results of this study were summarized previously.[2]

Comparison of the time dependence of the effects of 27-MHz and 2450-MHz CW RF radiation on glioma proliferation indicated differences in the cellular kinetic responses to these RF frequencies. Comparing 3-day to 5-day postexposure data revealed that glioma exposed to 27-MHz RF at SARs of 50 W/kg or greater exhibited a 45% increase in ^{3}H-TdR incorporation rate and a 54% increase in ^{3}H-UdR incorporation during this 2-day postexposure period. Over this same SAR range, a comparison of 3-day versus 5-day ^{3}H-TdR and ^{3}H-UdR incorporation rates in glioma exposed to 2450-MHz CW RF radiation indicated 13% and 19% reductions, respectively. Although 27-MHz and 2450-MHz CW RF radiation had qualitatively similar effects on glioma proliferation, these data indicated that there were frequency-dependent differences in the cell kinetic responses.[24]

TABLE 3 summarizes the effect of a 2-h 5-W/kg isothermal exposure of glioma to CW or PM 2450-MHz radiation on glioma ^{3}H-TdR incorporation rates. Exposure to either CW or PM 2450-MHz radiation resulted in statistically significant increased ^{3}H-TdR incorporation at 3 or 5 days postexposure. TABLE 4 indicates the effects of 27-MHz CW and PM exposure on ^{3}H-TdR incorporation rates in glioma at the same SAR (5 W/kg). Continuous wave (CW) RF exposure resulted in statistically significant increased incorporation rates at 3 or 5 days after exposure. There was a statistically significant 50% increase in ^{3}H-TdR uptake at 3 days after PM exposure, with no effect on day 5 postexposure.

The effects of 27- and 2450-MHz CW and PM RF radiation, at a time-averaged SAR of 0.5 W/kg, on glioma proliferation at 1, 3, or 5 days after a 2-h isothermal exposure were also determined. Exposure to CW 2450-MHz radiation increased

TABLE 3. ^{3}H-TdR Incorporation in Glioma^a at 3 or 5 Days after a 2-h Isothermal (37 ± 0.2 °C) Exposure to CW or PM 2450-MHz RF Radiation at an SAR of 5 W/kg (42.4 V/m)

| | SAR (W/kg) | | ^{3}H-TdR Ratio | ANOVA |
	Average	Maximum	Exposed/Sham	p-Value
3-Day postexposure	5 (CW)	5	1.42	0.0001
	5 (PM)	14.9×10^3	4.80	0.0001
5-Day postexposure	5 (CW)	5	1.49	0.0001
	5 (PM)	14.9×10^3	1.14	0.004

^{a}The CW data are for human glioma (LN71), whereas the PM data are for rat glioma (RT2).

^{3}H-TdR incorporation at 3 or 5 days postexposure, following suppression on day 1. A 17% decrease in uptake on day 1 was statistically significant ($p = 0.04$). Exposure to 2450-MHz PM RF radiation at 0.5 W/kg did not result in statistically significant effects on the glioma ^{3}H-TdR incorporation rates. However, the response pattern was the same as for CW exposure, namely, suppression on day 1 followed by stimulation of ^{3}H-TdR uptake at 3 and 5 days after RF exposure.

Statistically significant increases in ^{3}H-TdR occurred 3 days after exposure to CW or PM 27-MHz RF radiation ($p < 0.05$). A 26% increase in the ^{3}H-TdR incorporation rate at 5 days after CW exposure was not statistically significant, but log transformed data showed a significant increase ($p = 0.04$). Whereas there was a statistically significant decrease in ^{3}H-TdR at 1 day after exposure to PM radiation, this effect was reversed by day 3 (i.e., a statistically significant 112% increase). Five days after 27-MHz PM exposure at 0.5 W/kg, there was a nonstatistically significant 11% increase in the rate of glioma ^{3}H-TdR incorporation.

DISCUSSION

It is not feasible to use data derived from the studies of cellular effects of RF radiation to predict the *in vivo* effects resulting from exposure to NMRI or NMRS fields. There are a number of reasons for this, the most obvious being the differences in responses of complex integrated biological systems as compared to noninteracting

TABLE 4. ^{3}H-TdR Incorporation in Glioma^a at 3 or 5 Days after a 2-h Isothermal (37 ± 0.2 °C) Exposure to CW or PM 27-MHz RF Radiation at an SAR of 5 W/kg (50 V/m)

| | SAR (W/kg) | | ^{3}H-TdR Ratio | ANOVA |
	Average	Maximum	Exposed/Sham	p-Value
3-Day postexposure	5 (CW)	5	1.14	0.005
	5 (PM)	13.3	1.50	0.001
5-Day postexposure	5 (CW)	5	1.10	0.0002
	5 (PM)	13.3	0.87	0.34

^{a}The CW data are for human glioma (LN71), whereas the PM data are for rat glioma (RT2).

individual cells. Other factors include differences in RF frequency, intensity, modulation, and exposure duration, as well as the absence of static magnetic fields and magnetic field gradients. However, in spite of such limitations on extrapolation to *in vivo* systems, the data on *in vitro* RF cellular effects provide insight regarding the potential effects of NMRI and NMRS exposure.

The results of the studies summarized here provide evidence of direct nonthermal effects of RF radiation on cell proliferation. These results are consistent with the reported direct effects of RF radiation on cation fluxes and binding and on cell energy metabolism, reviewed here and elsewhere.[25]

In order to put the results of the studies of the effects of 27- or 2450-MHz radiation on cell proliferation into a proper context, the following should be considered:

(a) RF effects on lymphocyte proliferation occurred as a consequence of a single 2-h exposure under isothermal conditions at normal body temperature (37 °C). Because tissue exposure to RF at SARs of 5 W/kg or greater would generally involve radiation-induced temperature elevations, qualitatively and quantitatively different effects on cell proliferation *in vivo* could occur due to the interaction of RF radiation and tissue temperature. Studies of the interaction of RF radiation and cell heating are needed at temperatures higher than 37 °C.

(b) Statistically significant effects on ^{3}H-TdR and ^{3}H-UdR cellular incorporation rates occurred as early as 1 day after exposure and had a persistence of at least 5 days. There was evidence of time-dependent variation in the exposure effects, the nature of which may be related to RF frequency.

(c) Dose-fractionation data indicated the cumulation of exposure effects over a period of at least 1 day.

(d) Pulse modulation of 27- or 2450-MHz RF radiation resulted in qualitatively similar effects on cell proliferation, but there was evidence of differences in the dose response to those radiation modalities. Direct comparison of the effects of 27- and 2450-MHz PM is not appropriate due to differences in signal characteristics (i.e., 27-MHz RF modulation simulated occupational exposure to heat sealing devices; 2450-MHz RF modulation simulated the output of pulsed radar).

(e) Exposure of lymphocytes or glioma to 27- or 2450-MHz RF radiation at SARs of greater than 5 W/kg caused dose-rate-dependent biphasic effects on cell proliferation. Lymphocyte DNA synthesis was suppressed following exposure to 27- or 2450-MHz radiation at 5 W/kg, whereas it was increased in glioma. DNA synthesis decreased following lymphocyte exposure at 0.5 W/kg, with the exception of an increase in ^{3}H-TdR uptake after exposure to PM 27-MHz RF radiation. Exposure of glioma to 0.5-W/kg 27- or 2450-MHz radiation caused an increase in the incorporation rate of ^{3}H-TdR, with the exception of decreased uptake at 1 day postexposure to PM radiation.

(f) There was an inverse relationship between the variability of ^{3}H-TdR cellular uptake data and SAR, suggesting a detection threshold of approximately 0.5 W/kg for the effects of RF radiation on cell proliferation, under the acute exposure conditions used in these studies (namely, 2-h exposure at 37 ± 0.2 °C).

A more general assessment of the effects of low-intensity RF radiation on cell proliferation will require data on the effects of chronic or long-term exposure.

(g) Mechanisms for the effects of RF radiation on cell proliferation are not known. There are indications, however, that RF exposure may affect the mitotic cycle, resulting in time-dependent shifts in the relative number of cells in specific cycle phases.[23]

In conclusion, there is evidence of direct, nonthermal cellular effects of RF radiation in the general frequency, intensity, and exposure duration range employed in NMRI and NMRS. This indicates the need to consider factors other than tissue-induced heating in assessing the safety and fidelity of clinical uses of these modalities. Data are needed on the cellular effects of NMRI and NMRS fields under well-controlled experimental conditions.

REFERENCES

1. CLEARY, S. F. 1990. Cellular effects of radiofrequency electromagnetic radiation. *In* Biological Effects and Medical Applications of Electromagnetic Fields. Chapter 14. O. Gandhi, Ed. Prentice–Hall. Englewood Cliffs, New Jersey.
2. CLEARY, S. F., L. M. LIU & R. E. MERCHANT. 1990. Glioma proliferation modulated *in vitro* by isothermal radiofrequency radiation exposure. Radiat. Res. **121:** 38–45.
3. CLEARY, S. F., L. M. LIU & R. E. MERCHANT. 1990. Lymphocyte proliferation induced by radiofrequency radiation under isothermal conditions. Bioelectromagnetics **11:** 47–56.
4. SERPERSU, E. H. & T. W. TSONG. 1983. Stimulation of a ouabain-sensitive Rb^+ uptake in human erythrocytes with an external electric field. J. Membr. Biol. **74:** 191–201.
5. LIBURDY, R. P. & A. PENN. 1984. Microwave bioeffects in the erythrocyte are temperature and pO_2 dependent: cation permeability and protein shedding occur at the membrane phase transition. Bioelectromagnetics **5:** 283–291.
6. CLEARY, S. F., F. GARBER & L. M. LIU. 1982. Effects of X-band microwave (8.3 GHz) radiation on erythrocytes. Bioelectromagnetics **3:** 453–466.
7. ALLIS, J. W. & B. L. SINHA-ROBINSON. 1987. Temperature-specific inhibition of human red cell Na^+/K^+ ATPase by 2450-MHz microwave radiation. Bioelectromagnetics **8:** 203–212.
8. CLEARY, S. F., L. M. LIU & F. GARBER. 1985. Erythrocyte hemolysis by radiofrequency fields. Bioelectromagnetics **6:** 313–322.
9. BAWIN, S. M., L. K. KACZMAREK & W. R. ADEY. 1975. Effects of modulated VHF fields on the central nervous system. Ann. N.Y. Acad. Sci. **247:** 74–81.
10. BAWIN, S. M. & W. R. ADEY. 1976. Sensitivity of calcium binding in cerebral tissue to weak environmental electrical fields oscillating at low frequency. Proc. Natl. Acad. Sci. U.S.A. **73:** 1999–2003.
11. BLACKMAN, C. F., J. A. ELDER, C. M. WEIL, S. G. BENANE, D. C. EICHINGER & D. E. HOUSE. 1979. Induction of calcium ion efflux from brain tissue by radio-frequency radiation: effects of modulation frequency and field strength. Radio Sci. **14**(GS): 93–98.
12. BLACKMAN, C. F., S. G. BENANE, J. A. ELDER, D. E. HOUSE, J. A. LAMPE & J. M. FAULK. 1980. Induction of calcium ion efflux from brain tissue by radio-frequency radiation: effect of sample number and modulation frequency on the power-density window. Bioelectromagnetics **1:** 35–43.
13. BLACKMAN, C. F., S. G. BENANE, W. T. JOINES, M. A. HOLLIS & D. E. HOUSE. 1980. Calcium-ion efflux from brain tissue: power-density versus internal field-intensity dependence of 50-MHz RF radiation. Bioelectromagnetics **1:** 277–283.
14. SHEPPARD, A. R., S. M. BAWIN & W. R. ADEY. 1979. Models of long-range order in cerebral macromolecules: effects of sub-ELF and of modulated VHF and UHF fields. Radio Sci. **14**(GS): 141–145.
15. DUTTA, S. K., A. SUBRAMONIAM, B. GHOSH & R. PARSHAD. 1984. Microwave radiation-

induced calcium ion efflux from human neuroblastoma cells in culture. Bioelectromagnetics **5:** 71–78.

16. DUTTA, S. K., B. GHOSH & C. F. BLACKMAN. 1989. Radiofrequency radiation-induced calcium-ion-efflux enhancement from human and other neuroblastoma cells in culture. Bioelectromagnetics **10:** 197–202.

17. BLACKMAN, C. F., S. G. BENANE, D. E. HOUSE & W. T. JOINES. 1985. Effects of ELF (1–120 Hz) and modulated (50 Hz) RF fields on the efflux of calcium ions from brain tissue *in vitro.* Bioelectromagnetics **6:** 1–11.

18. BLACKMAN, C. F., S. G. BENANE, J. R. RABINOWITZ, D. E. HOUSE & W. T. JOINES. 1985. A role for the magnetic field in the radiation-induced efflux of calcium ions from brain tissue *in vitro.* Bioelectromagnetics **6:** 327–337.

19. GAVASAS-MEDICI, R. & S. R. DAY-MAGDALENO. 1976. Extremely low frequency, weak electric fields affect schedule-controlled behavior of monkeys. Nature (London) **261:** 256–259.

20. ADEY, W. R., S. M. BAWIN & A. F. LAWRENCE. 1982. Effects of weak amplitude modulated microwave fields on calcium efflux from awake cat cerebral cortex. Bioelectromagnetics **3:** 295–307.

21. SANDERS, A. P., W. T. JOINES & J. W. ALLIS. 1984. The differential effects of 200, 591, and 2450 MHz radiation on rat brain energy metabolism. Bioelectromagnetics **5:** 419–433.

22. SANDERS, A. P., W. T. JOINES & J. W. ALLIS. 1985. Effects of continuous-wave, pulsed, and sinusoidal-amplitude-modulated microwaves on brain energy metabolism. Bioelectromagnetics **6:** 89–97.

23. CLEARY, S. F. Unpublished observations.

24. CLEARY, S. F., L. M. LIU & G. CAO. 1990. Functional alteration of mammalian cells by direct high frequency electromagnetic field interactions. *In* Charge and Field Effects in Biosystems. Vol. 2: 211–221. Plenum. New York.

25. CLEARY, S. F. 1987. Cellular effects of electromagnetic radiation. IEEE Eng. Med. Biol. **EMB3-06:** 26–30.

26. CLEARY, S. F. 1991. *In vitro* studies: low frequency electromagnetic fields. *In* Proc. Scientific Workshop on the Health Effects of Electromagnetic Radiation on Workers. United States Department of Health and Human Services, CDC, National Institute for Occupational Safety and Health. Cincinnati, Ohio. In press.

Spatial Distribution of RF Power in Critical Organs during Magnetic Resonance Imaging

M. GRANDOLFO,[a] A. POLICHETTI,[a] P. VECCHIA,[a] AND
O. P. GANDHI[b]

[a] Physics Laboratory
National Institute of Health
00161 Rome, Italy

[b] Department of Electrical Engineering
University of Utah
Salt Lake City, Utah 84112

INTRODUCTION

With the rapid increase in the application of magnetic resonance imaging (MRI) as a diagnostic aid, progressively greater attention has been given to possible health risks for patients from exposure to the magnetic fields generated inside the apparatus.

Persons undergoing MRI examinations are subjected to three different magnetic fields, namely, a static field, a time-varying gradient field, and a radio-frequency field. In order to assess the biological effects resulting from the simultaneous exposure to these fields, it is necessary that the effects of each of them be well understood.

As regards radio-frequency (RF) fields, the interaction mechanism with a living body is well known, the primary effect being the heating of tissues, with consequent biological effects related to the thermally induced changes in the body. Safety aspects of exposure to RF fields have been covered in several reviews: a very comprehensive one has been issued by the World Health Organization.[1]

Limits of exposure to RF electromagnetic fields have been recommended by a number of national and international bodies, such as the American National Standards Institute (ANSI), the American Conference of Governmental Industrial Hygienists (ACGIH), and the International Radiation Protection Association (IRPA).[2] Deliberate exposures of patients undergoing medical treatment or diagnosis are out of the scope of the above standards. However, specific recommendations for safe exposure during MRI examinations have been issued by the Center for Devices and Radiological Health in the United States, by the National Radiological Protection Board in the United Kingdom, by the Federal Health Office in Germany, by Health and Welfare Canada, by the Health Council of the Netherlands, and by the Italian Ministry of Health;[3] a document of the IRPA on the protection of patients undergoing magnetic resonance examinations is also in the process of being published.[4]

In all the aforementioned standards, basic limits are expressed in terms of the specific absorption rate (SAR), which gives the rate of RF energy imparted to a unit body mass. Most of them, both general and specific to MRI, include limits for the whole-body SAR as well as for the local SAR; the latter is intended as a value averaged over any given quantity of mass (typically 1 g or 100 g) inside the body. Therefore, the knowledge of the SAR distribution is essential to ascertain the compliance with most standards.

The distribution of RF power inside the body is not uniform due to the different electrical characteristics of tissues. The pattern of energy absorption can be evaluated through measurements on phantoms or by numerical techniques that make use of realistic models of the human body.

In this communication, a computational technique known as the impedance method is presented and its application for the evaluation of RF power absorption in MRI examinations is discussed.

THE IMPEDANCE METHOD

In the frequency region currently used in MRI diagnostic procedures, the absorption of RF energy is almost completely associated with the magnetic field. The energy dissipation depends on the frequency, on the strength of the incident field, on the coupling efficiency between the RF coil and the specimen, and on several properties such as the mass density, size, and orientation of the specimen relative to the field polarity.

In the impedance method,[5,6] the SAR is calculated from these data, using a realistic model of the human body composed of a given number of cells, each one fully characterized, from the electrical point of view, by its impedance. The latter is calculated from the known permittivity and conductivity of the tissues composing the cell. In this way, the body is replaced by a three-dimensional network of impedances.

The complex currents along each cell's loop can be calculated from both the cell impedance and the electromotive force (EMF) induced around the loop due to the time-varying magnetic field. The EMF for each loop around a cell face of area A is given by Faraday's law of induction:

$$\text{EMF} = -\frac{d}{dt} \int_A \vec{B} \cdot d\vec{s},\tag{1}$$

where $\vec{B}$ is the magnetic flux density at the cell and $d\vec{s}$ is the differential area directed normal to the cell face. By applying equation 1 to each cell face and by requiring the current continuity for each cell in the network, a system of equations is obtained that can be solved for the induced currents. From these equations, the SAR can be calculated for individual cells and for different organs based on the knowledge of tissue percentages in each cell.

APPLICATION TO MRI PROCEDURES

We have applied the impedance method for the evaluation of the SAR in a human torso subjected to MR tomography in different procedures. A similar analysis has already been performed for a particular polarization of the RF field,[7] whereas in

TABLE 1. Values of the Relative Dielectric Constant Used for Calculation of Cell Impedances and SAR

Tissue	Frequency (MHz)			
	0.45	13.56	30	64
muscle	1×10^4	128	103	72
fat, bone	8×10^3	29	29	8.5
blood	2.4×10^3	150	100	80
intestine	5×10^3	60	60	40
cartilage	8×10^3	29	29	8.5
liver	6.4×10^3	165	130	88
kidney	9.8×10^3	250	200	115
pancreas	1.1×10^4	265	200	130
spleen	1.1×10^4	265	200	130
lung	3.3×10^3	40	34	27
heart	3×10^5	250	200	100
nerve	8×10^3	210	150	100
skin	1×10^4	128	103	72

this study the dependence of the pattern of the energy absorption on the field direction is also investigated.

For modeling purposes, the torso was enclosed in an ideal parallelepiped divided into $18 \times 12 \times 23 = 4968$ cubic cells of a 2.6-cm edge. It was considered to be composed of 13 different tissues, whose distribution inside each cell was obtained through a digital scanning of the anatomic diagrams of the cross sections of the torso.[5]

The complex impedances were calculated from permittivity and conductivity data found in the literature. The values for individual tissues at the frequencies of interest for this discussion are reported in TABLES 1 and 2. It is to be noted that, for the lung, we assumed 33% lung tissue and 67% air, and the values listed in TABLES 1 and 2 are obtained by dividing the literature data for deflated tissue by a factor of three.

TABLE 2. Values of Conductivity (S/m) Used for Calculation of Cell Impedances and SAR

Tissue	Frequency (MHz)			
	0.45	13.56	30	64
muscle	0.51	0.63	0.75	0.80
fat, bone	0.034	0.04	0.04	0.06
blood	0.20	0.28	0.28	0.80
intestine	0.25	0.30	0.30	0.35
cartilage	0.034	0.04	0.04	0.06
liver	0.33	0.48	0.52	0.58
kidney	0.54	0.74	0.80	0.90
pancreas	0.33	0.62	0.70	0.80
spleen	0.33	0.62	0.70	0.80
lung	0.18	0.22	0.17	0.24
heart	0.30	0.52	0.65	0.60
nerve	0.19	0.31	0.46	0.47
skin	0.51	0.63	0.75	0.80

The numerical calculations give SARs resulting from exposure to continuous waves. Because pulsed fields are employed in all MRI procedures, the data are to be scaled for the duty cycle, D, of the specific pulse sequence. Imagers can generally be programmed to produce several pulse sequences and the patterns of energy deposition strongly depend on the chosen sequence, which can vary greatly in the number and type of pulses.

For the sake of simplicity, we assume that one pulse, at an angle θ, dominates within the chosen sequence. If the pulse sequence contains a number N_p of θ pulses, the duty cycle is multiplied by N_p. In the case of multislice imaging, a further correction for the number N_s of slices simultaneously scanned is needed, so the general expression for the duty cycle is

$$D = N_p N_s \frac{t}{T}, \tag{2}$$

where t is the time length of the pulse and T is the repetition period of the pulse sequence.

In equation 2, rectangular pulses are assumed. In the case of Gaussian or sine wave modulated RF energy, the effective duty cycle is obtained through multiplication by suitable coefficients, as indicated by Bottomley *et al.*[8]

As an example of an application of the impedance method, results are shown relative to an exposure similar to that hypothesized by Bottomley and Edelstein.[9] These investigators estimated the surface absorption of the RF energy for a human head and torso imaged by nuclear magnetic resonance. The torso, which is of interest for our results, was approximated by a homogeneous cylinder of radius R. The permittivity (ϵ), conductivity (σ), and mass density (ρ) of the tissue inside the cylinder were assumed equal to those of muscle. The calculation was performed over a circular loop with radius R intersected by a spatially uniform RF magnetic field perpendicular to the loop and parallel to the torso axis.

For this model, it can be shown[9] that, in the case of $\pi/2$ pulses of sinusoidal waves of frequency f, the surface SAR is given by

$$SAR = (6.80 \times 10^{-26}) \frac{\sigma f^2 R^2}{\rho t T}. \tag{3}$$

In our calculations, we assumed a torso of maximal cross section of 46.8 × 31.2 × 59.8 cm along the x, y, and z axes, corresponding to the right-to-left, front-to-back, and up-to-down directions in the torso, respectively. To obtain results for realistic situations, we assumed $\pi/2$ pulses of 5-ms duration and 100-ms repetition period, that is, a duty cycle of 5×10^{-2}, as frequently used in fast imaging. The magnetic field strength B_{rf} was obtained by the basic equation of

$$2\pi\gamma B_1 t = \theta, \tag{4}$$

where γ is the gyromagnetic ratio (for protons, $\gamma = 42.58$ MHz/T) and $B_1 = 0.5 B_{rf}$ is the magnitude of the rotating component of the RF field.

In FIGURE 1, the average SARs in individual tissues versus frequency are shown for a B field polarized along the torso axis (i.e., the z direction). The curves were obtained by connecting the points corresponding to the frequencies of 0.45, 13.56, 30, and 64 MHz for which the dielectric constants were available and then the calculations were performed. Thanks to the fairly constant slope, the curves seem to be suitable for the estimation of the SAR in organs at any frequency in the range of 0.45–64 MHz.

As already stated, the impedance method allows the evaluation of the SAR distribution among the individual tissues and organs. Data shown in FIGURE 2 for the particular frequency of 30 MHz allow a comparison with the results of Bottomley and Edelstein for the same frequency, polarization, and duty cycle. The average SAR in the skin is ~ 7 mW/kg, which compares with a value of ~ 20 mW/kg given for the surface SAR by these investigators. The discrepancy can be accounted for by the different dimensions of our realistic torso and the simplified model adopted by

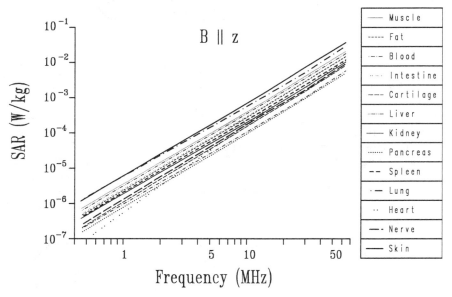

FIGURE 1. Average SAR in different tissues of the torso versus frequency for a homogeneous RF magnetic field parallel to the torso axis.

Bottomley and Edelstein: the radius of the latter equals in fact the maximal cross dimension of our torso, allowing higher values of the SAR in outer tissues.

The dependence of the average SAR on the polarization of RF fields has been proven for exposure to plane waves on simple models such as prolate spheroids. In order to evaluate the effect of polarization in the exposure conditions specified earlier, we performed calculations for the magnetic field directed along the x and y direction. FIGURES 3 and 4 show the frequency dependence of the SAR in individual tissues, whereas results for the particular frequency of 30 MHz are reported in more detail in FIGURES 5 and 6. It is clear that field polarization affects not only the values of average SAR in the torso, but also its relative magnitude in different tissues.

In all cases, the distribution of the energy deposition within each cross section perpendicular to the torso axis shows a general increase with the distance from the

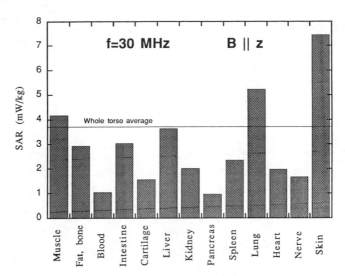

FIGURE 2. Distribution of the SAR in tissues for rectangular $\pi/2$ pulses of 30-MHz frequency ($B_0 = 0.7$ T). The homogeneous RF magnetic field is parallel to the torso axis. Pulse duration = 5 ms; repetition period = 100 ms.

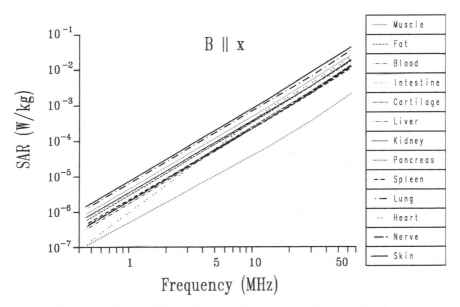

FIGURE 3. Average SAR in different tissues of the torso versus frequency for a homogeneous RF magnetic field parallel to the right-to-left direction of the torso.

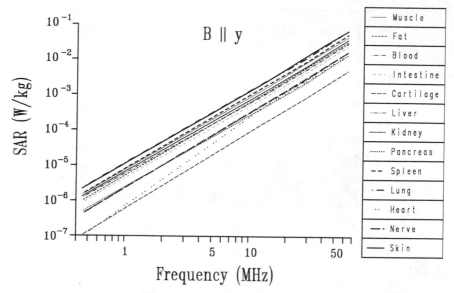

FIGURE 4. Average SAR in different tissues of the torso versus frequency for a homogeneous RF magnetic field parallel to the front-to-back direction of the torso.

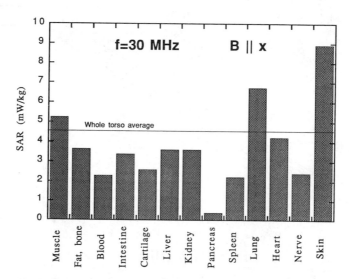

FIGURE 5. Distribution of the SAR in tissues for a homogeneous RF magnetic field parallel to the right-to-left direction of the torso. Experimental conditions are as in FIGURE 2.

center, which is expected[5] due to the larger current loops. This increase also explains the high value of the SAR in the skin compared with all other tissues, with the exception of the lung.

It is interesting to note that the ratio between the maximal value and the average SAR in the trunk ranges from 1.8 to 2.0 for different polarizations. These values agree well with the ratio of 2 expected in the case of a homogeneous tissue cylinder.

From the data of FIGURES 1, 3, and 4, the average SAR in the whole trunk was calculated for each frequency under consideration. To better describe the frequency dependence of the average SAR, a best-fit analysis was performed. We found an f^k dependence, with $k = 2.079, 2.081$, and 2.080 for the x, y, and z polarization, respectively.

The deviation of the exponents from the 2.0 value expected from the induction law is mainly due to the frequency dependence of the conductivity. A best-fit of the

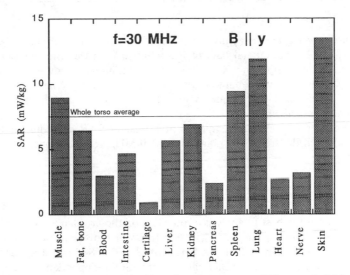

FIGURE 6. Distribution of the SAR in tissues for a homogeneous RF magnetic field parallel to the front-to-back direction of the torso. Experimental conditions are as in FIGURE 2.

average σ with an f^k function gives in fact $k = 0.09$. The small difference in our results is due to the frequency dependence of the permittivity.

From our results, we derived the following general equations that allow the calculation of the average SAR values in the whole trunk for any frequency between 0.45 and 64 MHz:

$$\text{SAR} = (2.66 \times 10^{-22})f^{2.079}\theta^2 \frac{N_p N_s}{tT} \qquad \text{B}\|\text{x}$$

$$\text{SAR} = (4.22 \times 10^{-22})f^{2.081}\theta^2 \frac{N_p N_s}{tT} \qquad \text{B}\|\text{y} \qquad (5)$$

$$\text{SAR} = (2.12 \times 10^{-22})f^{2.080}\theta^2 \frac{N_p N_s}{tT} \qquad \text{B}\|\text{z}.$$

TABLE 3. Whole-Torso Averaged SAR (W/kg) for Some Realistic MRI Procedures

MRI Procedure	Roeschmann (1987)[10]	Present Work
Spin echo, 1 echo, 1 π pulse, $t = 1$ ms, $T = 1$ s, B = 1.5 T, f = 64 MHz	0.028	0.038
Fast imaging, 1 echo, 1 π/2 pulse, $t = 5$ ms, $T = 0.1$ s, B = 0.7 T, f = 30 MHz	0.0027	0.0037
Inversion recovery, 4 echoes, 5 π pulses, 12 slices, $t = 0.5$ ms, $T = 1$ s, B = 1.5 T, f = 64 MHz	3.35	4.56

To further verify the reliability of the method, we also compared our theoretical results with the experimental data of Roeschmann[10] on the effective penetration depth and absorption of the RF frequency in the human body as a function of frequency. These data were mainly derived from bench measurements of the quality factor and of the resonance frequency shift due to the loading of the different types of coils under investigation.

According to Roeschmann's experimental data, the SAR in the human torso can be calculated, in the frequency range of 10–220 MHz, from the phenomenological equation:

$$\text{SAR} = (4.66 \times 10^{-23}) f^{2.15} \theta^2 \frac{N_p N_s}{tT}. \tag{6}$$

Moreover, if the best-fit analysis of our data on the average SAR in the torso is limited to the frequency range of 13.56–64 MHz, which overlaps that considered by Roeschmann, we obtain an f^k dependence with $k = 2.158$, 2.161, and 2.155 for the three polarizations, which is in fair agreement with the dependence deduced from the experiment.

To assess the potential hazard of MRI examinations, we made calculations for some realistic procedures, corresponding to different patterns of RF excitation. The results, relative to z polarization (magnetic field parallel to the body axis), are reported in TABLE 3 together with those obtained from Roeschmann's phenomenological equation under the same conditions.

DISCUSSION

The results shown in the previous section confirm the great potential of the impedance method for the evaluation of the SAR distribution in tissues. They show in particular that the SAR in individual organs depends on a number of factors, namely, the frequency and amplitude of the field, its orientation with respect to the body, the dielectric properties of the organs as well as those of the surrounding tissues, and the size, shape, and position of the organs.

The use of the quasi-static approximation over the whole frequency range under consideration could be questionable. This approach, which assumes that the magnetic field is not perturbed by the body and therefore remains uniform in tissues as in the free space, has in fact been criticized as not being sufficiently realistic for frequencies of more than 20–30 MHz.

To ascertain the validity range of our technique, we performed analytical calculations of the SAR inside a uniform, infinite cylinder of radius R (0.18 m). The comparison of the data obtained under the simplified assumption of a uniform field with the exact analytical solution is shown in FIGURE 7. It is seen that the quasi-static approximation, fairly adequate below 13.56 MHz, should be unacceptable for frequencies of the order of 60 MHz. These conclusions are in agreement with a similar comparative study performed by Gabriel.[11]

On the other hand, the experimental data by Roeschmann[10] suggest that the texture of the biological tissue (which consists of heterogeneously sized regions of relatively high values of conductivity and permittivity, but separated by regions with considerably lower values) allows the RF magnetic field to penetrate much deeper into the body than predicted by homogeneous models. Recent studies[12] actually indicate that the RF penetration limits are not likely to degrade the image quality at frequencies up to 100 MHz, well beyond the range of this study.

Lastly, however, the hypothesis of a uniform field leads to an overestimation of

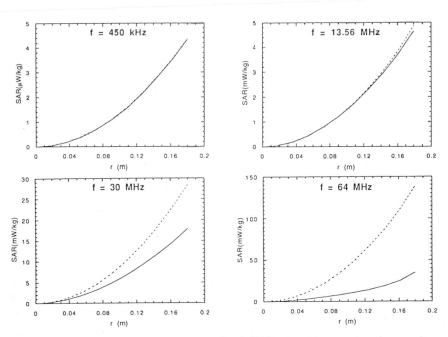

FIGURE 7. SARs calculated as an exact solution (solid lines) and in a quasi-static approximation (dotted lines) inside a homogeneous, infinite cylinder of muscle tissue as a function of the radial distance. Rectangular $\pi/2$ pulses of 5-ms duration and 100-ms repetition period are hypothesized.

the internal and average SARs and this could account for the discrepancies in TABLE 3.

CONCLUSIONS

The examples reported here show the great potential of the impedance method for the estimation of energy deposition in different organs, in particular for exposures during MRI examinations. This is of special importance in risk assessment because it has been recognized that, in certain cases, localized SARs could be higher than the recommended limits, especially at higher fields and in the case of multislice and multiecho pulse sequences.[13]

The aforementioned guidelines for safe exposure of patients during MRI examinations are based primarily on concerns about thermally induced biological effects. The recommended limit for the SAR, as averaged over the whole body, is 0.4 W/kg.[2,14] The guidelines for local maxima of the SAR are different in different countries, ranging from 2 to 5 W/kg.

The IRPA[4] recommends that the exposure to RF fields of persons without cardiovascular impairment be such that the absorbed energy, that is, the product of SAR and exposure time, does not exceed 120 W · min/kg (7.2 kJ/kg), provided the SAR does not exceed 8 W/kg, with both limits being averaged over the trunk.

Moreover, our results indicate that simple spin-echo procedures are not critical at all. However, procedures involving several slices and echoes at high static magnetic fields ($B_0 > 1.5$ T) could reach and even violate some of the existing guidelines. For instance, the inversion recovery procedure in TABLE 3 should not last more than 26 min to comply with IRPA limits.

It is to be reminded, though, that our data could be overestimated at higher frequencies. This would lead to conservative evaluations from the point of view of protection.

REFERENCES

1. WORLD HEALTH ORGANIZATION. 1981. Environmental Health Criteria 16: Radiofrequency and Microwaves. WHO. Geneva.
2. GRANDOLFO, M. & K. H. MILD. 1989. Worldwide public and occupational radiofrequency and microwaves protection guides. In Electromagnetic Biointeraction: Mechanisms, Safety Standards, Protection Guides. G. Franceschetti, O. P. Gandhi & M. Grandolfo, Eds.: 99–134. Plenum. New York.
3. MATHUR–DE VRÉ, R. 1987. Safety aspects of magnetic resonance imaging and magnetic resonance spectroscopy applications in medicine and biology. II. Recommendations for MR exposures in clinical practice. Arch. Belg. Med. Soc. Hyg. Med. Trav. Med. Leg. 45: 425–438.
4. INTERNATIONAL NON-IONIZING RADIATION COMMITTEE OF THE INTERNATIONAL RADIATION PROTECTION ASSOCIATION (INIRC/IRPA). Protection of the patient undergoing magnetic resonance examinations. Health Phys. In press.
5. DeFORD, J. F. & O. P. GANDHI. 1985. An impedance method to calculate currents induced in biological bodies exposed to quasi-static electromagnetic fields. IEEE Trans. Electromagn. Compat. 27: 168–173.
6. ORCUTT, N. & O. P. GANDHI. 1988. A 3-D impedance method to calculate power deposition in biological bodies subject to time-varying magnetic fields. IEEE Trans. Biomed. Eng. 35: 577–583.

7. GRANDOLFO, M., P. VECCHIA & O. P. GANDHI. 1990. Magnetic resonance imaging: calculation of rates of energy absorption by a human-torso model. Bioelectromagnetics **11:** 117–128.
8. BOTTOMLEY, P. A., R. W. REDINGTON, W. A. EDELSTEIN & J. F. SCHENCK. 1985. Estimating radiofrequency deposition in body NMR imaging. Magn. Reson. Med. **2:** 336–349.
9. BOTTOMLEY, P. A. & W. A. EDELSTEIN. 1981. Power deposition in whole-body NMR imaging. Med. Phys. **8:** 510–512.
10. ROESCHMANN, P. 1987. Radiofrequency penetration and absorption in the human body: limitations to high-field whole-body nuclear magnetic resonance imaging. Med. Phys. **14:** 922–931.
11. GABRIEL, C. Private communication.
12. VOLLMAN, W. & M. H. KUHN. 1985. Throughput limitations in clinical MR imaging due to RF heating. *In* Magnetic Resonance Imaging and Spectroscopy. Proceedings of the First Congress of the European Society of Magnetic Resonance in Medicine and Biology (Geneva, 5–6 October 1984). M. A. Hopf & G. M. Bydder, Eds.: 292–298. European Society of Magnetic Resonance in Medicine and Biology. Geneva.
13. MATHUR–DE VRÉ, R. 1987. Safety aspects of magnetic resonance imaging and magnetic resonance spectroscopy applications in medicine and biology. I. Biomagnetic effects. Arch. Belg. Med. Soc. Hyg. Med. Trav. Med. Leg. **45:** 394–424.
14. INTERNATIONAL NON-IONIZING RADIATION COMMITTEE OF THE INTERNATIONAL RADIATION PROTECTION ASSOCIATION (INIRC/IRPA). 1988. Guidelines on limits of exposure to radiofrequency electromagnetic fields in the frequency range from 100 kHz to 300 GHz. Health Phys. **54:** 115–123.

Predicted Thermophysiological Responses of Humans to MRI Fields

ELEANOR R. ADAIR AND LARRY G. BERGLUND

John B. Pierce Laboratory
New Haven, Connecticut 06519

INTRODUCTION

We have described[1,2] a relatively simple computerized model of physiological thermoregulation, which can be used to predict the probable human response to radio-frequency (RF) energy deposited in the body during the magnetic resonance imaging (MRI) procedure. This model is based on the basic physiological processes by which thermal energy is exchanged between the body and the environment. In general, the model predicts that the thermoregulatory response to absorbed RF energy, under any given ambient conditions, is similar to that which would be expected during an increase in metabolic heat production (such as during exercise). A rise in skin blood flow (SkBF) produces an increase in thermal conductance, which is a measure of heat flow from the body core to the skin. With continued absorption of RF energy, sweating is initiated, the skin surface becomes increasingly wet, and thermal discomfort increases. If these mobilized responses are of insufficient magnitude to dissipate all of the heat generated in the body by the absorbed RF energy, heat will be stored in body tissues and the core temperature will rise. Our predictions have shown that the magnitude of this temperature rise is a function of the rate of whole-body RF energy absorption, or SAR.

We have found that the limiting response under a wide variety of imaging conditions[1] appears to be the rate of SkBF, even though sweating plays a significant role in preventing an excessive rise in core temperature (ΔT_{co}). It is important to note that these predictions apply to a healthy 70-kg patient ("standard man"), wearing light pajamas, whose metabolic heat production is at the resting level (1 met) during the MRI procedure. Obviously, as we have emphasized,[1,3] these idealized conditions would seldom exist in the clinic and variations therefrom should be considered in any attempt to apply the predictions. Use of added insulation (a blanket) and consideration of the pharmacological action of prescribed medication on normal thermoregulatory processes are examples of significant variations from the modeled conditions.

A more recent paper[2] has considered the evaluation of possible cardiovascular impairment that might preclude, in certain patients, the efficient transfer of heat from the body core to the periphery. The computer model was further adapted to simulate impaired cardiovascular function in patients undergoing MRI scans. Restrictions on the rate of SkBF, ranging from 1% to 89% of normal, were studied. Predictions of physiological heat loss responses in real time were generated as a function of the ambient temperature (T_a), the relative humidity (RH), and the rate of whole-body RF energy deposition (SAR). Under the conditions stated earlier that are desirable in the clinic, moderate restrictions (up to 67%) of SkBF yielded tolerable increases in core temperature ($\Delta T_{co} \leq 1$ °C) during MRI scans (SAR ≤ 4

188

W/kg) of 40 min or less. An increase of T_a above 20 °C or an increase of RH above 50% exacerbated the thermal stress from imposed RF energy. Severely impaired SkBF encouraged short MRI procedures (e.g., 20 min or less) at SARs $\leq$ 3 W/kg. In warm/humid environments, sweating was predicted to be profuse and evaporative cooling was curtailed, yielding a state of extreme thermal discomfort. The use of a blanket was discouraged because other calculations indicated that added insulation further exacerbated the hyperthermia. Some guidelines, based on the predictions of the model, were offered for tolerable MRI exposure conditions; these guidelines incorporated restrictions of SkBF, T_a, RH, and insulation.

Although a model of the human body, in terms of two concentric compartments, accurately predicts experimental observations of physiological responses in exercising humans under assorted ambient conditions,[4] it admittedly has certain limitations when applied to the MRI environment. The major limitation concerns the fact that typical MRI scans involve the head, the trunk, or an extremity, but seldom, if ever, the whole body. Far more complex, multiple-node, simulation models (e.g., see references 5 and 6) are required to predict changes in thermoregulatory responses during partial-body MRI scans. Nevertheless, certain other important variables can be explored to advantage with the simple two-node model and the accuracy of the model's predictions can be demonstrated in the clinical setting by careful measurements of the thermoregulatory responses in humans undergoing controlled MRI scans. These extensions of our earlier work form the content of this report.

FUNDAMENTALS OF THE TWO-NODE MODEL

The model considers the human body as two concentric thermal compartments (cf. figure 4 in reference 1) that represent the skin and core of the body. The skin compartment, simulating dermis and epidermis, has a thickness of about 1.6 mm. Its weight, about 10% of the total body weight, depends on the vasomotor state. The temperature in each compartment is assumed to be uniform, with temperature gradients existing only between compartments. Metabolic energy (M) is assumed to be generated only in the core compartment.

Heat can be lost directly from the core of the body through respiration. Heat can also flow passively from the core to the skin and, in the model, the physiologically controllable heat loss path is SkBF. This vasomotor response is modeled as depending on the skin and core temperature deviations from their respective set points.[2] Any limitation on SkBF will influence the convection of heat by the blood from the body core to the skin, the heat in the skin compartment that is derived from the core, and the relative size or fraction of the total body weight that is thermally skin.

The heat transported to the skin, and any heat generated in the skin from the absorption of RF energy, can be dissipated to the surrounding environment by conduction, convection, radiation, evaporation of sweat, and diffusion of water vapor through the skin. If there is clothing or other insulation, all heat and vapor flowing from the skin is assumed to pass through this resistance. The rate of regulatory sweating (REG_{sw}) can be predicted from the skin and core temperature deviations from their set points.

In the model, RF energy deposition per unit body weight during MRI of the whole body is reasonably assumed to be uniformly distributed over the entire body. The energy absorbed (A) in each compartment, core (co) and skin (sk), is assumed to be proportional to the compartment's weight and to the average SAR level (W/kg) for the whole body:

$$A_{co} = (1 - \alpha) \cdot Wt \cdot SAR \quad [W]$$

$$A_{sk} = \alpha \cdot Wt \cdot SAR \quad\quad [W]$$

where α represents the fraction of the total body weight (Wt) that is skin. Although peripheral energy deposition may predominate during MRI, theoretical considerations and experimental observations support our simplifying assumptions and reduce the possibility of local thermal hot spots.[7–10]

PARAMETERS VARIED IN THE PRESENT CALCULATIONS

In the present study, the two-node model was used to generate predictions of specific thermoregulatory responses as well as the perceived thermal comfort of a standard man exposed to RF energy during a 20-min simulated MRI scan. All predictions are for a 70-kg man at rest; thus, the metabolic heat production is set at the resting level (1 met = 58.2 W/m^2). The man wears pajamas, which have an insulation value of 0.4 clo. The air temperature (T_a) equals the mean radiant temperature (T_r) of the environment and is set at 20 °C; the relative humidity (RH) is set at 50%. The maximum skin blood flow ($SkBF_{max}$) is set at the normal level of 90 $L/h \cdot m^2$ and the rate of regulatory sweating (E_{rsw}) is limited to 1 $L/h \cdot m^2$ or 670 W/m^2. In the simulation, absorbed RF energy, expressed as SAR in W/kg, is averaged over the whole body and is added to the metabolic heat production. It is also assumed that the energy is being absorbed continuously rather than aperiodically as is actually the case during the imaging process. This is a reasonable simplification given the thermal inertia of body tissues and fluids.

METHODS

Effects of Precooling

The first part of this study examined the effects of a 20-min precooling of the patient to the prevailing ambient conditions on the thermoregulatory responses achieved at the end of a subsequent 20-min MRI scan. The specific values of relevant variables were as follows:

$T_a = T_r = 15$ or 20 °C,

RH = 50%,

v = 0.1 m/s (still air conditions),

1 met,

clo = 0.4,

$SkBF_{max} = 90$ $L/h \cdot m^2$ (normal),

SAR = 2, 4, and 8 W/kg.

No precooling was available during the control condition. Output was generated for all possible combinations of $T_a = T_r$ and SAR, with and without precooling. Each run consisted of a 20-min prescan period with no RF present, a 20-min MRI scan at a given SAR, and a 20-min postscan period with no RF present. Data were computed at 2-min intervals throughout each run. In the analysis of the data, particular attention was paid to the change in deep body temperature (T_{co}), skin blood flow (SkBF), the rate of sweat secretion (REG_{sw}), and the index of thermal discomfort (Disc), as these variables changed with or without precooling.

Effects of Added Insulation

The second part of the study examined the effects of added insulation in the form of a blanket (1 clo) placed over the whole body. The specific conditions modeled were as follows:

$$T_a = T_r = 20\ °C,$$
$$RH = 50\%,$$
$$v = 0.1\ m/s\ (\text{still air conditions}),$$
$$1\ met,$$
$$clo = 0.4\ and\ 1.4,$$
$$SkBF_{max} = 90\ L/h{\cdot}m^2\ (\text{normal}),$$
$$SAR = 2,\ 4,\ and\ 8\ W/kg.$$

Output was generated for all possible combinations of clo and SAR. Each run consisted of a 20-min prescan, a 20-min MRI scan at a given SAR, and a 20-min postscan recovery period. No blanket (insulation = 0.4 clo) was available in the control condition at each SAR. In the analysis of the predictions, particular attention was paid to the change in core temperature during the MRI scan.

Experimental Verification of Predictions

The third part of the study involved tests of two male subjects under specific conditions that had been used to predict thermoregulatory responses during MRI scans (subject H.B.: 20 years of age, 6' tall, 185 pounds; subject J.S.: 47 years of age, 5'8" tall, 170 pounds). The Yale G.E. Signa 1.5-T MR System was used for the tests, which were conducted under normal clinical conditions ($T_a = T_r = 20\ °C$; 50% RH; $v = 0.1\ m/s$). Each subject, clad only in shorts, was given a brief physical and was then instrumented with temperature probes from a Luxtron Model 3000 Fluoroptic Thermometer. Esophageal temperature (probe at the level of the right atrium) and four skin temperatures (chest, inner thigh, forehead, and umbilicus) were measured. In addition, sweat rate was determined from the changes in dew-point temperature (T_{dp}) of room air drawn through capsules attached to chest and thigh skin. During the tests, the subject's body was centered within the bore of the machine and the lower half was covered with a light sheet-blanket. Periodically, the subject was asked to report on his thermal sensations and thermal comfort.

All tests began with a minimum 30-min equilibration to the ambient conditions (air off within the bore). Two or three 20-min MRI scans were then conducted, with a minimum 30-min reequilibration between successive scans. The maximum power output of the system was used during each scan; this produced an SAR of about 1.2 W/kg. Temperature data were recorded every minute during the test and sweating was recorded continuously on strip charts. Data for individual scans on each subject were compared with trends predicted by the two-node model under the same conditions.

RESULTS

Predicted Effects of Precooling on Thermoregulatory Responses during a 20-min MRI Scan

As background data for our calculations, it was important to know the predicted responses of a normal person to a 20-min MRI scan under conditions that normally prevail in the clinic. Both skin and core temperatures change slightly during exposure to the prescan environment. The level at the end of the prescan period was determined for each measure and the minute-to-minute change from this level was calculated across an MRI scan of 40-min duration. Sample functions for the change in core and mean skin temperature, together with the associated sweat rate, are shown in FIGURE 1 for a patient with normal $SkBF_{max}$ (90 L/h · m²). The parameter in each panel is the imposed SAR, which varies from 1 to 4 W/kg. The associated change in predicted SkBF over time, for the same range of SAR, is shown in FIGURE 2. The figures indicate that the change in core temperature at the end of the first 20 min is insignificant at SAR = 1–3 W/kg and is still less than 0.5 °C at SAR = 4 W/kg. The mean skin temperature rises significantly at all SARs because of the rapid increase in SkBF, but it stabilizes before the end of 40 min, presumably as a result of the initiation of significant sweating. In general, the higher the SAR, the more vigorous the sweating and the less the rise in skin temperature.

From plots such as those in FIGURES 1 and 2, the predicted alteration in response produced by a 20-min precooling of the patient to either a 20 or 15 °C environment could be determined. FIGURE 3 illustrates a generalized pattern of response change induced by precooling, in this case the mean skin temperature. No precooling occurred under control conditions. The figure indicates that skin temperature falls gradually during precooling to a level determined by the ambient temperature, the air velocity, and the duration of precooling. However, the difference between precooled and control skin temperature is gradually eliminated during the MRI scan at a rate that depends on the SAR. During the postscan recovery period, further convergence takes place until the precooling advantage may be entirely lost.

From plots of the change in core temperature, sweating, and other responses, such as those shown in FIGURES 1 and 2, the predicted response changes were determined after specified MRI scans. FIGURE 4 summarizes the predicted changes in core temperature (ΔT_{co}), SkBF, sweating (REG_{sw}), and thermal discomfort (Disc) at the end of 20-min MRI scans in both 20 and 15 °C environments. The SAR, at values of 2, 4, and 8 W/kg, is coded in the figure by different hatching on the bars. The left bar of each pair indicates responses after no precooling, whereas the right bar indicates responses after 20 min of precooling to the prevailing ambient temperature. In the 20 °C ambient, little improvement in any predicted variable occurs as a result of precooling the patient for 20 min. Slightly greater improvement occurs in the 15 °C environment, especially for sweating rate and discomfort, but the gain is still small. A far greater effect on all variables is related to the shift from a 20 °C to a 15 °C environment, reinforcing our earlier conclusions that a cooler environment is more supportive of thermostability during MRI.[1] FIGURE 4 shows that SkBF is changed somewhat less by precooling than other responses in either environment, presumably because this response is mobilized vigorously at the onset

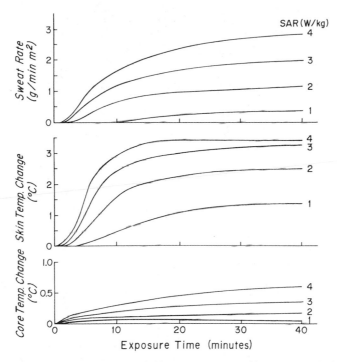

FIGURE 1. Predicted change in core and skin temperatures and in sweat rate during a 40-min MRI scan at SAR = 1–4 W/kg when skin blood flow (SkBF) is normal (90 L/h · m²). Ambient conditions are similar to those in the clinic: air temperature (T_a) and mean radiant temperature (T_r) are constant at 20 °C; relative humidity (RH) is constant at 50%; air movement (v) is constant at 0.1 m/s; metabolism is at resting level (1 met); clothing insulation is at 0.4 clo.

of the scan (cf. FIGURE 2). On the basis of these data, coupled with the fact that precooling is generally uncomfortable for the patient, this procedure would seem best avoided in the clinical setting.

Effects of Added Insulation

In an earlier study,[2] we examined the effects of added insulation (clo = 1.0) during MRI in warm and humid environments $(T_a = T_r = 27$ °C, RH = 80%). Under such ambient conditions, which are very unfavorable for adequate heat loss, we concluded from predictions of SkBF that the use of a light blanket would (i) increase the rapidity with which SkBF reached its maximum, (ii) limit the effectiveness of this vital response, and (iii) thereby exacerbate heat storage in the body. In addition, the added insulation would impede evaporative cooling from the skin surface.

Warm, humid conditions seldom occur in the clinical setting; however, light cotton blankets are commonly used to cover patients during MRI procedures. It is

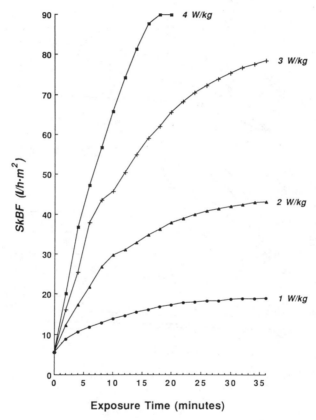

FIGURE 2. Predicted changes in skin blood flow (SkBF) during an MRI scan as a function of exposure duration under ambient conditions similar to those in the clinic (see legend to FIGURE 1). The parameter is SAR in W/kg.

important to know the consequences of this added insulation for the patient's thermoregulatory capability during the procedure. FIGURE 5 shows the predicted effect of a light blanket (clo = 1.0), added to the insulation of pajamas (clo = 0.4), on the elevation of core temperature at the end of a 20-min scan. These predictions, determined under conditions that normally prevail in the clinic, are plotted as a function of SAR (2, 4, and 8 W/kg). The open bars, ranging from 0.15 °C at SAR = 2

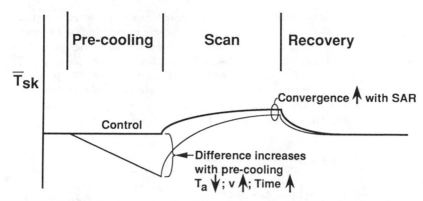

FIGURE 3. Schema showing a generalized response to precooling of a patient before initiation of an MRI scan. The response diagramed is the mean skin temperature (T_{sk}). The three phases represent the precooling period, the scan duration, and the recovery period.

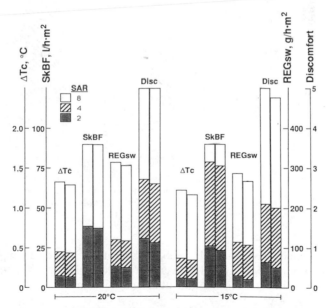

FIGURE 4. Predicted response changes at the end of a 20-min MRI scan at SAR = 2, 4, or 8 W/kg in two environments ($T_a = T_r = 20$ and 15 °C). The left bar of each pair represents no precooling; the right bar represents 20 min of precooling to the prevailing T_a. Individual responses are the change in core temperature (ΔT_{co}), skin blood flow (SkBF), sweat rate (REG$_{sw}$), and thermal discomfort (Disc). Other ambient conditions are similar to those in FIGURE 1.

W/kg to 1.3 °C at 8 W/kg, show the elevation in core temperature when only pajamas are worn. When a blanket covers the patient, these values are predicted to increase by 4% to 29% as SAR increases from 2 to 8 W/kg. The predictions shown in the figure incorporated a 20-min precooling of the patient to the prevailing 20 °C environment; other predictions, not shown here, indicate that the presence or absence of precooling matters little to the maximal elevation of core temperature achieved at the end of the scan. This result agrees with those reported in the previous subsection. In general, this analysis leads to the conclusion that use of a blanket

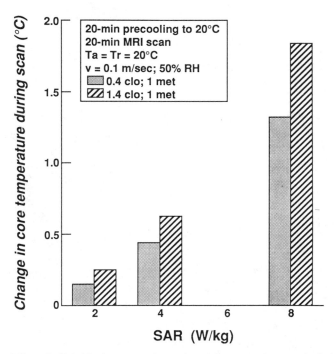

FIGURE 5. Effect of a light blanket over pajamas (1.4 clo) versus pajamas only (0.4 clo) on the change in core temperature at the end of a 20-min MRI scan under ambient conditions similar to those in the clinic (see legend to FIGURE 1). Predictions involve a 20-min precooling of the patient to the prevailing ambient conditions.

under normal clinical conditions always exacerbates the rise in core temperature to be expected during an MRI scan; however, the effect is minimal at the lower SARs that characterize the current generation of imaging machines.

Experimental Verification of Predictions

As detailed earlier, limited pilot experiments were conducted on two male subjects as a first attempt to verify in the clinical setting some of the predictions of the two-node model. Of particular interest was the measured increase in core temperature during individual and successive MRI scans, together with evidence for the mobilization of heat loss responses.

The most applicable predictions are those shown in FIGURE 1. However, some deviations from these modeled conditions should be noted. The model assumes that, during MRI, the RF energy will be uniformly deposited in the body, not localized to certain regions. In our pilot experiments, the subject's torso was centered within the bore, with head and lower legs protruding. Thus, we would expect maximal energy deposition in the trunk. Furthermore, the insulation, modeled as 0.4 clo, was slightly higher; although the subject wore only shorts, part of the body was covered by a light sheet-blanket. Finally, the scans were all of 20-min duration, whereas the predictions extended for 40 min. Although we were unable to measure SkBF, several skin temperatures were monitored that yield information on the nature of the surface heating that is characteristic of MRI in a 1.5-T system.[9]

Both subjects were highly experienced and in excellent health at the time that the measurements were taken. They had each recently completed a series of studies at the Pierce Laboratory that involved exposure to a variety of thermal environments (MRI absent), physiological measurements, and assessment of thermal sensation and thermal comfort.

FIGURE 6 shows representative data collected on subject J.S. during a succession of three 20-min MRI scans at an SAR of about 1.19 W/kg. The first scan was preceded by a 30-min period of equilibration to the prevailing ambient conditions and successive scans were separated by 35-min periods for reequilibration. The middle panel of the figure shows the sweat rate from thigh and chest, whereas the upper panel shows the associated judgments of thermal sensation. The lower panel gives the coincident changes in esophageal and two skin temperatures (chest and thigh). For simplicity, the changes in temperature of the other two sites are not plotted; umbilical temperature mirrored that of the chest, whereas forehead temperature changed minimally over the course of the experiment. For all temperatures, the changes are calculated from the level at the initiation of the first scan.

The figure shows that the esophageal temperature was remarkably stable throughout the 170-min duration of the experiment, varying at most 0.3 °C from the initial level. This stability occurred despite an overall rise of about 2.5 °C in skin temperature and periodic sweating of significant magnitude. A rough interpolation of the predictions in FIGURE 1 would yield, for SAR = 1.19 W/kg, a rise in core temperature of about 0.1 °C at the end of a single 20-min scan, just as was measured on this subject at the end of scan no. 1. It is of considerable interest that the elevation in esophageal temperature tends to increase slightly with each successive scan. This apparently results from the gradual overall increase in skin temperature that will decrease thermal conductance slightly, despite stabilization of the skin temperature after each individual scan.

FIGURE 1 predicts an increase in skin temperature of somewhat over 1 °C at the end of a single 20-min scan at this SAR. This is exactly what was measured at the end of any given scan on both subjects. However, as noted, there was little, if any, recovery between successive scans. In general, thigh temperature tended to rise less than chest temperature; this disparity was even more pronounced for the second subject. The fact that the thighs were located closer than the chest to the edge of the bore, where the RF field is less intense, may explain this finding.

Both subjects showed similar patterns of sweating, including differential recruitment at the two sites tested. The thigh skin exhibited sweating before the chest and consistently at a higher rate. Subject J.S. (FIGURE 6) did not sweat during scan no. 1, but exhibited an increased sweat rate partway through scan no. 2, as predicted in

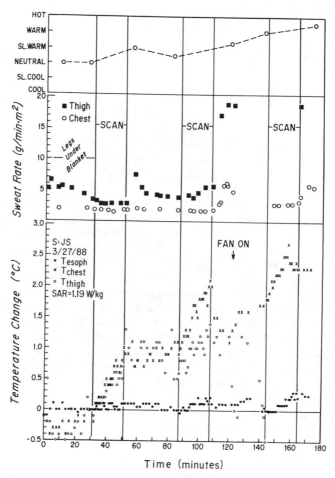

FIGURE 6. Changes in core and two skin temperatures (chest and thigh), sweat rate from two sites (chest and thigh), and judgments of thermal sensation when one subject underwent three successive 20-min MRI scans at SAR = 1.19 W/kg in a 1.5-T imaging system. Ambient conditions are similar to those normally found in the clinic. See text for details.

FIGURE 1. Subject H.B. (data not shown) exhibited increased thigh sweating halfway through scan no. 1 as was predicted and an increased sweat rate throughout the succeeding scan. Curiously, both subjects showed exaggerated sweating at the termination of each scan, a possible "rebound" response. Although we have not published predictions for such a sweating rebound, it may contribute to the recovery of both core and skin temperatures delineated in figure 9 of reference 1. It is clearly related to both the stability of esophageal temperature and the stabilization of skin temperature between scans in the present experiments. It is also related to the judgments of increased warmth expressed by each subject (cf. coded responses, top panel of FIGURE 6).

Taken as a whole, the limited measurements we have made in this study are encouraging indeed. All of the measured response changes were accurately predicted by the two-node model. It remains for future work to determine the accuracy of our predictions of response changes at higher SARs.

SUMMARY AND CONCLUSIONS

A relatively simple two-node model of human thermoregulation was developed to predict response changes during MRI procedures.[1] Subsequent modifications of the model simulated impairments in cardiovascular function in terms of altered skin blood flow.[2] In the present work, the model was programmed to predict the consequences of certain procedures used in the clinic, namely, precooling of the patient to the prevailing environment and covering the patient with a light blanket. Some of the fundamental predictions of the model during 20-min MRI scans at a low SAR were tested on two male subjects in the clinical setting. The following conclusions may be drawn:

(1) Precooling of the patient for 20 min to the prevailing ambient conditions, whether inadvertent or deliberate, has little value in terms of preventing a rise in body temperatures. At the conclusion of a subsequent 20-min MRI scan, even at SARs as low as 2 W/kg, the modest effects of precooling are all but eliminated. Thus, inadvertent precooling should be no cause for concern; deliberate precooling carries little advantage for the patient and wastes valuable time.

(2) Use of a blanket during an MRI scan should be discouraged in the normal clinical setting except when the SAR is 2 W/kg or less. At higher SARs, this added insulation impedes convective and radiative heat loss through evaporation of sweat. The result is an increase of heat storage in the body and a greater rise in core temperature than would occur otherwise.

(3) Clinical tests on two normal male subjects have provided limited confirmation of the predictions of the two-node model. During 20-min MRI scans at a whole-body SAR of 1.2 W/kg, core and skin temperatures, sweat rate, and judgments of thermal sensation and discomfort were very similar to predicted values. Unexpected findings of an incremental increase in core temperature with successive scans and a sweating rebound following each scan may be important for future investigation.

(4) Although pleased with the limited confirmation of our predictions, we are constantly aware of the limitations of the two-node model to accurately predict thermoregulatory responses of patients undergoing clinical MRI of various body parts. It is essential to keep in mind that the simulations are based on RF exposure of the whole body; thus, the predicted increase in core temperature will be proportionately higher than would be the case if only a

portion of the body were exposed within the MRI device. We recommend that any further predictions of this genre be undertaken with a model having many more nodes, such as that developed by Stolwijk.[11] Additionally, more experimental data are needed on well-instrumented subjects who are carefully equilibrated to the prevailing ambient conditions and who are tested at whole-body SARs from 1 to 4 W/kg. Continuous measurements should be made of an assortment of thermophysiological responses, including esophageal and several skin temperatures, sweat rate from several sites, skin wetness, skin blood flow, temperature sensation, and thermal discomfort.

ACKNOWLEDGMENTS

We are grateful to John Gore of the Yale MR Center for permission to use the 1.5-T Yale imaging system and to Robert Lange for his collaborative assistance in conducting the experiments at Yale, some dosimetry, and the SAR determinations. Without their help, we would not have been able to test our predictions in the clinical environment. We are also grateful to Kenneth Wickersheim of the Luxtron Corporation for loaning us the Luxtron Model 3000 Fluoroptic Thermometer used in these studies.

REFERENCES

1. ADAIR, E. R. & L. G. BERGLUND. 1986. On the thermoregulatory consequences of NMR imaging. Magn. Reson. Imag. **4:** 321–333.
2. ADAIR, E. R. & L. G. BERGLUND. 1989. Thermoregulatory consequences of cardiovascular impairment during NMR imaging in warm/humid environments. Magn. Reson. Imag. **7:** 25–37.
3. ADAIR, E. R. & L. G. BERGLUND. 1987. Reply to Shellock and Crues. Magn. Reson. Imag. **5:** 507.
4. BERGLUND, L. G. & J. A. J. STOLWIJK. 1978. The use of simulation models of human thermoregulation in assessing acceptability of complex dynamic thermal environments. *In* Energy Conservation Strategies in Buildings. J. A. J. Stolwijk, Ed.: 157–191. John B. Pierce Foundation Laboratory. New Haven, Connecticut.
5. STOLWIJK, J. A. J. & J. D. HARDY. 1966. Temperature regulation in man—a theoretical study. Pflügers Arch. Gesamte Physiol. Menschen Tiere **291:** 129–162.
6. WISSLER, E. H. 1988. Modeling exposure to thermal stress. *In* Environmental Ergonomics. E. W. Banister & J. B. Morrison, Eds.: 267–285. Taylor & Francis. London.
7. BOTTOMLEY, P. A., R. W. REDINGTON, W. A. EDELSTEIN & J. F. SCHENCK. 1985. Magn. Reson. Med. **2:** 336.
8. LAGENDIJK, J. J. W. 1987. Tissue temperature measurements and power deposition in NMR imaging. *In* Safety Assessment of NMR Clinical Equipment. K. H. Schmidt, Ed.: 7. Thieme. Stuttgart.
9. GUY, A. W. Unpublished data.
10. GANDHI, O. P. Unpublished data.
11. STOLWIJK, J. A. J. 1971. A mathematical model of physiological temperature regulation in man. NASA Report No. CR-1855. NASA. Washington, District of Columbia.

Session III Summary[a]

W. GREGORY LOTZ

Naval Aerospace Medical Research Laboratory
Pensacola, Florida 32508-5700

The session on high power, pulsed radio-frequency fields consisted of six papers that addressed issues of dosimetry, cellular effects, and thermophysiological effects that are associated with the radio-frequency (RF) signals used in nuclear magnetic resonance imaging (MRI) or spectroscopy (MRS). These papers provided a stimulating, insightful, up-to-date overview of this particular area of bioelectromagnetics. Four of the papers were concerned with theoretical dosimetry and employed numerical methods to predict the specific absorption rate (SAR) in the body during MRI. The other two papers were concerned with the biological responses to these fields in cells or in animals and humans where their effect on thermal physiology is of primary importance. The dosimetry papers included two presentations [(i) Gandhi and Chen and (ii) Grandolfo *et al.*] of research using numerical analysis of a complex, anatomically realistic model of the human body composed of several thousand individual cells or compartments (typically 1–1.5 cm in length). This modeling technique is known as the "impedance method" because each cell is characterized by its electrical impedance. Two other theoretical dosimetry papers [(i) Bottomley and Roemer and (ii) Boesiger *et al.*] were based on numerical analyses of simpler geometric models of spheres and cylinders. Initial work in the field of dosimetry of MRI used the simpler geometric models, whereas the application of the impedance method to MRI is a new contribution. The individual papers discussed the assumptions, strengths, and weaknesses of each method. These dosimetry methods are directed toward the analysis of the primary known effect of radio-frequency exposure, namely, heating of tissues. The techniques must take into account or make assumptions for the many complex factors affecting the absorption of RF energy by the body, including frequency, variations in time and space of the intensity of the magnetic field, coupling efficiency between the RF coil and the body, duty cycle and waveform of the specific pulse sequence used in imaging, electrical properties of different tissues, geometry, and orientation of the body with respect to the polarity of the field. All of the authors deal with both average and local (or peak) SARs for various MRI conditions. Considerations of local SARs in different regions of the body (e.g., skin) are the most difficult to determine and thus are the ones that received the most discussion.

The impedance method has the capability to provide much more detailed information about internal current distribution and local SAR than the simpler geometric models. However, one of the points that stimulated the most discussion, in this session, was the difference of opinion over the significance of eddy currents in determining the SAR. Bottomley and Roemer presented challenging arguments

---

[a]The views expressed in this article are those of the author and do not necessarily reflect the official policy or position of the Department of the Navy, the Department of Defense, nor the United States Government.

based on their simpler models that eddy currents represent a very important determinant in the SAR deposited during an MRI scan. Gandhi disagreed, though, both in his initial presentation and in the discussion that followed, as he presented his rationale for not including them in the factors of his model. This point was only one aspect of some lively discussion that indicated a need for additional research to improve our understanding of the distribution of RF energy deposited in the body during MRI and MRS.

Another point of particular interest in this session was the aspect of local SAR created by the interaction between decoupling surface coils and body coils, where both are employed. The papers by Bottomley and Roemer and by Boesiger *et al.* discussed at length the factors involved in the decoupling techniques, as well as the possibility that locally high SARs in excess of exposure guidelines may be generated. The paper by Boesiger *et al.* is somewhat unique among these dosimetry papers in that it combines numerical predictions with empirical measurements of a simple phantom to evaluate the influence on the SAR of coupling between the body coil and surface coil. A few comparisons to published data from measurements with patients have been made, but very little empirical data are available to evaluate the theoretical dosimetry predictions. This is clearly an area where more research needs to be conducted.

A distinctly different paper was presented by Cleary *et al.* Their work not only addressed biology rather than theoretical dosimetry research, but it raised the question of whether effects other than those caused by tissue heating might be important in evaluating the biological effects of MRI and MRS. Although data are limited, Cleary and co-workers present a summary of cellular effects that have been reported in the range of frequencies relevant to MRI. A large proportion of these data are from *in vitro* studies and raise questions of direct, field-related effects on cell function that may be independent of demonstrable heating of the tissue. The authors acknowledge that no mechanism is known to explain some of these findings, but the number of studies that have found cellular effects of RF exposure under isothermal conditions is compelling. In the discussion at the conference, Cleary was challenged to defend his conclusion that these cellular effects indicate a mechanism other than RF-induced heating, but no alternative explanation of the nature of these effects was offered by those who found his interpretation unacceptable. Cleary concluded with a useful summary of research needed to answer the questions raised by these reports.

In the final paper of the session, Adair and Berglund summarized work with a simple, two-dimensional model of the thermoregulatory system. Their analysis is directed towards clinically relevant situations, for example, precooling the patient, that would affect the thermoregulatory response. Their data are clear and allow them to make predictions of the expected temperature rises that are likely to occur in tissue (skin, fat, muscle) for specific MRI exposure conditions. An important consideration of the model they used was that it assumed uniform heat deposition by the MRI fields, which is not a valid assumption and which would be even further from the actual deposition pattern for higher frequency RF signals. In their conclusions, Adair and Berglund recommended additional research of this type using more complex models with a greater number of body compartments in order to deal more realistically with the heterogeneous nature of the SAR distribution in the body during MRI and MRS procedures.

Overall, this group of papers, although stemming from an area of the conference for which the most extensive background research probably exists (bioeffects of RF exposure), pointed out some serious limitations in our present knowledge and the resulting needs for future research in these aspects of nuclear magnetic resonance techniques. These research needs take on even greater significance when considering the prospect of increasing static magnetic field strengths in newer MRI devices, with associated shifts to higher RF frequencies. I have already mentioned the debate over the significance of eddy currents in predicting the SAR. There are also limitations with the modeling done thus far dealing with nonuniform power distribution within the body and particularly in predicting the SAR at frequencies above 60 MHz. The cellular bioeffects summarized in the report by Cleary *et al.* provide more questions than answers about the type of fields used in MRI and MRS. The levels of average SAR generated by present MRI devices are, by all accounts, below any standards yet promulgated. Potentially excessive local peak SARs must be investigated further. As a whole, more empirical data are required to confirm the models developed and to lead us to more conclusive data about the biological effects of strong pulsed radio-frequency fields associated with MRI and MRS.

An Overview of Electromagnetic Safety Considerations Associated with Magnetic Resonance Imaging

EMANUEL KANAL

Department of Radiology
University of Pittsburgh
Pittsburgh NMR Institute
Pittsburgh, Pennsylvania 15213

INTRODUCTION

The introduction of magnetic resonance imaging into the clinical patient care arena has enabled a marked expansion of the diagnostic capabilities of the radiologist. The field has continued to grow each year with significant improvements and advances in such areas as transmitter/receiver coil design, pulse sequence design and optimization, and technical advances in other MR-related hardware devices. This rapid growth, however, has not been accompanied by an equivalent dissemination and understanding of the potential, or real, safety considerations that might be associated with this modality. Although most who work in this environment are aware of the potential interactions between the magnetic field of the imaging system and ferromagnetic objects, there seems to be a relative lack of understanding of some of the other safety issues associated with the imaging environment and function of a magnetic resonance imaging system. The recent renewed awakening of public interest in safety considerations of electromagnetic fields in general and the recent appearance of several comprehensive MR safety review articles[1-5] have increased the timeliness of such a safety overview regarding electromagnetic and magnetic fields associated with magnetic resonance imaging, angiographic, and spectroscopic systems.

Clinical magnetic resonance imaging, as it is presently practiced, is associated with several types of potential health concerns that impact both the patient as well as the health practitioners themselves that work in and around this environment. These can be classified and subdivided into several major areas, with varying degrees of importance depending upon such issues as field strength, magnet design, etc. The more common issues include the following:

(1) Possible effects associated with the static magnetic and/or static gradient magnetic fields:
    (a) Potential biologic effects of the static magnetic fields and static magnetic field gradients.
    (b) Safety considerations pertaining to the attractive forces exerted by the static magnetic field on ferromagnetic material. These include torque and collision hazards as well as considerations of direct interactions between the static magnetic field and implanted devices.

(2) Possible effects from the time-varying magnetic fields associated with magnetic resonance imaging systems. These include the following:
  (a) Possible effects from the more slowly changing magnetic fields/magnetic field gradients:
    (i) Potential effects of electrical voltages and currents that might be induced within biologic tissue as a result of such gradient magnetic field switching inherent to the MR imaging process. These considerations are especially important as the much larger dB/dt values (rates of magnetic field change over time) used in such sequences as echo planar imaging become more commonly utilized and more generally available and accessible to the diagnostic radiologic community.
    (ii) Auditory considerations from the rapidly pulsed/cycled magnetic field gradients.
  (b) Possible effects from the rapidly (RF) changing magnetic fields:
    (i) Concerns that are associated with heat deposition and other potential biologic interactions within the patient as a result of the radio-frequency (RF) magnetic fields associated with MR imaging. This area incorporates concern over both diffuse power deposition/heating as well as inhomogeneous, or focal, heating that may result from such imaging sequences.
    (ii) Issues related to current induction, and eventual heating, of extraneous objects in the MR imaging device. This area includes power deposition into electrically conductive materials, such as EKG leads, plethysmographic gating wires, pulse oximeter leads, etc., that may themselves become heated during exposure to RF-oscillating magnetic fields. This heating may be so marked as to be sufficient to induce thermal injury via direct conductive heat transfer from the electrically conductive material itself to the patient with which it comes into contact.
    (iii) Although not technically a direct safety issue, there is an at least indirect issue of having the induced currents within electrically conductive material adjacent to the patient result in a distorted MR image that might be uninterpretable—or worse, misleading—in the anatomic region of interest.
    (iv) Possible biologic effects from exposure of patients and/or health practitioners to the time-varying magnetic field gradients inherent to magnetic resonance imaging processes. Included herein will also be possible effects from modulation, at extremely low frequency (ELF) ranges, of the baseline RF-oscillating magnetic fields associated with the resonance frequency of the individual imaging systems.
(3) Miscellaneous considerations:
  (a) Superconductive system concerns, including electrical and cryogenic considerations of a quench, and cryogen storage and handling issues.
  (b) Potential health considerations of any of various types of contrast agents utilized for clinical or research MR environments.
  (c) Issues of claustrophobia and anxiety related to exposure to such environments.

(As the scope of this review pertains to magnetic and electromagnetic fields, the third category of "miscellaneous considerations" will not be dealt with herein in any detail.)

There are thus numerous issues that need to be identified, considered, and addressed regarding the safety of a magnetic resonance examination vis-à-vis any particular patient, volunteer, or MR health care provider. The more knowledgeable that we are in recognizing and understanding these concerns, the more wisely we will be able to pursue a course of accurate diagnostic evaluation—and even interpretation—concerning magnetic resonance imaging examinations.

DISCUSSION

Static Magnetic Field Biologic Effects

Numerous studies into the possible safety effects of exposure of various organisms to static magnetic fields have yielded confusing and even conflicting results.[6-44] Some investigators have failed to reveal any detectable, clinically significant deleterious effects from static magnetic fields. On the other hand, other studies have demonstrated detectable biological (albeit not necessarily harmful) effects of static magnetic fields on various organisms.

Alteration in the shape of normal red blood cells and in the alignment of sickled red blood cells has been repeatedly demonstrated *in vitro* as has *in vitro* alignment of fibrin and fibrinogen in the presence of strong magnetic fields. Experientially, however, these do not seem to have an effect that is significant clinically in an *in vivo* setting.[45-49] Similarly, the known *in vitro* alignment of photoreceptor cells of the eye in the presence of magnetic fields of the strength used in clinical MR imaging systems does not seem to result in any detectable clinical effects.[50]

Electrocardiographic Alterations

It has been long known that electrocardiographic alterations can be observed when measured in the presence of a static magnetic field.[51] As a manifestation of flow potentials from motion of an electrical conductor, namely, blood, in the presence of such a magnetic field, this often results in variations, and often elevation, of especially the T wave segment of the electrocardiographic tracing. It should be noted that the magnitude of these changes is lower and therefore less apparent at lower magnetic field strengths. Although the current densities thus produced are not felt to be clinically significant, their existence should be recognized and should not be confused with signs of patient distress. Furthermore, there may rarely be sufficient elevation of the T wave segment to produce technical difficulties while attempting to gate or trigger the RF pulse timing of the MR imaging system relative to the timing of the QRS complex of the cardiac cycle.

Although no deleterious biologic effects from the static magnetic fields used in MRI have been definitively associated with this modality, it might be safely concluded that the answers may not all be in as of yet; hence, further research is continuing in this area.

Static Magnetic Field Physical Effects

The physical interaction between the static magnetic field of the MR imaging systems and ferromagnetic articles (i.e., used throughout this review to refer to objects capable of demonstrating attraction to magnetic fields/gradients) is one of the most significant and well-publicized safety considerations associated with MR imaging environments. This attraction can be quite substantial at the field strengths commonly utilized in diagnostic MR imaging systems. There are some rather prevalent and significant limitations of understanding, or even overt misconceptions, regarding the potential for harm resulting from exposure to various types of MR imaging systems. For example, is there a reason for concern for exposure to ultra low field imaging systems, with field strengths of only 200 to 600 gauss? Are magnetically shielded systems inherently more "safe" than nonshielded ones? Are systems with permanent magnets more immune to such considerations than are the superconducting ones? Is screening with a metal detector sufficient? The proliferation of multiple types of magnet hardware design and implementation makes dissemination of reliable data concerning this topic even more crucial to ensure that safe practices are being followed throughout the industry.

As background information, the forces experienced by a ferromagnetic object result from interactions between the magnetization of the object and the static magnetic field generated by the MR imaging system. Such forces result in rotational (torque) and/or translational (attractive) motion of the object. The exact nature and magnitude of the resultant force is itself dependent upon the configuration of the magnetic field and the shape/geometry and orientation of the object. Thus, ferromagnetic material in a spherical shape might have a markedly different set of forces acting upon it within the magnetic sphere of influence of the imaging magnet than would an identical mass of the same ferromagnetic material stretched into a linear, rodlike shape.

The tendency of an elongated ferromagnetic material to orient itself so that its long axis is parallel to the direction of the field is a manifestation of the torque experienced by the object. This can occur even in a homogeneous magnetic field. In contrast, a net attractive force that causes translational motion of the object is only encountered in an inhomogeneous magnetic field (i.e., a static field gradient). The attractive force exerted upon ferromagnetic objects is therefore dependent upon the magnitude of the static magnetic field gradient experienced by the object and their orientation relative to each other. In clinical imaging centers, these factors are themselves affected by such variables as the distance of the object from the center of the magnet, the strength of the magnet, the geometry of the object and its orientation relative to the static magnetic field gradient, and the configuration of the static magnetic field gradient itself. The latter refers to factors that might affect the three-dimensional configuration of the static magnetic field gradient, such as magnetic shielding.

It is also true that different objects may prove to possess various degrees of ferromagnetism. It is, for example, a serious misconception to believe that "surgical stainless" or "stainless steel" implies a nonferromagnetic nature to the material. Briefly, there are several major types of stainless steel, including ferritic, austenitic, and martensitic types.[52] The greater the degree of ferritic or martensitic composition of the particular type of metal or stainless steel, the greater the degree of ferromagnetism that will be exhibited by that metal. For example, all type 400 series stainless steels are strongly ferromagnetic, whereas most (but not all) of the 300 series stainless steels are austenitic and thus nonferromagnetic. It is, therefore, quite important to realize that not all stainless steel articles used, for example, in hospitals for medical care are necessarily magnet-safe.

A ferromagnetic metallic structure, when within the body, might be sufficiently attracted to or have a sufficient amount of torque exerted upon it by the magnetic field to create a hazardous situation for the patient or health practitioner. Examples of such foreign material would be certain types of intracranial aneurysm clips, shrapnel located in biologically sensitive areas such as near the spinal cord, intraorbital metallic foreign bodies, etc. Also included would be prosthetic limbs or other objects on the patient that might injure the patient if sufficient force is exerted upon them. These factors should be carefully considered before subjecting a patient with a ferromagnetic implant or material to MRI, particularly if it is located in a potentially dangerous area of the body where movement or dislodgment could injure the patient. The identified potential offending object should be then checked (after a positive identification is made) against a known list of tested objects for MR compatibility.[53-65]

It is also important to be cognizant of the necessity to appropriately screen everyone who will be approaching the static magnetic field for the possible presence of such ferromagnetic implants or "onplants". This requires screening of not only the patients being examined on such imaging systems, but also any accompanying family or professional health care personnel, including physicians, nurses, technologists, and physicists.

From a practical, clinical point of view, there are two categories of concern when dealing with interactions between static magnetic fields and ferromagnetic objects. One deals with forces that are exerted upon ferromagnetic objects that are located within, on, or distant from the patient and health practitioners when exposed to the static magnetic field. The other deals with those resulting from potential interactions between magnetically sensitive devices or equipment (either in or on the patient or health practitioner) whose integrity may be adversely affected by the magnetic field. When such malfunction could jeopardize the well-being of the patient (or health care provider), the latter category becomes even more of a contraindication. These two categories are now considered in more detail.

First, items that might be located either on or distant from the patient and health care personnel present a hazard that has come to be known as the so-called projectile, or missile, effect. This refers to the potential for ferromagnetic objects of virtually any size to gain sufficient speed during an attraction to the magnet that the accumulated kinetic energy could prove quite disastrous or even lethal if expended upon an intervening patient or health practitioner. TABLE 1 lists several examples of ferromagnetic objects that were inadvertently introduced into clinical or research magnetic resonance imaging environments.[1,66] The outcome of such exposures in the mishaps involving the objects in TABLE 1 ranged from minimal damage to severe injury and death.

Numerous studies have assessed the ferromagnetic qualities of various metallic implants and materials by measuring the deflection forces due to the static magnetic fields used for MRI. Most of these implants and onplants are indeed "magnet-safe", but there is an impressive list of such items that are to be considered unacceptable for such MR environments and that should be considered contraindications to such an examination if present.[59]

The second category of concern deals with magnetically sensitive equipment (either in or on the patient or health practitioner) whose integrity may be adversely affected by the magnetic field. When such malfunction could jeopardize the well-being of the patient (or health practitioner), this becomes even more of a contraindication.

The prime example of such a device would be that of a pacemaker (or a cousin of this device known as an automatic implantable cardioverter defibrillator).[67-71] There are several factors that combine to make the presence of a pacemaker in a patient a contraindication to undergoing an MR examination at any field strength. First, most modern pacemakers contain a reed switch that enables bypassing of the sensing mechanism of the pacemaker and asynchronous excitation. This switch is itself

TABLE 1. Objects Reported as Having Been Inadvertently Exposed/Attracted to an MRI Magnet

Fans	Forklift tines	"Sand" bags
Vacuum cleaner	Prosthetic limbs	Hairpins
Calculators	Keys	Tools
Insulin infusion pump	Watches	Cigarette lighters
Wheelchairs	Tile roller	Film magazines
Scissors	Pens/pencils/clips	Steel-tipped/heeled shoes
Chest tube stand	Pulse oximeters	Tile cutter
Buckets	Jewelry	Hearing aids
Assorted prosthetic devices/	Oxygen tanks	IV poles
surgical implants	Clipboards	Gurneys
Pacemakers	Stethoscopes	Knives
ID badges	Pagers	Mops
Nail clippers	Magnets	MR table parts
Shrapnel	Buffing machine	Gun

activated by holding a strong magnet over it. Furthermore, cardiac pacemakers are known to have their function adversely affected by field strengths as low as 17 gauss. Indeed, some of the more modern, smaller pacemakers contain less metal in their housing and thus possess less shielding as well. There are some recent data to suggest that such pacemakers might well have their normal function affected in fields as small as 5 to 7 gauss. There is thus no magnetic resonance imaging system at any currently utilized field strength that might be considered safe for imaging of patients with implanted cardiac pacemakers. The more dependent the patient is upon the continued uninterrupted function of the pacemaker, the more we should consider entry of such a patient into such an environment contraindicated. There are also several components within the pacemaker (including the lithium battery itself) that may be ferromagnetic and of sufficient mass to pose a possible hazard to the patient from a potential torque effect. Finally, the pacemaker leads themselves might serve as antennae, with the potential result being that the heart might be effectively paced during the MR examination at the frequency of the applied imaging pulses. This could have disastrous consequences in the form of secondary hypotension and possibly even fibrillation. At least two patients with cardiac pacemakers apparently experienced a cardiac arrest and expired while in an MR imaging system.[72] In at least one of these cases, the FDA statement reports that ". . . the coroner determined that the death was due to the interruption of the pacemaker by the MR system".[72] For all the aforementioned reasons, it is thus my strong opinion that patients with cardiac pacemakers be entirely restricted from not only undergoing MR examinations, but that they also be physically restricted to remaining at or outside of, at most, the 5-gauss line surrounding the MR imaging environment.

Magnetic Shielding and Permanent Magnet Systems

The three-dimensional configuration and strength of the fringe magnetic field associated with magnetic resonance imaging sites is extremely variable. Not only is this dependent upon the strength of the imaging system, but it is also dependent upon the presence or absence of magnetic shielding. There are vast differences in the degree, type, and even presence or absence of magnetic shielding in clinical and research MR imaging sites. With the relatively recent addition of intrinsic shielding to the types of shielding available, it is entirely possible for one new to the site to not be able to detect externally that the system is magnetically shielded by simply looking at it, as the shielding may be entirely located within the faceplate of the magnet housing itself. There are also permanent magnet designs wherein the fringe field is intrinsically very tightly constrained. Unfortunately, the very label of "shielding" seems to connote a higher level of safety. This may in actuality indeed be so for magnetically sensitive devices adjacent to the imaging system located outside of the shield. However, the presence of such sharply demarcated and rapidly, spatially, changing magnetic fields as may be found at the borders of such magnetic shields or permanent magnet designs may actually be of significant concern for those passing this threshold. As the amount of torque actually experienced by a ferromagnetic object is at least partially dependent upon the strength of the magnetic field gradient that it traverses, such "tight" fringe fields may certainly harbor every bit as much potential for projectile and/or torque effect as the same system without such shielding or such narrowly constrained fringe field contours. In some such systems, it is entirely possible to have an object traverse from background, subgauss magnetic field strengths to several hundred or even thousand gauss. Indeed, such a configuration might actually thus exert a force on the ferromagnetic object that might be even greater than it would have been had there been no shielding at all or had there been a more gradual tapering of the fringe static magnetic fields. Ironic as it may seem, shielded systems, their names notwithstanding, might present an even greater hazard to the patient/health practitioners than nonshielded ones, as they would provide less opportunity for a more gradual "warning" of attraction of a ferromagnetic object inadvertently being brought into this environment.

Permanent systems benefit from generally being restricted to lower magnetic field strengths than their superconductive counterparts. Nevertheless, their tightly constrained fringe fields can produce very significant static magnetic field gradients over space. There has been at least one incident whereby an insulin infusion pump on a patient was apparently knowingly permitted into the MR imaging system due to what appears to have been a misconception concerning the safety of a low field permanent magnet system.[66] Although this case luckily resulted in only minimal injury to the patient and damage to the pump, such incidents do serve to illustrate the need for increased safety education and awareness in the industry.

As a generalization, therefore, it is crucial to recognize that systems with magnetic shielding, or even permanent magnet systems, are by no means immune to the considerations of the interactions of the static magnetic field and its spatial gradient with ferromagnetic objects.

As an aside, it is my opinion that there is no real place for relying on the usage of metal detectors in magnetic resonance sites. These devices have variable sensitivity settings that can be set and that can be applied with varying degrees of skill by various operators or even the same operator at different times and with different patients. Perhaps most importantly, ferromagnetic objects or foreign bodies that may be in anatomically sensitive locations, such as the eye or spinal canal, may be of sufficiently small mass as to escape detection by such devices even when used appropriately by skilled operators, yet might still experience sufficient torque and/or attractive force as to result in significant injury. Thus, a positive metal detector screen should be considered significant, but a negative one is virtually worthless. It should certainly not be used as the only means of screening a patient or health care operator for entrance into the vicinity of the magnet. At best, its results (if used at all) should be combined with an adequate history and other available data prior to permitting access to the site.

Effects of Switched Magnetic Fields: Induced Voltages/Currents

Along with the transient repeated and rapid application of magnetic field gradients to which the patient is exposed during MR imaging comes the associated potential to induce voltages within the patient from Faraday's law. The current induced by such a voltage is itself dependent upon several factors, including the time rate of change of the magnetic field (dB/dt) (i.e., the induced voltage), the cross-sectional area of the conducting tissue loop, and the conductivity/resistance of the tissue. Hence, the induced currents will be generated during gradient rise/fall times. Biological effects of induced currents, if any, may result either from the power deposited by the induced currents (thermal effects) or from direct effects of the induced current (nonthermal effects). The thermal effects due to switched gradients used in MR imaging are negligible,[73-75] whereas those relating to current induction require more elaboration and investigation.

In typical multislice-mode whole-body MR imaging, magnetic field gradients of roughly 0.01 tesla/meter (T/m) are switched on or off in a time duration of 0.5–1.0 ms every few milliseconds. This corresponds to a field variation of 5.0 to 2.5 T/s at a distance of 25 cm from the center of the magnet. Human body tissue inhomogeneities, though, make accurate estimation of the induced current difficult. Furthermore, more recently developed and investigational sequences such as echo planar techniques utilize much greater time rates of change of the gradient magnetic fields used for imaging. Recent studies have reported what appears to have been peripheral muscle stimulation observed during such imaging techniques on humans beyond a threshold of 60 T/s.[76,77]

There is a strong frequency dependence in determining the threshold of current required to produce biological effects. This "biological-detectability" threshold is further dependent upon the duration of the induced current, the repetition rate of the study, and the waveform shape.[78] Nevertheless, once this threshold is passed, among the possible nonthermal effects of induced currents are stimulation of nerve or muscle cells, induction of ventricular fibrillation, increased brain mannitol space,[79] epileptogenic potential, stimulation of visual flash sensations (so-called "magnetophosphenes"), and bone healing. Of these, the threshold currents required for nerve stimulation or ventricular fibrillation are known to be much higher than those that are estimated to be induced at routine clinical MR imaging conditions. Although numerous seizures have been reported to have occurred during active clinical MR imaging examinations, there are no data that suggest that this is in any way secondary to induced voltages or currents and not, for example, related to the auditory or visual or other such excitatory stimuli associated with clinical MR examinations. Magnetophosphenes, as noted earlier, are felt to result from direct excitation of the optic nerve/retina by currents induced by rapid gradient magnetic field alterations or, alternatively, rapid eye motion within a static magnetic field.[80–82] These have not been reported to my knowledge at exposure to static magnetic fields of up to and including 1.95 teslas (i.e., those static field levels approved by the Food and Drug Administration), although they have been reported in volunteers working in and around a 4+ tesla research system.[83] In addition, a metallic taste and symptoms of vertigo seem to also be relatively reproducible symptoms associated with rapid motion within the static magnetic field of these 4+ tesla imaging/research systems.[83] It should be pointed out that the current densities necessary to elicit such a visual stimulus are several orders of magnitude below those estimated to be needed to induce nerve action potentials or even ventricular fibrillation.[1] Finally, although bone healing does indeed seem to occur at comparable current densities as those induced in clinical MR imaging examinations, repeated application of such current pulses over several days or weeks seems to be required to produce the desired positive effect.[1]

Auditory Considerations

Along with the currents that might be induced within patients from gradient switching comes another related phenomenon. As these gradient coils are being rapidly energized and de-energized dozens of times every second during the MR imaging process while in the presence of the static magnetic field of the imaging system, there are resultant forces that are produced from the interactions of the static magnetic field and the magnetic field associated with the changing current within the gradient coils. These forces result in motion or vibration of these gradient coils (and/or adjacent conductors), which produces a banging sound. The amplitude of this noise tends to remain between 65 and 95 dB,[84] but it can prove to be quite variable. The actual amplitude of the noise produced is dependent upon several factors including the physical configuration of the magnet itself, the pulse sequence type and its timing specifications, and the amount of current being passed through these coils (which itself is dependent upon other operator controllable scan parameters such as slice thickness, field of view, etc.).

Temporary and even permanent hearing loss as a result of the MR examination has been claimed and reported.[85] As magnet-safe headphones or earplugs are readily available, are quite low-cost items, and have been shown to prevent the temporary hearing loss associated with MR imaging, all sites should at least offer such hearing-protective devices to patients (and all others remaining within the scan room during imaging) prior to the onset of the MR examination. Furthermore, the amplitude of the noise so produced can be significantly greater than the more "typical" case with some of the more recently introduced or experimental sequences, such as many of the fast and ultra fast imaging techniques. In such cases, it is my recommendation that all such sequences be performed only on patients on whom such hearing-protective devices are in place.

In addition to attempting to improve the acoustical insulation of the magnet casing itself, a recently developed technique[86,87] aims at decreasing the actual amplitude of the perceived system noise. With this technique, a real-time Fourier analysis of the noise permits the summing of noise of similar amplitude, but of opposite phase to that produced by the imaging system. This phase cancellation technique serves to decrease the amplitude of the sound actually reaching the patient and thus holds considerable promise for clinical examinations.

Effects of the Radio-Frequency Time-varying Magnetic Fields

The energy absorbed by the resonant protons is dissipated as heat and is of such a small magnitude as to be of no biological concern.[88] The transmitted radio-frequency (RF) magnetic field used in the excitation phase of the MR process, on the other hand, does induce electrical currents within the tissues of the patient. These currents have the potential of producing either nonthermal or thermal biologic effects.

Whether there are, or are not, significant nonthermal effects from radio-frequency magnetic fields and/or ELF modulation of RF magnetic fields is extremely controversial. There have been numerous studies of late regarding possible biological effects of systems exposed to ELF magnetic fields (roughly at the 0–100 Hz range) or RF electromagnetic fields modulated at ELF frequencies. Time-varying ELF magnetic fields have been demonstrated to be associated with multiple effects, including clustering and altered orientation as well as increased mitotic activity of fibroblast growth, altered DNA synthesis, reduced fentanyl-induced anesthesia, and possible effects in multiple organisms, including man.[89-98] To be sure, there do not seem to be any articles to date that have demonstrated definitive associations between time-varying magnetic fields and the development of cancer of any type. Yet, there are several investigators who feel that such an association between the two is quite possible or even likely. An exhaustive review of the literature pertaining to this issue has been recently published;[98] the reader is referred to this source for further information regarding this rapidly changing field. Considering the rather confusing mix of results presently available from the studies performed in this area, though, it seems most appropriate to suggest that it might yet be too early to hazard an opinion at this time as to what association, if any, might exist between biologically detectable or harmful effects and exposure of humans (or other organisms) to ELF or ELF-modulated RF, as in the case of clinical MRI examinations.

The majority of the transmitted RF power to which the patient is exposed during the excitation phase of the MR sequence is transformed into heat within the patient's tissue(s) as a result of dielectric and resistive properties of the tissue(s). This differs from the case of induced currents secondary to gradient switching/pulsing due to variations in (i) the frequency of the oscillating magnetic fields, (ii) their waveform shape, and (iii) their magnitudes. RF pulses give rise to oscillating currents of high frequency (megahertz) and magnitude, whereas gradient switching produces low-amplitude current pulses at a low periodicity (< 1000 Hz).

Electrical currents induced from oscillating RF magnetic fields are unable to excite nervous tissue, as shown by d'Arsonval in 1893.[99] RF fields are, however, capable of heating tissues via dielectric and resistive losses experienced by these currents within biological tissues and implants. As opposed to the negligible thermal effects due to switched gradients, thermal effects do present a major concern from the RF pulses. In fact, the main biological effects associated with exposure to RF radiation are related to the thermogenic qualities of this RF magnetic field.[100-117]

The power deposited by RF pulses during MR examinations is dependent upon multiple factors, including the power and duration of the RF pulse (i.e., its RF excitation flip angle), the transmitted magnetic field frequency, the RF pulse time/density (i.e., the number of such RF pulses that are applied per unit time), the type and configuration of the RF transmitter coil used, the volume of tissue imaged, the electrical resistivity of the tissue, the configuration of the anatomical region imaged, etc. As a general rule of thumb, it is helpful to remember that the power deposition from an RF pulse increases with the square of the flip angle and with the square of its oscillation frequency (the latter being linearly dependent upon the field strength of the imaging system).

The absorbed power per unit time is only one of the factors that needs to be considered when determining the suitability of a patient for undergoing an MR examination. Another is the ability of the patient to handle this amount of extra energy deposition. Assuming intact thermoregulatory mechanisms, then, as this RF power or heat is deposited into the patient, she or he will attempt to lose this excess heat via any or all of four possible mechanisms as the body attempts to maintain a thermoregulatory homeostasis: convection, conduction, radiation, and evaporation. Indeed, if there is any appreciable increase in the core temperature of the patient, it is itself a manifestation of the failure of the body's compensatory thermoregulatory mechanisms to keep up with the rate at which power is being deposited into it.[118,119] The increase in tissue temperature, if any, caused by exposure to RF is itself dependent upon numerous physiological, physical, and environmental factors: the duration of exposure; the rate at which the energy is deposited; the ambient temperature, humidity, and airflow over and around the patient within the imaging magnet; the status of the patient's thermoregulatory system; and the number of insulating layers on/over the patient.

Relatively small amounts of quantitative data are available on the thermoregulatory responses of humans exposed to RF magnetic fields and only a small percentage of these data can be directly applied to MRI. It appears that, during MRI, tissue heating results primarily from magnetic induction. Thus, ohmic heating is maximal at the surface of the body and approaches zero at its center. Due to the increased ability of the skin to lose heat locally, the greatest actual temperature elevation would be theoretically expected to take place in the subcutaneous tissues. Predictive calculations and phantom and human MRI measurements support this distribution pattern.[73,107-111]

It is certainly safe to say that, for the vast majority of studies performed in this country, the total power/heat load to the patient, when viewed as a diffuse phenomenon, is not considered clinically significant at the FDA-approved imaging sequences and guidelines in force today.

Focal Heating Considerations

In a recent survey conducted of MR sites in this country,[66,72] there were several reports of first-, second-, and even third-degree burns (i.e., true tissue necrosis) that resulted from clinical MR examinations. These burns, quite rare in overall incidence, seem to occasionally be the result of a conductive loop inadvertently formed between some electrical conductor, such as electrocardiographic monitoring or gating leads, plethysmographic gating wire, or fingertip attachment, etc., and the patient's skin. Conversely, some of these may have resulted from heating of the electrically conductive lead (for example) and having the burn result secondary to the hot lead touching the patient's skin.[120,121] It is therefore recommended that several steps be followed in order to attempt to decrease the possibility of such a thermal injury. First, it is important to be sure that no unconnected imaging coils be left within the volume of the magnet system during imaging. Similarly, no (induced) current loops should be permitted to be formed that in any way directly involve the patient's tissues in an electrical current loop. For example, we must be sure that no obvious exposed wires/conductors are touching any portion of the patient during the examination. Indeed, loops of any kind of conductor (gating wires, surface coil leads, etc.) should be avoided within the imaging system during imaging and, if at all possible, thermally insulating material (such as air) should be interposed between the wires being led out of the magnet system and the patient so that they do not directly contact each other.

Certain human organs, such as the testis and eye, are particularly sensitive to heat due to reduced capabilities for heat dissipation or to intrinsic biologic heat intolerance.[114,116,117] These, therefore, are primary sites of potential harmful effects if RF exposures during MRI are excessive. Recent preliminary data suggest that scrotal temperature elevations from MRI examinations are below the threshold known to impair spermatogenesis.

At least one study revealed no discernible cataractogenic effects produced by MRI on the eyes of rats at exposures that exceeded typical clinical imaging levels.[117] Further studies involving patient corneal temperatures have revealed that the corneal temperature elevations produced by MRI examinations are well below those known to be of concern for cataractogenesis.[109] Any long-term effects of MRI on ocular tissues—and specifically what they are—are still somewhat of an unknown at this time and they remain to be determined.

Although not technically a safety issue in the strictest sense, the presence of focal hot spots in RF power deposition will, for all practical purposes, produce images with signal intensity inhomogeneities, as determined by the RF power distribution map of a particular slice and study. Aside from the focal power deposition problem noted earlier, this might indirectly be considered a safety issue insofar as it might lead to image artifact production and could possibly worsen the diagnostic potential of the image.

Superconductive System Concerns: Electromagnetic Consequences of a Quench

This of course pertains only to superconductive magnet systems. Although a discussion of this topic (especially insofar as the cryogen considerations per se are concerned) is beyond the scope and intended purpose of this review, it should be noted that the loss of a magnetic field associated with a system quench is also associated with questions regarding electrical, induced voltages and/or currents that may be induced in biologic tissues. In one study where physiologic monitoring of a pig and environmental measurements were performed during an intentional quench from 1.76 T, there did not seem to be any significant effect upon the blood pressure, pulse, temperature, EEG, and ECG measurements of the pig during or immediately following such a quench.[122] Although such a single observation does not, of course, prove safety for humans undergoing exposure to a quench, the data do suggest that there is good reason to presume that the experience would indeed be similar and that, in all likelihood, no deleterious electrical effects would be experienced by humans undergoing a similar experience and exposure.

Pregnancy

The issue of the safety of magnetic resonance imaging environments for pregnancy, for that of the health care practitioner or the patient, is one that has been the focus of much attention for several years now. Unfortunately, there has been a paucity of data available to date for such populations as MR technologists and nurses that examined this population as a whole, as opposed to attempting to examine the effects of static fields, time-varying fields, etc., individually. However, an attempt at a true epidemiologic study of MR technologists in the United States has been recently conducted.[123] Even though the data are still preliminary at this point, they are reassuringly negative against any statistically significant elevations of spontaneous abortion rates, infertility, low birth weight, and premature delivery, among other associated risk factors that were examined for this population. Although far from conclusive, the results are reassuring from this first attempt at such an epidemiologic study involving this population of health care providers and MRI.

RECOMMENDATIONS

Although it should be stressed that not all the facts are yet available for many of the areas discussed herein, the following are several recommendations that reflect the safety recommendations and practices I have implemented at my own institution.

First, all patients should be screened prior to being permitted into the MR imaging environment for possible ferromagnetic objects in or on their person. When suspected, plain film radiography for such areas of the body as the orbit can be obtained to help exclude the presence of such objects. No patients with pacemakers or other such contraindicated devices should be permitted into the scanner, regardless of the static field strength of the MR imaging system being considered. Data are available for determining if the specific object in question is magnet-compatible. If it is not an item that has been cleared as being "magnet-safe", we do not permit it into the MR environment until further testing can be performed for such factors as its attractability to the magnetic fields of the MR imager. We personally test and maintain our own data base of surgical devices, clamps, clips, etc., that are used in our own inpatient sites to help us identify those objects that may be a relative contraindication to MR. Because of their uncertain safety status, we do not scan patients that have been prospectively identified as having epicardial pacer leads or Swan-Ganz thermistor catheters in place. A powerful hand magnet is used to help check the status of superficial metallic foreign bodies in prospective patients. No metal detectors of any kind are used at any time.

Second, pregnant patients are scanned in any stage of the pregnancy if the alternatives involve exposing the patient to ionizing radiation. This applies to examinations that utilize the head, body, or any other transmitting RF coil and/or anatomic region of interest. If ultrasonography is appropriate and available, we opt for it preferentially if equivalent diagnostic information is expected to be available from either study. We treat each case individually and each request for an MR examination for a pregnant patient requires a specific approval by the attending radiologist, who will make the final assessment as to the appropriateness of the examination and the acuteness of the diagnostic need. In general, we will examine any pregnant patient if it can be demonstrated that the outcome of the MR study might well change patient care during that pregnancy.

Third, pregnant personnel are advised that there are no known data to suggest that there is any quantifiable level of harm experienced by exposing the fetus to the static magnetic field of the imaging system. Nevertheless, due to a lack of sound data upon which to claim safety, we still recommend that pregnant personnel not be exposed to the time-varying RF or gradient magnetic field of the imaging system on any routine basis. In our site(s), this translates into our pregnant technologists being able to prep the patient, as well as to scan, archive, film, and hang the case on the multiviewer, but it would not permit them to remain in the scan room with the patient (e.g., for monitoring or real-time contrast agent injection purposes) during scanning. Similar guidelines are applied for our nursing staff.

Fourth, we do permit family members, after they have been similarly and appropriately screened for contraindications, to remain within the scan room during imaging if that is requested by the patient or family member or if it appears to be advisable, as in the case of, for example, a pediatric patient.

Fifth, all unused electrically conductive materials (e.g., unused surface coils) are removed from the bore of the imaging system during scanning. Care is taken to check the insulation of the wires of our surface coils, EKG leads, plethysmographic gating device leads, pulse oximeter wires, etc., after each usage and before being used on the subsequent patient. If possible, we attempt to keep all electrically conductive material, even if appropriately electrically insulated, off of exposed patient skin. Under no circumstances are multiple wires to be permitted to cross/touch each other within the bore of the system during imaging.

Sixth, earplugs are offered to all of our patients should they desire them to help alleviate the acoustical noise problem. If fast imaging techniques are to be performed, the patient must have hearing protection in place before such an exam is performed.

Last and perhaps most importantly, all of our technologist, nursing, and physician employees and staff, as well as any staff that may likely respond to emergencies or calls to the MR suite, are taught about safety considerations of the magnetic resonance imaging environment.

CONCLUSIONS

Despite the fact that there are several areas of potential safety concern for patients undergoing MR examinations and although the answers are not all in as of yet, MRI examinations, when applied with common sense and within FDA-approved guidelines, do indeed appear to be a low-to-minimal risk procedure. Ongoing studies continue to elucidate more information about the potential hazards regarding magnetic and electromagnetic fields associated with clinical magnetic resonance imaging examinations.

REFERENCES

1. BUDINGER, T. F. 1981. Nuclear magnetic resonance (NMR) *in vivo* studies: known thresholds for health effects. J. Comput. Assist. Tomogr. **5**(6): 800–811.
2. KANAL, E., F. SHELLOCK & L. TALAGALA. 1990. Safety considerations in MR imaging. Radiology **176**: 593–606.
3. TENFORDE, T. S. & T. F. BUDINGER. 1986. Biological effects and physical safety aspects of NMR imaging and *in vivo* spectroscopy. *In* NMR in Medicine: Instrumentation and Clinical Applications. Medical Monograph No. 14. S. R. Thomas & R. L. Dixon, Eds.: 493–548. Amer. Assoc. Phys. Med. New York.
4. PERSSON, B. R. R. & F. STAHLBERG. 1989. Health and Safety of Clinical NMR Examinations. CRC Press. Boca Raton, Florida.
5. SHELLOCK, F. G. 1989. Biological effects and safety aspects of magnetic resonance imaging. Magn. Reson. Q. **5**: 243–261.
6. LIBURDY, R. P. 1982. Carcinogenesis and exposure to electrical and magnetic fields. N. Engl. J. Med. **307**: 1402.
7. GONET, B. 1985. Influence of constant magnetic fields on certain physiochemical properties of water. Bioelectromagnetics **6**: 169–175.
8. WOLFF, S., L. E. CROOKS, P. BROWN, R. HOWARD & R. B. PAINTER. 1980. Tests for DNA and chromosomal damage induced by nuclear magnetic resonance imaging. Radiology **136**: 707–710.
9. WOLFF, S., T. L. JAMES, G. B. YOUNG, A. R. MARGULIS, J. BODYCOTE & V. AFZAL. 1985. Magnetic resonance imaging: absence of *in vitro* cytogenetic damage. Radiology **155**: 163–165.
10. GEARD, C. R., R. S. OSMAK, E. J. HALL, H. E. SIMON, A. A. MAUDSLEY & S. K. HILAL. 1984. Magnetic resonance and ionizing radiation: a comparative evaluation *in vitro* of oncogenic and genotoxic potential. Radiology **152**: 199–202.
11. COOKE, P. & P. G. MORRIS. 1981. The effects of NMR exposure on living organisms. II. A genetic study of human lymphocytes. Br. J. Radiol. **54**: 622–625.

12. SCHWARTZ, J. L. & L. E. CROOKS. 1982. NMR imaging produces no observable mutations or cytotoxicity in mammalian cells. Am. J. Roentgenol. **139:** 583–585.
13. KALE, P. G. & J. W. BAUM. 1982. Genetic effects of strong magnetic fields on *Drosophila melanogaster.* Mutat. Res. **105:** 79.
14. WITHERS, H. R., K. A. MASON & C. A. DAVIS. 1985. MR effect on murine spermatogenesis. Radiology **156:** 741–742.
15. SUTHERLAND, R. M., J. P. MARTON, J. C. F. MACDONALD & R. HOWELL. 1978. Effect of weak magnetic fields on growth of cells in tissue culture. Physiol. Chem. Phys. **10:** 125–131.
16. BELLOSSI, A. & L. TOUJAS. 1982. The effect of a static uniform magnetic field on mice. Radiat. Environ. Biophys. **20:** 153–157.
17. VOGL, T., A. FUCHS, K. KRIMMEL, W. PAULUS & J. A. LISSNER. 1988. Influence of high-field MR imaging on evoked potentials and nerve conduction in humans. Abstract No. 848 Presented at the Annual Meeting of the Radiological Society of North America (Chicago, November/December 1988).
18. GULCH, R. W. & O. LUTZ. 1986. Influence of strong static magnetic fields on heart muscle contraction. Phys. Med. Biol. **31**(7): 763–769.
19. DOHERTY, J. U., G. J. R. WHITMAN, M. D. ROBINSON, A. H. HARKEN, M. B. SIMSON, J. F. SPEAR & M. E. JOSEPHSON. 1985. Changes in cardiac excitability and vulnerability in NMR fields. Invest. Radiol. **20:** 129–135.
20. OSSENKOPP, K-P., N. K. INNIS, F. S. PRATO & E. SESTINI. 1986. Behavioral effects of exposure to nuclear magnetic resonance imaging: I. Open-field behavior and passive avoidance learning in rats. Magn. Reson. Imag. **4:** 275–280.
21. INNIS, N. K., K-P. OSSENKOPP, F. S. PRATO & E. SESTINI. 1986. Behavioral effects of exposure to nuclear magnetic resonance imaging: II. Spatial memory tests. Magn. Reson. Imag. **4:** 281–284.
22. MARSH, J. L., T. J. ARMSTRONG, A. P. JACOBSON & R. G. SMITH. 1982. Health effects of occupational exposure to steady magnetic fields. Am. Ind. Hyg. Assoc. J. **43**(6): 387–394.
23. RAMIREZ, E., J. L. MONTEAGUDO, M. GARCIA-GARCIA & J. M. R. DELGADO. 1983. Oviposition and development of *Drosophila* modified by magnetic fields. Bioelectromagnetics **4:** 315.
24. GORCZYNSKA, E. & R. WEGRZYNOWICZ. 1983. The effect of magnetic fields on platelets, blood coagulation, and fibrinolysis in guinea pigs. Physiol. Chem. Phys. Med. NMR **15:** 459–468.
25. STRAND, J. A., C. S. ABERNETHY, J. R. SKALSKI & R. G. GENOWAY. 1983. Effects of magnetic field exposure on fertilization success in rainbow trout, *Salmo gairdneri.* Bioelectromagnetics **4:** 295.
26. ODINTSOV, Y. N. 1974. The effect of a magnetic field on the natural resistance of white mice to *Listeria* infection. Report No. JPRS-62865. National Technical Information Service.
27. BEISCHER, D. E. & J. C. KNEPTON. 1972. The electroencephalogram of the squirrel monkey (*Saimiri sciureus*) in a very high magnetic field. Report No. NAMI-972. Naval Aerospace Medical Institute (Pensacola, Florida).
28. TOROPTSEV, I. V. 1974. Pathologicoanatomic characteristics of changes in experimental animals under the influence of magnetic fields. Report No. JPRS-63038. *In* Influence of Magnetic Fields on Biological Objects. Y. Kholodev, Ed. National Technical Information Service.
29. ARDITO, G., L. LAMBERTI, P. BIGATTI & G. PRONO. 1984. Influence of a constant magnetic field on human lymphocyte culture. Boll. Soc. Ital. Biol. Sper. **LX**(7): 1341–1346.
30. JOSHI, M. V., M. Z. KHAN & P. S. DAMLE. 1978. Effect of magnetic field on chick morphogenesis. Differentiation **10:** 39–43.
31. UENO, S., K. HARADA & K. SHIOKAWA. 1984. The embryonic development of frogs under strong DC magnetic fields. IEEE Trans. Magn. **MAG-20**(5): 1663–1665.
32. GROSS, L. 1962. Effect of magnetic fields on tumor immune responses in mice. Nature **195:** 662–663.

33. HAYEK, A., C. GUARDIAN, J. GUARDIAN & G. OBARSKI. 1984. Homogeneous magnetic fields influence pancreatic islet function *in vitro*. Biochem. Biophys. Res. Commun. **122**(1): 191–196.

34. JEHENSEN, P., D. DUBOC, T. LAVERGNE, L. GUIZE, F. GUERIN, M. DEGEORGES & A. SYROTA. 1988. Change in human cardiac rhythm induced by a 2 tesla static magnetic field. Radiology **166**: 227–230.

35. HONG, C-Z., D. HARMON & J. YU. 1986. Static magnetic field influence on rat tail nerve function. Arch. Phys. Med. Rehabil. **67**: 746–749.

36. NAKAGAWA, M. & Y. MATSUDA. 1988. A strong static-magnetic field alters operant responding by rats. Bioelectromagnetics **9**: 25–37.

37. SHIVERS, R. R., M. KAVALIERS, G. TESKEY, F. S. PRATO & R-M. PELLETIER. 1987. Magnetic resonance imaging temporarily alters blood-brain barrier permeability in the rat. Neurosci. Lett. **76**: 25–31.

38. GORCZYNSKA, E. & R. WEGRZYNOWICZ. 1986. Magnetic field provokes the increase of prostacyclin in aorta of rats. Naturwissenschaften **73**: 675–677.

39. GORCZYNSKA, E. 1986. Dynamics of the thrombolytic process under conditions of a constant magnetic field. Clin. Phys. Physiol. Meas. **7**(3): 225–235.

40. GORCZYNSKA, E. & R. WEGRZYNOWICZ. 1986. Effect of chronic exposure to static magnetic field upon the serum glutamic pyruvic transaminase activity GPT and morphology of the cardiac muscle, skeletal muscles, kidneys, cerebellum, and lung tissue in guinea pigs. J. Hyg. Epidemiol. Microbiol. Immunol. **30**(3): 275–281.

41. GORCZYNSKA, E. 1987. A magnetic field generates morphological changes in guinea pig bone marrow. Folia Morphol. **35**(1): 40–45.

42. SHEPPARD, A. R. 1978. Magnetic effects on mammals. *In* Magnetic Field Effect on Biological Systems (Based on the Proceedings of the Biomagnetic Effects Workshop, Lawrence Berkeley Laboratory, University of California, 6–7 April 1978). T. Tenforde, Ed. Plenum. New York.

43. HUDRY-CLERGEON, G. & J-M. FREYSSINET. 1983. Orientation of fibrin in strong magnetic fields. Ann. N.Y. Acad. Sci. **408**: 380–387.

44. FREYSSINET, J-M., J. TORBET & G. HUDRY-CLERGEON. 1984. Fibrinogen and fibrin in strong magnetic fields: complementary results and discussion. Biochemie **66**: 81–85.

45. MURAYAMA, M. 1965. Orientation of sickled erythrocytes in a magnetic field. Nature **206**: 420–422.

46. BRODY, A. S., M. P. SORETTE, C. A. GOODING, J. LISTERUD, M. R. CLARK, W. C. MENTZER, R. C. BRASCH & T. L. JAMES. 1985. Induced alignment of flowing sickle erythrocytes in a magnetic field: a preliminary report (AUR Memorial Award). Invest. Radiol. **20**: 560–566.

47. LEITMANNOVA, A., R. STOSSER & R. GLASER. 1977. Changes in the shape of human erythrocytes under the influence of a static homogeneous magnetic field. Acta Biol. Med. Ger. **36**: 931–934.

48. TAKASHIMA, S., S. CHANG & T. ASAKURA. 1985. Shape change of sickled erythrocytes induced by pulsed RF electrical fields. Proc. Natl. Acad. Sci. U.S.A. **82**: 6860–6864.

49. BRODY, A. S., S. H. EMBURY, W. C. MENTZER, M. L. WINKLER & C. A. GOODING. 1988. Preservation of sickle cell blood-flow patterns during MR imaging: an *in vivo* study. Am. J. Roentgenol. **151**: 139–141.

50. STARR, S. J. & M. W. GROCH. 1988. Magnetochemical stress in the human retina and the safety of MR imaging. Abstract No. 849 Presented at the Annual Meeting of the Radiological Society of North America (Chicago, November/December 1988).

51. BEISCHER, D. E. & J. C. KNEPTON, JR. 1964. Influence of strong magnetic fields on the electrocardiogram of squirrel monkeys (*Saimiri sciureus*). Aerosp. Med. **October:** 939–944.

52. AMERICAN SOCIETY FOR METALS COMMITTEE FOR WROUGHT STAINLESS STEELS. 1961. Wrought stainless steels. *In* Metals Handbook (8th Edition). T. Lyman, H. Boyer, P. Unterweiser, J. Foster, J. Hontas & H. Lawton, Eds. Amer. Soc. Metals. Metals Park, Ohio.

53. PERSSON, B. R. R. & F. STAHLBERG. 1989. Other hazards in clinical NMR examinations.

In Health and Safety of Clinical NMR Examinations. Chapter 6, p. 93–94. CRC Press. Boca Raton, Florida.

54. DUJOVNY, M., N. KOSSOVSKY, R. KOSSOWSKY, R. VASLDIVIA, J. SUK, F. G. DIAZ, S. BERMAN & W. CLEARY. 1985. Aneurysm clip motion during magnetic resonance imaging: *in vivo* experimental study with metallurgical factor analysis. Neurosurgery **17**(4): 543–548.

55. NEW, P. F. J., B. R. ROSEN, T. J. BRADY, F. S. BUONANNO, J. P. KISTLER, C. T. BURT, W. S. HINSHAW, J. H. NEWHOUSE, G. M. POHOST & J. M. TAVERAS. 1983. Potential hazards and artifacts of ferromagnetic and nonferromagnetic surgical and dental materials and devices in nuclear magnetic resonance imaging. Radiology **147**: 139–148.

56. SHELLOCK, F. G. & J. V. CRUES. 1987. High-field MR imaging of metallic biomedical implants: an *in vitro* evaluation of deflection forces and temperature changes induced in large prostheses. Radiology **165**: 150.

57. SHELLOCK, F. G. 1989. *Ex vivo* assessment of deflection forces and artifacts associated with high-field MRI of "mini-magnet" dental prostheses. Magn. Reson. Imag. **7**(S1): P38.

58. SHELLOCK, F. G. & J. V. CRUES. 1988. High-field MR imaging of metallic biomedical implants: an *ex vivo* evaluation of deflection forces. Am. J. Roentgenol. **151**: 389–392.

59. SHELLOCK, F. G. 1988. MR imaging of metallic implants and materials: a compilation of the literature. Am. J. Roentgenol. **151**: 811–814.

60. HUTTENBRINK, K. B. & W. GROBE-NOBIS. 1987. Experimentelle Untersuchungen und theoretische Betrachtungen uber das Verhalten von Stapes-Metall-Prosthesen im Magnetfeld eines Kernspintomographen. Laryng. Rhinol. Otol. **665**: 127–130.

61. BECKER, R., J. NORFRAY, G. TEITELBAUM, W. BRADLEY, J. JACOBS, L. WACASER & R. RIEMAN. 1988. MR imaging in patients with intracranial aneurysm clips. Am. J. Neuroradiol. **9**: 885–889.

62. RANDALL, P. A., L. J. KOHMAN, E. M. SCALZETTI, N. M. SZEVERENYI & D. M. PANICEK. 1988. Magnetic resonance imaging of prosthetic cardiac valves *in vitro* and *in vivo*. Am. J. Cardiol. **62**: 973–976.

63. ROMNER, B., M. OLSSON, B. LJUNGGREN, S. HOLTAS, H. SAVELAND, L. BRANDT & B. PERSSON. 1989. Magnetic resonance imaging and aneurysm clips. J. Neurosurg. **70**: 426–431.

64. AUGUSTINY, N., G. VON SCHULTESS, D. MEIER & P. BOESIGER. 1987. MR imaging of large nonferromagnetic metallic implants at 1.5 T. J. Comput. Assist. Tomogr. **11**: 678–683.

65. TEITELBAUM, G. P., W. G. BRADLEY & B. D. KLEIN. 1988. MR imaging artifacts, ferromagnetism, and magnetic torque of intravascular filters, stents, and coils. Radiology **166**: 657–664.

66. KANAL, E., F. G. SHELLOCK & D. SONNENBLICK. 1988. MRI clinical site safety survey: phase I results and preliminary data. Magn. Reson. Imag. **7**(S1): 106 (abstract no. IT-03).

67. PAVLICEK, W., M. GEISINGER, L. CASTLE, G. BORKOWSKI, T. MEANEY, B. BREAM & J. GALLAGHER. 1983. The effects of nuclear magnetic resonance on patients with cardiac pacemakers. Radiology **147**: 149–153.

68. HAYES, D. L., D. R. HOLMES, J. E. GRAY, J. G. FETTER, G. C. ARAM, P. TARJAN & L. PRECHTER. 1986. The effects of nuclear magnetic resonance (NMR) on implantable pulse generators. JACC **2929**: 3A.

69. HOLMES, D. R., JR., D. L. HAYES, J. E. GRAY & J. MEREDITH. 1986. The effects of magnetic resonance imaging on implantable pulse generators. PACE **9**: 360–370.

70. FETTER, J., G. ARAM, D. R. HOLMES, JR., J. E. GRAY & D. L. HAYES. 1984. The effects of nuclear magnetic resonance imagers on external and implantable pulse generators. PACE **7**: 720–727.

71. MANOLIS, A. S., H. RASTEGAR & M. ESTES III. 1989. Automatic implantable cardioverter defibrillator: current status. J. Am. Med. Assoc. **262**: 1362–1368.

72. FDA. 1989 (December). Report: CDRH MR Product Reporting Program and Medical Device Report Program.

73. BOTTOMLEY, P. A. & W. A. EDELSTEIN. 1981. Power deposition in whole body NMR imaging. Med. Phys. **8**(4): 510–512.
74. SCHAEFER, D. J. 1988. Safety aspects of magnetic resonance imaging. *In* Biomedical Magnetic Resonance Imaging: Principles, Methodology, and Applications. Chapter 13. F. W. Wehrli, D. Shaw & B. J. Kneeland, Eds.: 553–578. VCH Pub. New York.
75. PERSSON, B. R. R. & F. STAHLBERG. 1989. Extremely low frequency (ELF) magnetic fields. *In* Health and Safety of Clinical NMR Examinations. Chapter 3, p. 49. CRC Press. Boca Raton, Florida.
76. FISCHER, H. 1989. Physiologic effects by fast oscillating magnetic field gradients. Radiology **173**(P): 382.
77. COHEN, M., R. WEISSKOFF, R. RZEDZIAN & H. KANTOR. 1990. Sensory stimulation by time-varying magnetic fields. Magn. Reson. Med. **14**(2): 409–414.
78. SAUNDERS, R. D. 1982. Biological hazards of NMR. *In* Proceedings of the International Symposium of Nuclear Magnetic Resonance Imaging. R. L. Witcofski, N. Karstaedt & C. L. Partain, Eds.: 65–71. Bowman Gray School of Medicine of Wake Forest University. Winston-Salem, North Carolina.
79. GARBER, H. J., W. H. OLDENDORF, L. D. BRAUN & R. B. LUFKIN. 1989. MRI gradient fields increase brain mannitol space. Magn. Reson. Imag. **7**(6): 605–610.
80. BECKER, R. O. 1963. The biological effects of magnetic fields—a survey. Med. Electron. Biol. Eng. **1**: 293–303.
81. BARLOW, H. B., H. I. KOHN & E. G. WALSH. 1947. Visual sensations aroused by magnetic fields. Am. J. Physiol. **148**: 372–375.
82. LOVSUND, P., S. E. G. NILLSON, T. REUTER & P. OBERG. 1980. Magnetophosphenes: a quantitative analysis of thresholds. Med. Biol. Eng. Comput. **18**: 326–334.
83. REDINGTON, R. W., C. L. DOMOULIN, J. F. SCHENCK, P. B. ROEMER, S. P. SOUZA, O. M. MUELLER, D. R. EISNER, J. E. PIEL & W. A. EDELSTEIN. 1988. MR imaging and bioeffects in a whole body 4.0 tesla imaging system. *In* Book of Abstracts 1988 of the Society of Magnetic Resonance in Medicine. Abstract No. 20, p. 4.
84. FDA. 1988. Data obtained from FDA MR product reclassification documents and product summary data sheets submitted by various MR manufacturers.
85. BRUMMETT, R. E., J. M. TALBOT & P. CHARUHAS. 1988. Potential hearing loss resulting from MR imaging. Radiology **169**: 539–540.
86. NOISE CANCELLATION TECHNOLOGIES (Great Neck, New York).
87. GOLDMAN, A. M., W. E. GOSSMAN & P. C. FRIEDLANDER. 1989. Reduction of sound levels with antinoise in MR imaging. Radiology **173**: 549–550.
88. KRAMER, D. M. 1984. Basic principles of magnetic resonance imaging. Radiol. Clin. North Am. **22**(4): 765–778.
89. MARTIN, A. H. 1988. Magnetic fields and time dependent effects on development. Bioelectromagnetics **9**: 393–396.
90. SCHUETZ, P. W., J. C. BARBENEL & J. P. PAUL. 1985. Effects of time-varying magnetic fields on fibroblast growth. Clin. Phys. Physiol. Meas. **6**(2): 155–160.
91. LIBOFF, A. R., T. WILLIAM, JR., D. M. STRONG & R. WISTAR, JR. 1984. Time-varying magnetic fields: effect on DNA synthesis. Science **223**: 818–820.
92. TESKEY, G. C., F. S. PRATO, K-P. OSSENKOPP & M. KAVALIERS. 1988. Exposure to time-varying magnetic fields associated with magnetic resonance imaging reduces fentanyl-induced analgesia in mice. Bioelectromagnetics **9**: 167–174.
93. VYALOV, A. M. 1974. Clinico-hygienic and experimental data on the effects of magnetic fields under industrial conditions (JPRS-63038). *In* Influence of Magnetic Fields on Biologic Objects. Y. Kholodev, Ed.: 163–174. Joint Publication Research Service.
94. MILHAM, S., JR. 1982. Mortality from leukemia in workers exposed to electrical and magnetic fields. N. Engl. J. Med. **307**(4): 249.
95. BERMAN, E., D. E. HOUSE, W. E. KOCH, J. TEAL, A. H. MARTIN, G. MARTUCCI, K. H. MILD & L. C. MONAHAN. 1988. The henhouse project: effect of pulsed magnetic fields on developing chick embryos. Tenth Annual Meeting, Bioelectromagnetics Society, Stamford, Connecticut (p. 72).
96. MCROBBIE, D. & M. A. FOSTER. 1985. Pulsed magnetic field exposure during pregnancy

and implications for NMR fetal imaging: a study with mice. Magn. Reson. Imag. **3:** 231–234.

97. ADEY, W. R. 1981. Tissue interactions with nonionizing electromagnetic fields. Physiol. Rev. **61:** 435–514.

98. BEERS, G. J. 1989. Biological effects of weak electromagnetic fields from 0 Hz to 200 MHz: a survey of the literature with special emphasis on possible magnetic resonance effects. Magn. Reson. Imag. **7:** 309–331.

99. D'ARSONVAL, M. A. 1893. Action physiologique des courants alternatifs a grande frequence. Arch. Physiol. **5:** 401.

100. SHUMAN, W. P., D. R. HAYNOR, A. W. GUY, G. E. WESBEY, D. J. SCHAEFER & A. A. MOSS. 1988. Superficial and deep tissue temperature increases in anesthetized dogs during exposure to high specific absorption rates in a 1.5-T MR imager. Radiology **167:** 551–554.

101. GORDON, C. J. 1987. Normalizing the thermal effects of radiofrequency radiation: body mass versus total body surface area. Bioelectromagnetics **8:** 111–118.

102. GORDON, C. J. 1988. Effect of radiofrequency radiation exposure on thermoregulation. ISI Atlas Sci. Plants Anim. **1:** 245–250.

103. BOTTOMLEY, P. A., R. W. REDINGTON, W. A. EDELSTEIN & J. F. SCHENCK. 1985. Estimating radiofrequency power deposition in body NMR imaging. Magn. Reson. Med. **2:** 336–349.

104. ADAIR, E. R. & L. G. BERGLUND. 1986. On the thermoregulatory consequences of NMR imaging. Magn. Reson. Imag. **4:** 321–333.

105. ADAIR, E. R. & L. G. BERGLUND. 1989. Thermoregulatory consequences of cardiovascular impairment during NMR imaging in warm/humid environments. Magn. Reson. Imag. **7:** 25–37.

106. NCRP. 1986. Biological effects and exposure criteria for radiofrequency electromagnetic fields. Report No. 86. National Council on Radiation Protection and Measurements (Bethesda, Maryland).

107. SHELLOCK, F. G. & J. V. CRUES. 1987. Temperature, heart rate, and blood pressure changes associated with clinical MR imaging at 1.5 T. Radiology **163:** 259–262.

108. SHELLOCK, F. G., D. J. SCHAEFER, W. GRUNDFEST & J. V. CRUES. 1986. Thermal effects of high-field (1.5 T) magnetic resonance imaging of the spine: clinical experience above a specific absorption rate of 0.4 W/kg. Acta Radiol. Suppl. **369:** 514–516.

109. SHELLOCK, F. G. & J. V. CRUES. 1987. Corneal temperature changes induced by high-field-strength MR imaging with a head coil. Radiology **167:** 809–811.

110. SHELLOCK, F. G. & J. V. CRUES. 1988. Temperature changes caused by clinical MR imaging of the brain at 1.5 tesla using a head coil. Am. J. Neuroradiol. **9:** 287–291.

111. SHELLOCK, F. G., C. J. GORDON & D. J. SCHAEFER. 1986. Thermoregulatory responses to clinical magnetic resonance imaging of the head at 1.5 tesla: lack of evidence for direct effects on the hypothalamus. Acta Radiol. Suppl. **369:** 512–513.

112. KIDO, D. K., T. W. MORRIS, J. L. ERICKSON, D. B. PLEWES & J. H. SIMON. 1987. Physiologic changes during high field strength MR imaging. Am. J. Neuroradiol. **8:** 263–266.

113. SHELLOCK, F. G., D. J. SCHAEFER & J. V. CRUES. 1989. Alterations in body and skin temperature caused by MR imaging: is the recommended exposure for radiofrequency radiation too conservative? Br. J. Radiol. **62:** 904–909.

114. SHELLOCK, F. G., B. ROTHMAN & D. SARTI. 1988. Scrotal heating produced by high field strength MR imaging. Radiology **168**(P): 375.

115. ABART, J., G. BRINKER, W. IRLBACHER & J. GREBMEIER. 1989. Temperature and heart rate changes in MRI at SAR levels of up to 3 W/kg. Abstract Presented at the Eighth Annual Scientific Meeting of the Society of Magnetic Resonance in Medicine (12–18 August 1989, Amsterdam). Book of Abstracts, Vol. 2: 998.

116. BERMAN, E. 1984. Reproductive effects. *In* Biological Effects of Radiofrequency Radiation. EPA-600/8-83-026A.

117. SACKS, E., B. V. WORGUL, G. R. MERRIAM & S. HILAL. 1986. The effects of nuclear magnetic resonance imaging on ocular tissues. Arch. Ophthalmol. **104:** 890–893.

118. HAMMEL, H. T. 1970. Concept of the adjustable set temperature. *In* Physiological and

Behavioral Temperature Regulation. Chapter 46. J. D. Hardy, A. P. Gagge & J. A. J. Stolwijk, Eds.: 676–683. Thomas. Springfield, Illinois.

119. GORDON, C. J. 1984. Thermal physiology. *In* Biological Effects of Radiofrequency Radiation. EPA-600/8-83-026A, p. 4-1 to 4-28.

120. SHELLOCK, F. G. & G. SLIMP. 1989. Severe burn of the finger caused by using a pulse oximeter during MR imaging. Am. J. Roentgenol. **153:** 1105 (letter to the editor).

121. KANAL, E. & F. G. SHELLOCK. 1990. Burns associated with clinical MR examinations. Radiology **175**(2): 585.

122. BORE, P. J., G. J. GALLOWAY, P. STYLES, G. K. RADDA, G. FLYNN & P. R. PITTS. 1986. Are quenches dangerous? Magn. Reson. Med. **3:** 112–117.

123. KANAL, E., F. G. SHELLOCK & D. A. SAVITZ. 1991. Survey of reproductive health among female MR operators. Abstract Presented at the Seventy-seventh Annual Meeting of the Radiological Society of North America (Chicago, 1–6 December 1991).

Dosimetry and Effects of MR Exposure to RF and Switched Magnetic Fields

DANIEL J. SCHAEFER

General Electric Medical Systems
Milwaukee, Wisconsin 53201

INTRODUCTION

As magnetic resonance (MR) technology evolves, the need for more detailed knowledge of the safety implications of larger and faster gradients and higher average radio-frequency (RF) power scans grows. It is imperative to protect patient safety during MR scans. It is also imperative to avoid overly restrictive safety standards that might compromise patient health by unnecessarily restricting use of beneficial pulse sequences. The purpose of this report is to explore gradient and radio-frequency dosimetry and effects.

GRADIENT DOSIMETRY AND EFFECTS

In MR imaging, time-varying magnetic field gradients spatially encode the anatomy of the patient, generating acoustic noise in the process. Typically, the time rate of change of gradient magnetic fields is below 20 T/s. However, echo-planar techniques could exceed 20 T/s. The time-varying magnetic field associated with gradients will induce electric fields in the human body and may stimulate nerves and even the heart.[1,2] Because ventricular fibrillation is life-threatening, safety standards are designed to ensure that gradient-induced fields are far below ventricular fibrillation thresholds. A physiological early warning sign of high induced electric fields is peripheral nerve stimulation.[3,4] Note that peripheral nerve stimulation is not considered life-threatening. It may, however, become unpleasant.

The amplitude of the gradient-induced electric field, $\overline{E}$, depends upon the time rate of change of the flux:[5]

$$\oint (\overline{E} \cdot d\overline{l}) = \int \left(-\frac{d\overline{B}}{dt} \right) \cdot d\overline{A}. \tag{1}$$

In equation 1, $\overline{B}$ is the magnetic field strength, $\overline{A}$ is the area, and t is the time. For the ideal Z-gradient coil (assuming the static field points in the Z direction), there will be two axial planes in which the magnitude of the gradient magnetic field is maximal. If the body is modeled as a cylinder with a radius R and if the area-weighted average magnetic field strength is B_{ave}, then the induced electric field may be expressed as

$$E = \left(\frac{\pi R^2}{2\pi R} \right) \left(\frac{-d B_{ave}}{dt} \right) = \left(\frac{R}{2} \right) \left(-\frac{d B_{ave}}{dt} \right). \tag{2}$$

Now, consider the case for an ideal transverse-gradient coil. If we examine an

225

axial slice near the isocenter, we find that the flux in the Z direction is less than half the worst-case Z-gradient coil value. Although it is tempting to assume that the lower flux leads to higher transverse stimulation thresholds, geometry compensates for the lower flux. For transverse gradients, the flux turns in the $\pm Y$ direction near the center of each coil. The sign of the flux is positive near the coil pair in the positive Z direction and is negative near the other coil pair. Induced electric fields from each coil pair point in the same direction halfway between the coils and add. The result is that transverse-gradient coils produce stimulation thresholds comparable to those from the Z coils.

For this study, a mathematical model of a whole-body, Maxwell-pair, Z-gradient coil was devised. The model consisted of a pair of single-turn coils with radii of 0.327 meters. A transverse-gradient set was also designed with four single-turn saddle coils with radii of 0.327 meters. The Biot-Savart law was used to calculate the magnetic fields near the patient, assuming sufficient current to produce 1-gauss/cm gradients. Gradient current rise and fall times of 500 μs were used to calculate dB/dt for both types of gradient coils. Induced electric fields were calculated from

$$\nabla \times \vec{E} = -\frac{d\vec{B}}{dt}. \tag{3}$$

The results are that the Z-gradient induced a peak electric field magnitude of 0.56 volts/m in a 20-cm-radius cylinder, whereas the transverse-gradient coil induced a peak electric field magnitude of 0.82 volts/m. Clearly, the induced fields are comparable in magnitude.

The experimental stimulation data in TABLE 1 indicate that transverse- and Z-gradient-induced stimulation thresholds are nearly identical. Bourland et al.[6] with single capacitor discharges obtained somewhat lower values than Fischer,[7] Budinger et al.,[8] and Cohen et al.,[9] but it is well known that the waveform and number of pulses alter the threshold. Theory and experiment thus appear to agree.

EFFECT OF PULSE WIDTH ON STIMULATION

Peripheral nerve and cardiac stimulation thresholds vary with the induced waveform pulse width, t, to form a strength-duration curve. An approximate representation of this curve is given by[1]

$$\frac{dB}{dt} = \frac{\left(\frac{dB}{dt}\right)_0}{1 - \exp^{-t/\tau}}. \tag{4}$$

In equation 4, τ is a time constant and the subscript o designates the dB/dt threshold for infinite pulse width. Note that if $t \ll \tau$ and if the gradient waveform is trapezoidal, then

$$\left(\frac{dB}{dt}\right)t \approx \left(\frac{dB}{dt}\right)_0 \tau = B_{max}. \tag{5}$$

TABLE 1. Gradient Stimulation Data[a]

Investigator	Waveform	Coil	Pulse Width (μs)	Peak Nerve Threshold (T/s)
Bourland[6]	discharge	Z	228–1189 [485]	10–333 [56]
Cohen[9]	sine	X	357[b]	93
Fischer[7]/Budinger[8]	sine	Z & trans	400[b]	60

[a]None of the investigators reported cardiac stimulation.
[b]Half-period of the sine wave.

In equation 5, B_{max} is the stimulation threshold gradient magnetic field strength for the given conditions.

In TABLE 2, calculated Z-gradient stimulation thresholds are listed as functions of induced pulse width. Also tabulated are threshold gradient strengths for stimulation. Maximum gradient strengths were calculated assuming a 40-gauss peak field from the 1-gauss/cm Maxwell pair. Fast imaging techniques may require increased bandwidth and gradients for a fixed field of view. Assuming current limits on dB/dt,[3,4] the peripheral nerve gradient limits in TABLE 2 should be divided by three to arrive at practical limits.

Reilly[1,2] estimates that the $(dB/dt)_o$ for both peripheral nerve stimulation and cardiac stimulation (for the most sensitive 1% of the population) is 62.5 T/s, that the peripheral nerve stimulation time constant is 120 μs, and that the cardiac stimulation time constant is 3000 μs. For gradients with rise and fall times less than about 600 μs, equation 5 becomes an excellent approximation for equation 4. Under these conditions, Z-gradient coils with trapezoidal gradient waveforms, whose maximum field is less than $62.5 \times 0.003 = 0.1875$ T, should be incapable of cardiac stimulation, regardless of the pulse width of the induced field. This formulation could simplify safety criteria.

Safety standards that set upper bounds on dB/dt by dividing the peripheral nerve stimulation threshold by a factor of three may be excessive. Assuming a Gaussian distribution for cardiac stimulation, at an induced pulse width of 1000 μs, the probability of inducing cardiac stimulation at the peripheral nerve stimulation threshold is only one chance in $10^{-15.625}$; in contrast, at ⅓ peripheral nerve threshold, the probability is $10^{-133.009}$ (note that the population of the world $< 10^{10}$). For shorter induced pulse widths, the probability diminishes until it is only $10^{-351.133}$ at 100 μs

TABLE 2. Z-Gradient Stimulation Thresholds

Rise/Fall Time (μs)	Nerve Threshold (T/s)	Cardiac Threshold (T/s)	Nerve Max G (g/cm)	Cardiac Max G (g/cm)
50	183	3781	2.3	47.3
100	110	1906	2.8	47.7
200	77	969	3.9	48.5
400	65	501	6.5	50.1
800	63	321	12.5	53.4

($10^{-3147.064}$ for $\frac{1}{3}$ peripheral nerve threshold). Safety standards with limits closer to peripheral nerve stimulation levels should be safe and may permit echo-planar-type scans.

Another confusing point is where to measure the peak field. Fields near conductors become very large compared to the average. Expressing safety criteria in terms of flux seen by the cylindrical patient model could reduce confusion. Hence, a Z-gradient coil with a trapezoidal waveform, whose Z flux component is less than $0.1875 \times \pi \times 0.2^2 = 0.024$ Wb, should be incapable of producing cardiac stimulation. Safety standards formulated in this fashion may be more easily understood and would also apply to local gradient coils. Appropriate safety factors to account for stimulation threshold as a function of gradient waveform should be included as well.

RF DOSIMETRY

MR scanners use resonant RF fields for imaging. The resonant frequency is 42.57 MHz/T. The peak RF amplitude is calibrated by the tip angle. The average RF power is proportional to the number of images per unit time. Patient geometry, RF waveform, tip angle, and whether the system is quadrature during transmission determine the peak power. Quadrature excitation lowers the RF power requirements by a factor of two and "stirs" any field inhomogeneities. Both mechanisms lower the local specific absorption rate (SAR).

To a first approximation, patient power absorption during an MR scan can be derived from quasi-static analysis assuming the electric field to be zero.[10] Such analysis shows that the peak power deposition for a homogeneous sphere is 2.5 times the average.[10] RF deposition in MR is peripheral. For the spherical model, 87% of the power deposition is in the outer third of the sphere. The peripheral nature of the RF deposition facilitates its dissipation to the environment.

Schenck and Hussain[11] developed a most useful model for studying the effects of inhomogeneities on local power deposition. They demonstrated (using spherical models) that production of power deposition "hot spots" depends upon both the dielectric constants and the conductivities of the media. In this paper, their derivations are made explicit in terms of tissue electrical properties and limits are used to find the conditions for and the magnitudes of the worst-case local power deposition amplification. A small sphere (sphere no. 1) with permittivity ϵ_1 and conductivity σ_1 is placed either outside sphere no. 2 at the pole (tangential electric field location) or at the equator (normal electric field location) of sphere no. 2 or inside sphere no. 2. Sphere no. 2 is a large, homogeneous sphere of "standard tissue" representing the body. Sphere no. 2 has a permittivity ϵ_2 and a conductivity σ_2. The amplification A_p of the local power deposition when sphere no. 1 is near the pole of sphere no. 2 may be expressed as

$$A_p = \frac{9(\sigma_1^2 + \omega^2 \epsilon_1^2)}{(\sigma_1 + 2\sigma_2)^2 + \omega^2(\epsilon_1 + 2\epsilon_2)^2}. \tag{6}$$

The amplification A_e of the local power deposition when sphere no. 1 is located near the equator of sphere no. 2 may be expressed as

$$A_e = \frac{9(\sigma_2^2 + \omega^2\epsilon_2^2)}{(\sigma_1 + 2\sigma_2)^2 + \omega^2(\epsilon_1 + 2\epsilon_2)^2}. \tag{7}$$

When sphere no. 1 is located within sphere no. 2, the amplification A_s of the local power deposition may be expressed as

$$A_s = \frac{9\sigma_1(\sigma_2^2 + \omega^2\epsilon_2^2)}{\sigma_2[(\sigma_1 + 2\sigma_2)^2 + \omega^2(\epsilon_1 + 2\epsilon_2)^2]} = \left(\frac{\sigma_1}{\sigma_2}\right)A_e. \tag{8}$$

In equations 6, 7, and 8, all terms are positive. Only the properties of the small sphere (sphere no. 1) can be adjusted to find the conditions for the maximum amplification of the local power deposition. Maximal power deposition amplification near the pole, A_p, will occur when sphere no. 1 is a perfect conductor ($\sigma_1 \approx \infty$). Under these conditions, $A_p = 9$ and the peak SAR at the pole is equal to $9 \times 2.5 = 22.5$ times the SAR averaged over sphere no. 2. This situation may be approximated by metallic leads (perhaps from monitoring equipment) placed in contact with the skin of a patient. Note that there is almost no power deposition amplification if sphere no. 1 is a radius or more away from sphere no. 2. Hence, care must be taken to keep conductors well away from patients.

An interesting case involves a void near the equator. In equation 7, the largest amplification of local power deposition takes place when the electrical properties of sphere no. 1 are minimal; that is, $\sigma_1 = 0$ and $\epsilon_1 = \epsilon_0$ (free space value). Under these worst-case conditions, which would be valid for an air bubble, $A_e = 2.25$. Fat or bone at the equator produces slightly smaller amplifications. As a result, the worst-case local SAR near the equator occurs when a low conductivity sphere is located near the outer edge of a larger (conductive) sphere and is limited to 5.625 times the average SAR. Finally, for the case of the small sphere embedded inside the large sphere, the highest amplification of the local SAR occurs in the unlikely case that $\sigma_1 = 2\sigma_2$ and $\epsilon_1 = 2\epsilon_2$. For this case, $A_s = 1.125$ and the highest local SAR is $2.5 \times 1.125 = 2.8125$ times the local average SAR.

The previous discussion of the effects of inhomogeneities assumes excitation of the RF coil in the linear mode. With quadrature excitation, the local power deposition amplification is reduced. The reason is that quadrature causes eddy current loops to rotate in space, effectively causing sphere no. 1 to alternate between being an equatorial sphere and a polar sphere. In fact, the worst-case local power deposition amplification for quadrature (assuming inhomogeneous biology) turns out to be $0.5(0 + 5.625) = 2.8125$. This value results when the electrical properties of sphere no. 1 approach those of a void. If quadrature can be maintained in the presence of a conductor, the worst-case local power deposition amplification would be $0.5(0 + 22.5) = 11.25$. A further consideration is that, in a living patient, thermal diffusion and blood flow act to thermodynamically "stir" the system. The result is that higher power deposition regions are not necessarily higher temperature regions. The thermal effects of blood flow are given in TABLE 5 (see later) and in the section on local temperature rise.

THERMAL PHYSIOLOGY REVIEW

RF fields are too high in frequency to stimulate excitable tissues electrically. The only well-established mechanism for RF bioeffects is heating. Proteins denature at about 45 °C.[12] Guy *et al.*[13] showed that the SAR threshold for cataractogenesis is 100 W/kg. The highest safe core temperature for workers is 39.4 °C.[14,15] The teratogenic effects threshold core temperature for pregnant women is 38.9 °C.[16] During a day, core temperature fluctuates 1 °C.[17] Skin temperature fluctuates over a range of 15 °C.[18] The skin pain threshold is 43 °C.[19] Finally, the resting metabolic rate is 1.3 W/kg, whereas during vigorous exercise it may be as high as 18 W/kg.[14]

WHOLE-BODY TEMPERATURE RISE

To gain insight into the temperature rise due to RF power deposition, consider an insulated tissue section. The insulated tissue, when exposed to an SAR of 1 W/kg, will rise approximately 1 °C in one hour. It would rise to infinite temperature in infinite time at any finite SAR. Such a situation is not physical.

The outer surface of a body whose temperature T_{sk} is warmer than the ambient temperature T_a will radiate to its surroundings. Such a body, when exposed to RF, will increase in temperature until steady state develops in which power is lost and gained at the same rate. The temperature increases until it levels off to a final steady state value. The temperature time course may be expressed as

$$\Delta T = \Delta T_0 (1 - \exp^{-t/\tau}). \tag{9}$$

In equation 9, τ is a constant, ΔT is the temperature rise at any time t, and ΔT_0 is the steady state temperature rise. Note that an infinite duration exposure to the RF power level results in a finite, nonlinear temperature rise. If σ is taken as the Stefan-Boltzmann constant and if A is the surface area of the body, then the radiated power P may be expressed as

$$P = \sigma A (T_{sk}^4 - T_a^4) \approx 4\sigma A T_a^3 \Delta T. \tag{10}$$

For example, consider a hypothetical, uninsulated human (70 kg with 2 m² of surface area) who is constrained to lose energy to the environment only by radiation. Also assume that the ambient temperature is 25 °C and the thermal neutral (steady state) temperature of the skin is 33 °C. In steady state, the hypothetical human would radiate about 1.4 W/kg, which is replaced by his/her own metabolic energy at the same rate. The result is no change in temperature.

Next, consider the same hypothetical human, but this time his/her skin temperature has risen to 38 °C (vasodilatation of skin blood vessels may permit the skin to reach the core temperature). Now, the hypothetical human radiates energy at a rate of 2.4 W/kg, which is 1 W/kg above his/her metabolic rate. This hypothetical human might experience a 1 °C rise in temperature in one hour when exposed to 2 W/kg, demonstrating the importance of ambient temperature to core temperature rise.

Adair and Berglund[20,21] have utilized a mathematical thermal model of the body, based on the widely accepted Gagge model,[22] to predict the effects of SAR, ambient temperature, impairment of blood flow, relative humidity, clothing, and scan time on core temperature rise. Their summarized results can be approximated with a simple program.[21] For this paper, the Adair program was used to predict the effect of ambient temperature on the core temperature rise (FIGURE 1). For the plot, it was assumed that clothing = 0.2 clo, relative humidity was 50%, blood flow impairment was 40%, and the scan duration was 60 min. Note that a 40% reduction in cardiac output is life-threatening.[23] From the plot, it is clear that an exposure to 4 W/kg for one hour should result in only a 1 °C core temperature rise when T_a = 19 °C. However, if T_a = 25 °C, then 3 W/kg is needed. A one-hour exposure to 1 W/kg, even at T_a = 27 °C, should result in no temperature rise. Clearly, ambient temperature plays an important role in core temperature rise.

Humans can dissipate energy through conduction, convection, and evaporation as well as by radiation. In an experimental study on human volunteers exposed to 4 W/kg for 20 min, the average temperature rise was 0.3 °C[24] rather than the 1 °C rise predicted by our simple radiating human model. In experiments on anesthetized, unshorn, and intubated sheep,[25] the core temperature rose roughly one-third as fast as the insulated tissue model. A 60-min, 2-W/kg scan would raise the core temperature by 0.76 °C. An SAR of 2.75 W/kg would raise the temperature by 1 °C in 60 min of scanning even in this "worst-case" animal model. In subsequent experiments,[26] humans were exposed for 30 min to SAR levels ranging from 2.8 to 4 W/kg (the average was 3.35 ± 0.504 W/kg). Body core temperature increased a statistically insignificant 0.1 °C during the 30-min scan, well within safe exposure levels.

Febrile patients thermoregulate with higher set points than 37 °C.[17] As a result, febrile body core temperature rises during MRI will behave much as those for normal patients. Absolute core temperatures of febrile patients after scanning may be higher than normal.

Overall, it is clear that the core temperature rise depends on SAR, wall temperature, air temperature, airflow rate, relative humidity, and patient insulation. Low ambient temperatures may cause drops in the core temperature during MR scans.[27] MR scanning seems to have little effect on heart rate, breathing rate, metabolism,[24] and blood pressure. Using thermographic imaging on patients exposed to SAR levels of 0.5 to 1.3 W/kg, Shellock et al.[28] noted significant elevations in the temperatures of the hand, of skin proximal to the positioning isocenter, and of the cornea; however, the temperatures never approached hazardous levels. The oral temperature increased 0.2 °C.

POWER DEPOSITION AND CARDIAC STRESS

Can RF power deposition in cardiac-compromised patients place potentially unsafe stresses on their cardiovascular systems? For example, could a scan cause an increase in the skin blood flow rate resulting in potentially unsafe changes in either heart rate or blood pressure? At some SAR, this thermal stress is likely to be a problem. The maximum blood flow rate to the skin in a 63-kg adult is 150 mL/100 g/min[17] or 5400 mL/min total. If the skin temperature is 4 °C below the body core temperature, then blood can dissipate 1296 W (or 20.6 W/kg) to the skin during maximal blood flow. TABLE 3 shows the calculated results for 60-min scans at various SAR levels assuming that the body core temperature may rise 1 °C for both normal

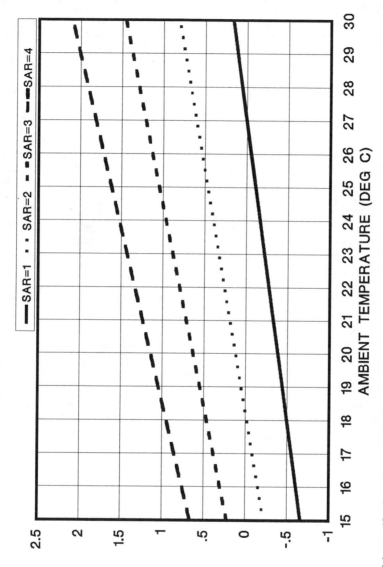

FIGURE 1. Effects of the specific absorption rate (SAR) and ambient temperature on the human core temperature during 60-min MR scans. The plot is based on the Adair thermal model assuming a relative humidity of 50%, clothing = 0.2 clo, and a 40% impairment of blood flow at various SAR levels and ambient temperatures.

TABLE 3. Power Deposition and Cardiovascular Stress—Theory

SAR_{net} (W/kg)	C_{out}	Heart Rate (bpm)	Compromised C_{out}	Compromised Heart Rate (bpm)
0	1.00	69.0	0.60	115
1	1.02	70.1	0.61	117
2	1.03	71.3	0.62	119
3	1.05	72.4	0.63	121
4	1.07	73.6	0.64	123

subjects and cardiac-compromised subjects. Note that an exposure, for example, to 2 W/kg, elevates cardiac output by only 2.7%. To accommodate this increased cardiac output, the heart rate must increase 2.7%, for example, from 69 to 71.3. Such an increase is not likely to pose a safety problem for the patient because eating increases cardiac output by 30%.[17]

Experimental data (TABLE 4) are available on humans exposed to SAR levels of 4 W/kg for up to 20 min[24] that show that the heart rate increased a statistically insignificant 5.7%. In this study, breathing rate also increased a statistically insignificant amount, whereas blood pressure dropped a statistically insignificant amount. Abart et al.[29] found that subjects exposed to 3 W/kg at an ambient temperature of 24 °C experienced core temperature rises averaging 0.3 °C. Moreover, the heart rate increased 29%. This increase may have been due to the higher ambient temperature, which may have led to higher skin temperatures. For example, if the skin were only 1 °C lower than the core, then the theoretical model would predict a 20% elevation in heart rate. The skin/core temperature differential is likely to be highest in cardiac-compromised patients.

In another study, Shellock and Crues[30] found that patients subjected to SAR levels of 0.5 to 1.2 W/kg increased body temperature by 0.2 °C with no accompanying changes in heart rate and blood pressure. Shellock et al.[26] exposed humans for 30 min to SAR levels ranging from 2.8 to 4 W/kg. The body temperature increased a statistically insignificant 0.1 °C during the 30-min scan. Blood flow increased from 1.00 mL/min/100 g to 2.04 mL/min/100 g (roughly 1.3% of the maximum rate).

Finally, in a clinical study,[27] groups of patients were studied at ambient temperatures of 19.6 °C ($n = 509$) and 22.4 °C ($n = 362$) at SAR levels ranging from 0.1 to 1.6 W/kg. In head coil scans at the lower temperature, the core temperature dropped 0.14 °C, the heart rate dropped 1.6 beats/min, and the mean blood pressure rose 0.9

TABLE 4. Power Deposition and Cardiac Stress—Data

Investigator	SAR (W/kg)	Time (min)	T_a (°C)	ΔHR (%)	ΔBP (%)	ΔT (°C)
Abart[29]	3	20	24	29	—	0.3
Barber[25]	4	82	19	—	—	2.0
Kanal[27]	0.1–1.6	clinical	20/22	—/—	2/2	−0.1/0
Schaefer[24]	4	20	19	5.7	0	0.3
Shellock[30]	0.5–1.2	clinical	20–24	0	0	0.2
Shellock[26]	2.8–4.0	30	21	—	—	0

mmHg. In head coil scans at the higher temperature, there was no change in the core temperature or the mean blood pressure, but there was a similar decrease in the heart rate. In body scans at the lower temperature, there was a decrease in the core temperature of 0.07 °C, no change in the heart rate, and a slight elevation in the mean blood pressure. In body scans at the higher temperature, there were no changes in the core temperature or the heart rate, but there was a similar elevation in the mean blood pressure. Although two patients experienced angina during scanning, these incidents were termed "likely to be coincidental". Again, these levels are not likely to prove stressful to the cardiovascular systems of the patients.

LOCAL THERMAL DOSIMETRY

An issue that often arises in RF bioeffects work is whether localized regions of heating or "hot spots" might exist and, if so, what their biological impact might be.

TABLE 5. Maximum Local SAR Level for a Local Temperature Rise of 1 °C for Various Perfused Organs[a]

Organ	Mass (kg)	Blood Flow (mL/kg/min)	Maximum SAR (W/kg)[b]	Maximum T (°C)[c]
liver	2.6	577	33.4	0.12
kidneys	0.3	4200	243.2	0.02
brain	1.4	540	31.0	0.13
skin-normal	3.6	128	7.4	0.54
skin-vasodilation	3.6	1500	86.9	0.05
heart muscle	0.3	840	48.3	0.08

[a]Data calculated from Ganong.[17]

[b]Maximum local SAR level that would cause a local temperature rise of 1 °C ignoring vasodilation or any increases in cardiac output (increased cardiac output could increase this number by a factor of 3.3 and vasodilation could increase it by an order of magnitude).

[c]Maximum local temperature rise for local SAR exposures of 4.0 W/kg assuming no vasodilation and no increase of cardiac output (increased cardiac output could reduce this number by a factor of 3.3 and vasodilation could reduce it by an order of magnitude).

The issue is complicated because models often must be relied upon and the distinction between temperature hot spots and power deposition hot spots is often confused. The thermal impact of local power deposition is reduced by thermal diffusion and blood flow, which thermodynamically stir the system. The result is that the local temperature rise will generally not correlate well with the local power deposition in a living subject.

Consider now a region with a small mass m cooled by blood flowing from a cooler, more massive region. Under steady state conditions, the SAR that is dumped to the more massive region depends upon an energy constant K, the specific heat C, the temperature difference between the massive and small region ΔT, and the mass rate of blood flow $d\mathrm{M}/dt$; it may be expressed as

$$\mathrm{SAR} = \left(\frac{KC\Delta T}{m}\right)\left(\frac{d\mathrm{M}}{dt}\right). \tag{11}$$

Equation 11 was used to calculate the SARs required for a maximum temperature rise of 1 °C. These values are listed for various organs in TABLE 5. TABLE 5 demonstrates the ability of blood flow to homogenize temperature "hot spots" in the body. The blood flow to each organ[17] was used to calculate the SAR required for that organ to reach a steady state temperature of 1 °C over the surrounding body and to calculate the steady state (maximum) temperature rise when exposed to 4 W/kg. Athey[31] has shown similar theoretical results demonstrating the improbability of significant thermal "hot spots".

CONCLUSIONS

Transverse-gradient stimulation and Z-gradient stimulation are accurately predicted by simple models. More data are needed on cardiac and peripheral stimulation (including thresholds and time constants) to improve our understanding of these phenomena. A simple gradient safety standard based on minimum flux required for cardiac stimulation appears possible. More experimental research (including blood pressure, heart rate, skin temperature, core temperature, and skin blood flow) on cardiac-compromised patients and their reaction to RF power deposition would be useful.

REFERENCES

1. REILLY, J. P. 1989. Peripheral nerve stimulation by induced electric currents: exposure to time-varying magnetic fields. Med. Biol. Eng. Comput. 27: 101–110.
2. REILLY, J. P. 1989. Cardiac sensitivity to electrical stimulation. United States Food and Drug Administration Report No. MT 89-101.
3. FDA (Department of Health and Human Services). 1988. Magnetic resonance diagnostic device. Panel recommendation and report on petitions for MR reclassification. Docket nos. 87P0214/CP through 87P0214/CP0013. Fed. Regist. 53(46): 7575–7579.
4. FDA (Department of Health and Human Services). 1989. Recommendation and report on petitions for magnetic resonance reclassification and codification of reclassification (final rule, 21 CFR part 892). Fed. Regist. 54(20): 5077–5088.
5. RAMO, S., J. R. WHINNERY & T. VAN DUZER. 1965. Fields and Waves in Communication Electronics. Wiley. New York.
6. BOURLAND, J. D., J. A. NYENHUIS, G. A. MOUCHAWAR, L. A. GEDDES, D. J. SCHAEFER & M. E. RIEHL. 1990. Human peripheral nerve stimulation from z-gradients. Abstracts of the SMRM—Works in Progress, p. 1157.
7. FISCHER, H. 1989. Physiological effects by fast oscillating magnetic field gradients. Abstr. Radiol. Soc. North Am., p. 382.
8. BUDINGER, T. F., H. FISCHER, D. HENTSCHEL, H. E. REINFELDER & F. SCHMITT. 1990. Neural stimulation thresholds for frequency and number of oscillations using sinusoidal magnetic field gradients. Abstracts of the SMRM, p. 276.
9. COHEN, M. S., R. WEISSKOFF & H. KANTOR. 1989. Evidence of peripheral stimulation by time-varying magnetic fields. Abstr. Radiol. Soc. North Am., p. 382.
10. BOTTOMLEY, P. A. & E. R. ANDREW. 1978. RF magnetic field penetration, phase shift, and power dissipation in biological tissue: implications for NMR imaging. Phys. Med. Biol. 23: 630.
11. SCHENCK, J. F. & M. A. HUSSAIN. 1984. Power deposition during magnetic resonance: the effects of local electrical inhomogeneities and field exclusion. General Electric Corporate Research and Development Labs, NMR Project Memo No. 84-199.
12. ELDER, J. E. 1984. Special senses. In Biological Effects of Radiofrequency Radiation.

Section 5. J. E. Elder & D. F. Cahill, Eds.: 64–78. EPA-600/8-83-026F. United States Environmental Protection Agency. Research Triangle Park, North Carolina.

13. GUY, A. W., J. C. LIN, P. O. KRAMER & A. F. EMERY. 1975. Effect of 2450 MHz radiation on the rabbit eye. IEEE Trans. Microwave Theory Tech. **MTT-23:** 492–498.

14. DURNEY, C. H., C. C. JOHNSON, P. W. BARBER et al. 1978. Radiofrequency Radiation Dosimetry Handbook. USAF School of Aerospace Medicine Report No. SAM-TR-78-22 (Second Edition). Brooks Air Force Base, Texas.

15. GOLDMAN, R. F., E. B. GREEN & P. F. IAMPIETRO. 1965. Tolerance of hot wet environments by resting men. J. Appl. Physiol. **20**(2): 271–277.

16. SMITH, D. A., S. K. CLARREN & M. A. S. HARVEY. 1978. Hyperthermia as a possible teratogenic agent. Pediatrics **92**(6): 878–883.

17. GANONG, W. F. 1973. Review of Medical Physiology (Sixth Edition). Lange Med. Pub. Los Altos, California.

18. CARLSON, L. D. & A. C. L. HSIEH. 1982. Control of Energy Exchange, pp. 56, 73, and 85. Macmillan & Co. London.

19. BENJAMIN, F. B. 1952. Pain reaction to locally applied heat. J. Appl. Physiol. **4:** 907–910.

20. ADAIR, E. R. & L. G. BERGLUND. 1986. On the thermoregulatory consequences of NMR imaging. Magn. Reson. Imag. **4:** 321–333.

21. ADAIR, E. R. & L. G. BERGLUND. 1989. Thermoregulatory consequences of cardiovascular impairment during NMR imaging in warm/humid environments. Magn. Reson. Imag. **7:** 25.

22. GAGGE, A. P. 1980. The new effective temperature (ET)—an index of human adaptation to warm environments. In Environmental Physiology: Aging, Heat, and Altitude. S. Horvath & M. Yousef, Eds.: 59–77. Elsevier. Amsterdam/New York.

23. HURST, J. W., Ed. 1978. The Heart. McGraw–Hill. New York.

24. SCHAEFER, D. J. 1988. Safety aspects of magnetic resonance imaging. In Biomedical Magnetic Resonance Imaging: Principles, Methodology, and Applications. Chapter 13. F. W. Wehrli, D. Shaw & J. B. Kneeland, Eds.: 553–578. VCH Pub. New York.

25. BARBER, B. J., D. J. SCHAEFER, C. J. GORDON, D. C. ZAWIEJA & J. HECKER. 1990. Thermal effects of MR imaging: worst-case studies on sheep. Am. J. Roentgenol. **155:** 1105–1110.

26. SHELLOCK, F. G., D. J. SCHAEFER & J. V. CRUES. 1990. Alterations in body and skin temperatures caused by MR imaging: is the recommended exposure for radiofrequency radiation too conservative? Br. J. Radiol. **62:** 904–909.

27. KANAL, E. & G. L. WOLF. 1987. Heat deposition effects in nuclear magnetic resonance imaging in 550 patients. Personal communication.

28. SHELLOCK, F. G., D. J. SCHAEFER, W. GRUNFEST & J. V. CRUES. 1987. Thermal effects of high-field (1.5 tesla) magnetic resonance imaging of the spine: clinical experience above a specific absorption rate of 0.4 W/kg. Acta Radiol. Suppl. **369:** 514–516.

29. ABART, J., G. BRINKER, W. IRLBACHER & J. GREBMEIR. 1989. Temperature and heart rate changes in MRI at SAR levels up to 3 W/kg (poster presentation). SMRM Book of Abstracts, p. 998.

30. SHELLOCK, F. G. & J. V. CRUES. 1987. Temperature, heart rate, and blood pressure changes associated with clinical magnetic resonance imaging at 1.5 tesla. Radiology **163:** 259–262.

31. ATHEY, T. W. 1989. A model of the temperature rise in the head due to magnetic resonance imaging procedures. Magn. Reson. Med. **9:** 177–184.

Development of Dosimetry Monitors for MRI Staff and Patients[a]

RICHARD G. OLSEN

Bioengineering Division
Naval Aerospace Medical Research Laboratory
Pensacola, Florida 32508-5700

INTRODUCTION

Clinical MRI devices have a very high radio-frequency (RF) power output capability. Common systems can generate RF pulses with peak powers of up to 15 kW and average powers of hundreds of watts. This pulsed RF energy is focused on the patient and is an integral part of MRI. Fortunately, built-in safeguards such as RF power monitors and system software checks serve to protect MRI patients and, to some extent, MRI staff from overexposure. These built-in protective measures have a good track record with respect to patient protection,[1] but there is presently no independent means to routinely verify patient RF energy dosage or staff exposure. Potentially hazardous tissue temperature increases are possible with clinical MRI systems when safeguards are bypassed or fail;[2] therefore, a dosimetry system that is entirely independent of the MRI system is needed, especially as the present devices age and require maintenance and/or rework.

Unfortunately, a practical, convenient personal dosimeter for nonionizing radiation, particularly radio waves and microwaves, has not been developed. The problem is not trivial because irradiation at such wavelengths cannot be treated like clinically used X rays or other ionizing radiation. The propagation of RF energy is affected by the presence of the human body and the body's orientation with respect to the electric-field (E-field) and magnetic-field (H-field) vectors that define the irradiation. A mere sampling of the E- or H-fields near the body during MRI irradiation cannot, per se, indicate the specific absorption rate (SAR), the now-accepted quantity of RF absorption that is measured in W/kg. No SAR meter exists even though the localized SAR is proportional to the (linear) in-tissue heating rate as well as to the square of the internal E-field magnitude.

The implied invasive nature of measuring the SAR has been a significant obstacle to the development of a dosimeter. For a time, it was thought that the technology of bubble-dosimetry could be applied in the RF and microwave spectra. Bubble-type dosimeters have been found to be highly sensitive and useful in the quantitation of neutron and gamma-ray radiation.[3] We found, however, that bubble formation during microwave irradiation was secondary to the relatively insensitive process of heating the media.[4]

[a]This research was sponsored by the Naval Medical Research and Development Command under Work Unit No. 63706N-M0096.004-7011. The views expressed in this article are those of the author and do not reflect the official policy or position of the Department of the Navy, the Department of Defense, or the United States Government.

A prominent feature of RF dosimeter operation that emerged during our study of bubble-type devices was the previously described degree to which E-fields were excluded from the interiors of dosimeters that were composed of high-permittivity, tissue-equivalent phantom materials.[5,6] Dosimetric studies at the Naval Aerospace Medical Research Laboratory have used such materials for years to simulate animal and human models,[7-9] but no previous consideration was given to using the material as a dosimetric medium itself. We now believe that state-of-the-art, miniaturized RF detection technology can be combined with the use of tissue-equivalent materials to produce a practical dosimeter for use by MRI patients and staff and for use in other occupational situations involving nonionizing radiation.

This report gives localized SARs obtained in a full-size, muscle-equivalent human model exposed to realistic imaging protocols on 1.0-T and 1.5-T MRI systems. During some irradiations, special conditions such as implanted wire loops, external pickup coils, and a metal prosthesis were used. Localized SARs were further measured in a muscle-equivalent prototype dosimeter that was placed on the full-size model in order to specify the sensitivity needed by the RF detector to adequately record the exposure.

MATERIALS AND METHODS

The 69-kg, 167-cm-tall human model was contained in a sewn bag of reinforced plastic.[10] For the range of frequencies to be used, the model was composed of 10.36% gelling agent (TX-151 from Oil Center Research, Lafayette, Louisiana), 0.42% sodium chloride, 2.72% aluminum powder, and 86.50% water. As previously determined, the 70-MHz electrical properties of this mixture exhibited a relative dielectric constant of 85 and a conductivity of 0.76 S/m.[11] The human model rested supine as a normal human patient undergoing MRI diagnostic procedures. On separate days, two different systems were used. The first system was a 1.5-T (General Electric) machine with which both spin-echo (SE) and inversion recovery spin-echo (IRSE) modes were used, whereas the second system was a 1.0-T (Siemens) device with which the SE mode was used exclusively. Both systems had the capability to predict the whole-body average SAR for each irradiation, but the 1.0-T system, in addition, had the ability to predict a localized SAR for the body region being imaged.

Localized SAR was calculated from temperature-rise data obtained from an electromagnetically nonperturbing temperature probe (Luxtron 750).[2] Typically, a 5-min temperature baseline was recorded (at 30-second intervals) for a given location. An imaging sequence lasting 4 to 5 min was then commenced during which temperatures were also recorded. Regression lines were obtained from the baseline and irradiation temperature data. SAR was then calculated as the product of the irradiation-induced net change in slope multiplied by the specific heat of the material. As time permitted, repeat runs were conducted and the SARs for a given location and depth were averaged.

We focused attention on the head and central torso regions because MRI scans are often conducted there. We furthermore obtained most SARs near the surface rather than deep within the model because they were higher near the surface and therefore represented the worst-case localized exposure. In order to study SAR under a variety of possible conditions, we implanted loops of 24-gauge stainless steel wire in the model along with a stainless steel hip joint prosthesis. We also calculated SAR near external pickup coils (one resonant and one not) that were placed on the model during irradiation.

A prototype dosimeter was constructed with about 180 g of the same material that comprised the human model. The muscle-equivalent material was placed in a sandwich-sized self-sealing plastic bag. As used, the material had assumed the shape of a disk with a 10-cm diameter and a 15-mm thickness. Localized SAR near the center of the disk was calculated from two irradiations (1.0-T system only) as it rested atop the human model.

RESULTS

Results from the 1.5-T system (64-MHz) scans are given in TABLE 1 along with the predicted average, whole-body SARs. The IRSE mode produced higher SARs

TABLE 1. SAR Results with a 1.5-T (64-MHz) MRI Device

Location	Depth (mm)	Special Conditions	Predicted Average SAR (W/kg)	Measured Localized SAR (W/kg)
	30	spin-echo (SE) mode	0.56	1.2 ($N = 2$)
	3	SE mode	0.56	2.6
	3	inversion recovery spin-echo (IRSE) mode	0.66	8.4
Abdomen, at navel	7	IRSE mode, 14-cm-diam. wire implanted below surface, axial plane	0.66	4.3
	7	IRSE mode, 8-cm-diam. wire implanted below surface, coronal plane	0.66	4.1
Head, midfacial surface	5	IRSE mode	0.05	7.0
	5	IRSE mode, 2-cm-diam. wire implanted below surface, coronal plane	0.05	4.8 ($N = 2$)

than the SE mode with more than 8 W/kg at the abdomen and 7 W/kg in the head. No large SARs were seen near the implanted wire loops. Results from the 1.0-T system (42-MHz) scans are given in TABLE 2 along with the predicted localized SARs. In general, the SARs were lower than those shown in TABLE 1 except when the external pickup coils were present; a resonant pickup coil tripled the localized SAR near the surface. No large SARs were seen near the implanted metal hip joint prosthesis. TABLE 2 also shows that SAR in the prototype dosimeter was about the same as that measured near the model surface for that location.

DISCUSSION

These results show that the localized SAR in MRI is a relatively minor problem under nominal clinical conditions, given the current regulatory guidelines. Localized

SARs notwithstanding, the observed thermal accumulation in the model indicated the need to keep MRI scan time to a minimum. Deep-tissue SARs were, in general, less than surface SARs for a given location in contrast to what was seen in dogs.[2] The system-generated estimates of the localized SAR were not exactly the same as we calculated, but they were not too much different to be considered useless.

Near the implanted wire loops, SARs were relatively low. It must be emphasized, however, that the loops were not configured as commonly used; that is, they were not holding bones together. The presence of bones could alter the SAR picture by the introduction of subsurface dielectric boundaries that tend to greatly distort internal E-fields.

The problem of placing external electronic circuits on MRI patients needs continued attention. Our results showed that the localized SAR was significantly enhanced by the presence of the resonant pickup coil. Such enhancement implied

TABLE 2. SAR Results with a 1.0-T (42-MHz) MRI Device[a]

Location	Depth (mm)	Special Conditions	Predicted Localized SAR (W/kg)	Measured Localized SAR (W/kg)
Abdomen, at navel	5	—	4.8	3.2 ($N = 2$)
	5	nonresonant coil circuit over probe	5.3	6.7
	5	resonant coil circuit over probe	6.0	9.1
Head, midfacial surface	5	—	1.3	2.5
Near hip joint prosthesis	50	near ball end	2.9	1.4
	50	near pointed end	2.7	0.75 ($N = 2$)
Abdomen, at navel	—	probe in tissue-equivalent bolus resting on abdomen	6.2	3.1 ($N = 2$)

[a]All irradiations used the spin-echo (SE) mode.

that the circuitry was strongly interacting with the applied RF energy and was probably carrying a high RF voltage potential. A sufficiently high RF voltage could burn an actual patient at a small-area skin contact point. Care should be taken, therefore, to always provide adequate separation between the patient and any external circuitry (including connecting cables). It might not be sufficient to simply use the patient's clothing as a dielectric barrier.

The fact that localized SAR in the prototype dosimeter was not much different than SAR in the model suggests that a useful dosimeter (for MRI use, at least) could be constructed as a miniaturized E-field recorder embedded in a mass of tissue-equivalent material. For the SARs measured, the average E-field intensities were about 60 V/m; therefore, a detector capable of sensing pulsed signals in that range and further capable of registering the presence of those signals over time is needed.

Such a device would prove to be invaluable should an unscrupulous patient or MRI staff member allege an RF overexposure.

CONCLUSIONS

In conclusion, SARs produced by today's MRI apparatus are sufficient to warrant a dosimetry modality that is independent of the MRI system itself. There is increased public awareness and concern over exposure to electromagnetic fields and the trend of this concern appears to be increasing. Effort to produce a practical MRI dosimeter should therefore be expended to head off a potential stumbling block to progress in this technology. This discussion has attempted to provide some guidance in this effort.

ACKNOWLEDGMENT

I am grateful to Jeffrey R. Fitzsimmons for providing the access to and the expert operation of the two MRI systems.

REFERENCES

1. KANAL, E., F. G. SHELLOCK & L. TALAGALA. 1990. Safety considerations in MR imaging. Radiology **176:** 593–606.
2. SHUMAN, W. P., D. R. HAYNOR, A. W. GUY, G. E. WESBEY, D. J. SCHAEFER & A. A. MOSS. 1988. Superficial- and deep-tissue temperature increases in anesthetized dogs during exposure to high specific absorption rates in a 1.5-T MR imager. Radiology **167:** 551–554.
3. ING, H. & H. C. BIRNBOIM. 1984. A bubble-damage polymer detector for neutrons. Nucl. Tracks **8:** 285–288.
4. OLSEN, R. G. 1990. Radiofrequency detection by bubble dosimeter technology. Radiat. Prot. Dosimetry **33:** 381–384.
5. BOTTOMLEY, P. A. & E. R. ANDREW. 1978. RF magnetic field penetration, phase shift, and power dissipation in biological tissue: implications for NMR imaging. Phys. Med. Biol. **23:** 630–634.
6. MURPHY-BOESCH, J. 1984. Sensitivity improvement via coil and probe design. In Biomedical Magnetic Resonance. T. L. James & A. R. Margulis, Eds.: 47–61. Radiat. Res. Educ. Foundation. San Francisco.
7. OLSEN, R. G. & T. A. GRINER. 1987. Specific absorption rate (SAR) in models of man and monkey at 225 and 2000 MHz. Bioelectromagnetics **8:** 377–384.
8. OLSEN, R. G. & T. A. GRINER. 1982. Partial-body absorption resonances in a sitting rhesus model at 1.29 GHz. Radiat. Environ. Biophys. **21:** 33–43.
9. OLSEN, R. G. & T. A. GRINER. 1982. Electromagnetic dosimetry in a sitting rhesus model at 225 MHz. Bioelectromagnetics **3:** 385–389.
10. OLSEN, R. G. & T. A. GRINER. 1989. Outdoor measurement of SAR in a full-sized human model exposed to 29.9 MHz in the near field. Bioelectromagnetics **10:** 161–171.
11. CHOU, C. K., G. W. CHEN, A. W. GUY & K. H. LUK. 1984. Formulas for preparing phantom muscle tissue at various radiofrequencies. Bioelectromagnetics **5:** 435–441.

Current FDA Guidance for MR Patient Exposure and Considerations for the Future[a]

T. WHIT ATHEY

Center for Devices and Radiological Health
Food and Drug Administration
Rockville, Maryland 20857

INTRODUCTION

In contrast to standards authorities in many other countries, the Food and Drug Administration (FDA) does not usually issue general safety standards to which users of medical equipment must adhere. Rather, the FDA puts requirements on the manufacturers of medical devices to present valid scientific evidence to the Agency that will substantiate claims that the device is reasonably safe and effective for its intended use. Manufacturers may approach safety questions in different ways, resulting in some differences in patient risk levels. For example, one company may take a very conservative approach and limit its device to performance that has safety factors of several orders of magnitude, whereas another company may be less conservative, but still make a convincing case that its device can be operated safely. By law, the FDA would have to give its approval to both devices from a safety point of view.

In this report, the regulatory approach that the FDA takes for medical devices is briefly reviewed, along with the specific history of the FDA's regulation of magnetic resonance (MR) devices. The FDA's current guidance on the safety aspects of MR devices is discussed, along with its rationale. Finally, several new studies have provided results that may have an impact on standards and guidelines for MR devices and these will be discussed.

FDA's REGULATION OF MR DEVICES

The FDA classifies medical devices into three classes, based in part upon the potential risk from use of the device.[2] The three classes of devices receive proportionate levels of regulatory attention. Class I devices require only general controls to assure reasonable safety and effectiveness. Class II devices have some risks associated with their use, but these risks are sufficiently understood that they can be managed by general controls plus special controls such as specific standards or guidelines. Class III devices are those with the highest risks or those that are new

---

[a]Portions of this report have been adapted from reference 1 by P. Czerski and T. W. Athey. P. Czerski is now deceased after playing a leading international role in electromagnetic bioeffects for many years.

devices whose risks may be incompletely understood, as was the case initially for magnetic resonance (MR) devices. Class III devices require a premarket approval (PMA) application to be approved by the FDA before the company may market the device. Data to support a device application to the FDA will usually be collected in clinical trials of the device and an investigational device exemption (IDE) is required before clinical trials are undertaken.

IDEs may be handled by the local institutional review board (IRB) for device studies that are considered by the sponsor and the IRB to involve "nonsignificant risk". If the local IRB cannot concur with the sponsor's finding of nonsignificant risk or if the FDA declares a device to represent a "significant risk", then the IDE application must be considered by the FDA.

Because MR devices presented IRBs with safety issues that were usually unfamiliar to them and in order to avoid requiring unnecessary IDEs to be considered by the FDA, the FDA issued in 1982 a document entitled "Guidelines for Evaluating Electromagnetic Risk for Trials of Clinical NMR Systems".[3] The document was intended to facilitate the introduction of MR technology by indicating the magnetic and electromagnetic field levels that would generally be considered safe. The guidelines were set conservatively in the interest of issuing them without delay. Most early MR devices operated within these guidelines anyway, so the conservatism did not initially hinder development of the technology.

By 1987, the MR technology had matured to the point where the safety and effectiveness issues were somewhat better understood. At that point, the FDA began to review and process the 13 reclassification petitions submitted by manufacturers to determine whether a subset of MR devices could be regulated as Class II medical devices. To help define this subset of MR devices, a new safety analysis was carried out by the FDA and this resulted in the issuance in 1988 of a set of "Safety Parameter Action Levels", contained as an attachment to Guidance on MR 510(k) Applications,[4] which an MR device would have to meet to be considered Class II. This Guidance is the latest available on MR safety levels from the FDA.

RATIONALE FOR FDA GUIDANCE

There are three types of magnetic field exposure to patients in MR examinations that are of concern: static magnetic fields, rapidly switched spatial gradient magnetic fields, and radio-frequency magnetic fields. Before the 1988 Guidance was issued, the world literature on bioeffects existing in 1987 was reviewed to determine appropriate safety levels. A fourth area of concern is acoustic noise generated by the gradient coils, but this subject was not covered in the literature review. The FDA Guidance for acoustic noise simply defers to the guidance from other Federal regulatory or standards setting organizations such as the Occupational Safety and Health Administration (OSHA) or the American Conference of Government and Industrial Hygienists (ACGIH).

A complete understanding of the biophysics, bioelectrochemistry, and mechanisms of interaction of electromagnetic fields with living systems would provide a basis for a predictive theory for evaluation of MR safety, but such a comprehensive theory is not available. Certain classes of interactions are well established and understood, and some effects can be predicted on that basis. This has to be supplemented by considerations derived from *in vitro* and animal experiments and such human data as are available. Allowances have to be made for areas of uncertainty.

Diagnostic MR examinations usually can be completed within one hour. Therefore, the considerations to be presented next were focused on effects of exposure for periods of up to one hour with emphasis on immediate (acute) adverse reactions. It should be stressed that the discussion here does not apply to occupational or public exposure limits.

Static Magnetic Fields

In 1987, most MR devices used static magnetic fields with flux densities of 0.5 to 1.5 tesla (T), although some small bore spectroscopy systems employed fields up to 10 T and large bore imaging systems using 4-T fields were under development. The patient is exposed to the main field and levels up to 900 mT are expected at the mouth of the bore and up to 250 mT in the imaging room and adjoining areas.

Because the magnetic permeability of most biological materials relative to free space is about 1, the magnetic fields inside the body can be considered as equal to incident fields. There are three classes of magnetic field interactions:[5] (1) electrodynamic and magnetohydrodynamic effects, (2) magnetomechanical effects, and (3) interactions at the atomic and nuclear levels.

The first class involves interactions of applied magnetic fields with ionic currents according to the Lorentz force law, which relates the force exerted on a charge to its velocity, local electric field strength, and magnetic flux density. From physical and biophysical considerations, relationships can be derived and calculations can be made to predict effects arising out of these interactions.[4] Experimental data agree with theoretical expectations.

Interaction of magnetic fields with ionic currents through the Lorentz force law may influence the propagation of action potentials along peripheral nerve fibers and loops in the central nervous system. Wikswo and Barach[6] calculated that a field of 24 T may induce, under conservative assumptions, a 10% reduction in nerve conductivity. No measurable effects are expected on the bioelectric properties of isolated neurons exposed to fields of up to 2 T, an expectation confirmed by experimental findings.[7] Therefore, no significant effects are expected on the function of peripheral nerves. This is not necessarily the case where complex neural networks, such as occur in the central nervous system, are concerned.

Perturbations in the EEG patterns were observed by Beischer and Knepton[8] in squirrel monkeys and by Kholodov[9] in rabbits exposed to fields ranging from 0.1 to 9.1 T. The changes were induced upon the application of the field and disappeared after removal of the field. In humans, changes in amplitude and latency periods of evoked acoustic potentials were seen during exposure to 0.35-T fields.[10] These changes disappeared over 20 to 30 minutes following termination of exposure. Following exposures to 2-T fields, the pattern of evoked acoustic potentials reverted to preexposure levels during three hours.[11]

Electrodynamic interactions also result in flow potentials during the flow of an electrolyte solution through a static magnetic field. The magnitude of the induced potential is linearly related to the magnetic flux density and diameter of the vessel and also depends upon the flow velocity and the orientation of the flow relative to the field.[12] From this, it can be predicted that the largest potentials will be associated with blood flow into the aorta because of its diameter and the velocity of blood flow. The induced potentials can be calculated and studied experimentally using ECG surface electrodes.[13] The magnetically induced flow potentials appear in the ECG superimposed on the T wave. Their occurrence and their dependence upon exposure parameters were studied in rats, rabbits, and baboons.[14] Biological effects can be expected when the induced flow potentials reach values at which interference with the function of cell membranes of heart muscle fibers and the impulse conduction system may occur. Mansfield and Morris[15] calculated the maximum aortic flow potential for an adult (diameter of 2.5 cm, peak flow of 63 cm/s) as 16 mV per tesla. Using a different model, Kinouchi et al.[16] calculated the induced current density at 1 T as 0.05 A/m^2 on the vascular wall and as 0.02 A/m^2 in the vicinity of the sinoatrial node, compared to the 50% response level for ventricular fibrillation of about 1.7 A/m^2. Such calculations were the basis for the limitation of the static magnetic flux density to 2.5 T in the British (NRPB) MR safety recommendations.[17,18]

Electrodynamic interactions with the flow of electrolyte solution lead to magneto-hydrodynamic effects, resulting in the retardation of axial flow and an increase in intra-aortic pressure. Experimental studies by Tenforde et al.[19] of cardiovascular function in Macaca monkeys exposed to static magnetic fields up to 1.5 T showed negligible increase in blood pressure. Whereas negligible hemodynamic effects occur during exposure to 2-T fields, 50 T could reduce the aortic flow velocity by 7%. (Previous calculations of the blood flow reduction have contained an error of a factor of ten according to the presentation by Budinger at this conference.)

Magnetomechanical effects include magneto-orientation and magnetomechanical translation. Diamagnetic and paramagnetic molecules are subject to a torque force, which leads to an orientation in the field that minimizes their free energy. These effects are reviewed by Czerski and myself[1] and by WHO-UNEP-IRPA.[20] Several biological macromolecular structures have diamagnetic anisotropies and are subject to orientation in magnetic fields. One example of such a structure in mammals is the array of photopigments in retinal rod disk membranes.

Spatial gradients of static magnetic fields exert forces on paramagnetic and ferromagnetic structures that lead to a translation motion. This effect is of limited significance in mammalian systems, which contain little magnetic material. Magneto-mechanical effects are, however, important if metallic inclusions or implants are present. Displacement or reorientation of such objects in the presence of magnetic fields may lead to injury.

Interactions at the atomic and nuclear levels may affect charge transfer reactions. Experimental data at flux densities below 2 T[19] indicate that, in biological systems, these effects are transient, can be compensated for by living systems, and do not lead to perturbations or irreversible effects on growth, reproduction, prenatal and postnatal development, or behavioral and physiological parameters.

In summary, the principal factors limiting exposure to static magnetic fields for periods up to one hour are effects on the nervous and cardiocirculatory systems relatable to electrodynamic and magnetohydrodynamic interactions. No adverse reactions are likely at flux densities up to 2 T. Exposure of extremities to fields up to 5

T is not likely to affect the function of peripheral nerves or blood vessels. As exposure fields approach 10 T, the uncertainties increase and theoretical considerations seem to indicate the possibility of a range of adverse reactions. Based on the aforementioned considerations, the FDA selected, for its 1987 Guidance, limits of 2 T for whole-body exposure and 5 T for extremities (see Appendix in this volume).

Time-varying (Switched Gradient) Magnetic Fields

Time-varying fields induce electric potentials and circulating currents in accord with Faraday's law. In a simplified case of a circular loop (such as the circumference of the head, trunk, or heart) intersected by a uniform time-varying magnetic field, the magnitude of the average induced electric field depends on the radius of the loop and on dB/dt (i.e., the rate of change in the magnetic flux density). The induced current density in tissue of a given conductivity can be derived from Ohm's law. As a rough approximation, the greater the radius and dB/dt, the greater is the likelihood of inducing effects. However, other parameters, such as fundamental frequency, maximum and average flux densities, waveform (sinusoidal, square, or variously shaped pulsed), and polarity of the signal, have to be taken into account. A more sophisticated treatment of these dependencies is presented in the papers by Bernhardt,[21-23] Reilly,[24] and Silny.[25]

The energy of induced fields and currents is dissipated in the tissue at a rate that depends on the local electric field strength and conductivity and can be quantified in units of watts per cubic meter (W/m^3). Knowing the specific density of tissue, this can be converted to specific absorption rate (SAR) units of W/kg used to quantify RF field exposure. From the SAR and thermal characteristics of the tissue, heating effects associated with currents can be calculated. However, heating effects become more limiting than electrophysiological effects only at frequencies above about 100 kHz, as will be discussed later.

There is a large body of evidence indicating that a wide range of cellular functions are affected at induced current densities slightly above the level of those occurring naturally.[19] The effects are frequency-dependent. With increasing frequency, higher current densities are required to produce an effect. Waveform shape also plays a role. According to the WHO-UNEP-IRPA review,[20] no effects can be considered as established at current densities below 1 mA/m^2 and only minor inconsequential effects were reported in the range between 1 and 10 mA/m^2 at frequencies below 300 Hz, where biological systems appear to be the most sensitive.

At current densities between 10 and 100 mA/m^2, well-established effects occur, the best-known example being the induction of phosphenes. These are light flashes perceived during exposure of the head (frontal part or the eye) to time-varying fields at frequencies less than 100 Hz, with maximum susceptibility at about 20 Hz. The threshold magnetic flux density was reported variously as 5 to 10 mT with rise times of 2 to 3 ms. Threshold values of dB/dt may vary among individuals. Tenforde and Budinger[26] indicated values ranging from 1.3 to 1.9 T/s; however, pulses of shorter duration than about 0.9 ms did not induce visual sensations at 12 T/s. Effects disappear upon cessation of exposure and do not affect visual acuity. Thus, apart from an unusual sensation, magnetophosphenes experienced for a short period do not seem to pose health hazards. Note, though, that current densities above 1 A/m^2

pose immediate health hazards, associated with the increasing possibility of inducing cardiac fibrillation and continuous (tetanic) muscle contractions.[19]

As mentioned earlier, induced current densities depend on the radius of the loop, on tissue conductivity, and on dB/dt. A very useful rule of thumb was suggested by Budinger:[27,28] assuming a radius of 10 cm and an average tissue conductivity of 0.2 siemens per meter (S/m), he obtains 10 mA/m^2 per 1 tesla per second (1 T/s). The assumed radius is larger than the average values for the human adult heart or head, estimated as 6 cm[25] and 7.7 cm,[21] and in the British MRI safety guidelines.[17,18] Bernhardt[21] used also a higher value for the conductivity, that is, 0.25 S/m. Considerations on peripheral nerve stimulation (see later discussion) are based on an assumption of a 20-cm radius and a conductivity of 0.2 S/m. This leads to a rule of thumb of an induced current density of 20 mA/m^2 per 1 T/s. Such current densities are expected at the periphery of the body of an unusually large person with a trunk circumference of 125.7 cm or about 49.5 inches. In theory, the induced current density decreases to zero at the center of the loop. In the case of an inhomogeneous conductor with different realistic conductivities (blood, muscle, lung, bones, fat), complex eddy current formations occur in the body. In view of the scarcity of empirical data and due to the lack of precise numerical solutions for current distributions in a realistic human body model, a large area of uncertainty exists and safety factors become necessary.

Animal studies[29,30] indicate that time-varying magnetic fields induce skeletal muscle contractions at dB/dt levels at which no disturbances in cardiac function occur. Because of this consideration and because the highest current densities are induced at the periphery of the body, thresholds for peripheral neuromuscular stimulation are a convenient end point for the evaluation of the levels of exposure.

Based on physical and electrophysiological data, a model for the excitation of myelinated nerves, which are characterized by lower excitation thresholds than nonmyelinated ones, was developed.[31,32] This spatially extended nonlinear node (SENN) model was applied by Reilly[24] for analysis of neuromuscular effects of MR exposure. As shown in FIGURE 1, for single pulses of a duration above 0.3 ms, the threshold for peripheral nerve stimulation is approximately 62 T/s for an inductive loop radius of 20 cm and a nerve fiber of 20-μm diameter. The threshold value increases with decreases in the inductive loop diameter and the diameter of the fiber considered and it is also higher for pulses shorter than 0.3 ms. The frequency dependence of the SENN model predictions as compared to experimental data is shown in FIGURE 2.

The threshold for cardiac fibrillation is also derived from animal studies and a few human studies on the effects of currents delivered through electrodes applied to the heart. There is a consensus that the best approximation is the value of 3 A/m^2,[21,28,33] although Saunders and Orr[34] mention unpublished data indicating a lower value of 1.5 A/m^2. British MR safety recommendations[17] require that the current densities induced in any part of the body should be ten times less than the cardiac fibrillation threshold. Assuming a value of 3 A/m^2, a radius of 15 cm, and a conductivity of 0.2 S/m, this corresponds to 20 T/s. The NRPB[17] allows an increase in dB/dt for pulses shorter than 10 ms according to the formula,

$$(dB/dt)^2 \times \tau < 4,$$

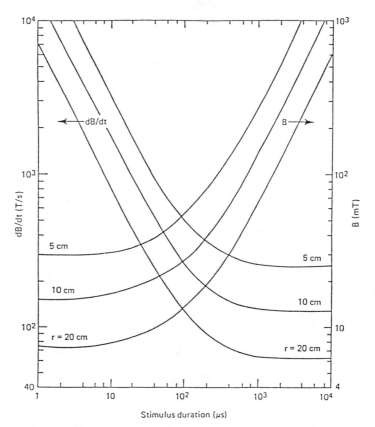

FIGURE 1. Strength/duration curves for peripheral stimulation by a single magnetic field pulse; 20-μm neuron. The r indicates the maximum induction loop radius, the left axis gives the dB/dt thresholds, and the right axis gives the B thresholds. (From Reilly.[24])

where dB/dt is the rms value of the rate of change of magnetic flux density in T/s and τ (in seconds) is the half-period for a sinusoidal wave or the duration of the rate of change for other waveforms.

Reilly's data[24] indicate that, under worse-case assumptions, exposures of the trunk (whole body) to pulses longer than 0.12 ms (FIGURE 2) of fields with a dB/dt not exceeding 20 T/s incorporate a safety factor of about three for peripheral nerve stimulation and of at least ten (in all likelihood much higher) for ventricular fibrillation. The same value of 20 T/s may be used for limiting exposure of the head. The smaller radius of the inductive loop, that is, about 6 cm for the brain and 7.7 cm for the circumference of the head, provides an additional factor to account for uncertainties of exposure related to effects on the nervous system or to realistic current distributions inside the body.[24,35] In the case of exposures involving only extremities, dB/dt may be increased by a factor obtained by dividing 20 cm (the "worst-case" radius for the trunk) by the radius (centimeters) of the bore of the magnet used for exposure, for example, by a factor of two for a bore radius of 10 cm or four for a 5-cm radius.

In summary, the FDA chose to limit exposure to switched gradient fields to a dB/dt of 20 T/s for pulses longer than 0.12 ms (frequencies below 1 kHz). Higher dB/dt values are allowed for shorter pulses and higher frequencies (see Appendix in this volume) and the acceptability of a given value may also be demonstrated with valid scientific evidence.

Radio-Frequency (RF) Fields

Several mechanisms of interaction of RF fields with living systems have been proposed, but the established and noncontroversial mechanism for acute exposures is dielectric heating. There is a wide consensus that limits for human exposure at frequencies above 100 kHz have to be derived primarily from thermal considerations.[36] Effects of short-term exposure correlate with increases in temperature, whereas effects not associated with heating and having possible health implications were reported following long-term (days, months) continuous or intermittent exposures.[19,37-39] Therefore, the assessment of health consequences of exposures of up to one hour should primarily take into account the physiological consequences of increases in temperature.

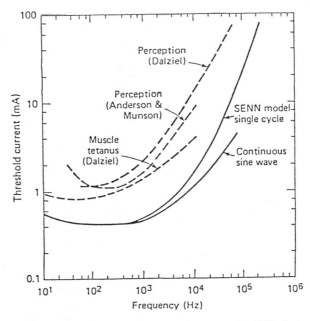

FIGURE 2. Strength/frequency curves for sinusoidal current stimuli. Dashed curves are from experimental data. Solid curves apply to the SENN model. The experimental curves have been shifted vertically to facilitate comparisons. (From Reilly.[24])

The average normal core temperature is about 37 °C with diurnal variations of ±0.5 °C. Normal values vary among individuals. Shimada and Stitt[40] quote oral temperatures in normal, healthy individuals ranging from 35.9 to 37.4 °C, with a mean of 36.7 °C. Moderate exercise or environmental heat can result in increases of 1 °C. Emotion may lead to the same effect. Active children may exhibit temperatures of 38 °C for hours. Thus, normal temperatures cover a range of values. Diurnal variations span a range of 1 °C and increases of 1 °C above the initial temperature within the zone of comfort in environmental conditions are not accompanied by any evident disturbances in function in healthy individuals.[41,42]

Exercise-induced heat loads accompanied by a 1 °C rise in temperature do not impose a significant stress on the thermoregulatory system in healthy individuals.[43] The metabolic rate increases 10% for a 1 °C rise, an inconsequential change. Studies of animals exposed to RF fields indicate that a 1 °C increase in core temperature over 40–60 minutes correlates with a threshold for disruption of operant behavior based on an observing task, with a return to preexposure baseline within a few minutes after extinction of the field.[44]

The aforementioned considerations indicate that an increase of 1 °C in core temperature will not pose immediate health hazards to healthy individuals, that is, those with an unimpaired blood flow from the core to the skin and within the skin, as well as having normal evaporative heat loss through respiration and sweating. Moreover, ambient conditions influence heat dissipation. This is enhanced under conditions expected in an examination room, that is, about 20–22 °C air temperature, a 30–50% relative humidity, and a lightly clothed (light pajamas) patient. A moderate airflow of 0.8 m/s would further facilitate heat loss.

An increase of less than 0.5 °C in core or brain temperature remains within diurnal variation and is predicted to be below the threshold for a response from the hypothalamic thermoregulatory center.[45] NRPB MR safety recommendations state that the body temperature during MRI examinations should not increase by more than 1 °C.[17] The ACGIH in its "Threshold Limit Values (TLVs) for 1985–86" recommends that work in hot environments should be interrupted when the temperature of the body exceeds 38 °C, assuming an initial value of 37 °C.[46]

Upper levels of tolerance to core temperature increases are not clearly defined. Michaelson and Schwan[47] quote 39.2 °C as a useful criterion for setting the limit for clinical trials, or an increase of 2.2 °C over one hour in rectal temperature, assuming 37 °C before exposure. Note that 41 °C is indicated as the temperature at which a healthy person is likely to develop a heat stroke.[41]

Nonuniformity of RF energy absorption may lead to an increase of temperature over a limited volume (hot spots) not accompanied by core temperature elevation. Thresholds for injury by local hyperthermia range from 41 °C for the induction of cataracts in the rabbit eye[48] to 43 °C used as a minimum effective temperature for heat cell killing in cancer therapy.[47] This has to be compared with the 41 °C required as a minimum for therapeutic action of RF diathermy applied for 20 to 30 minutes.[36] One hour at 42 °C leads to desquamation and erythema in human skin.

In summary, an increase in core temperature of up to 0.5 °C is within the limits of physiological oscillations. No adverse reactions are expected to be associated with increases of up to 1 °C, except for patients with significant impairment of cardiovascular function and/or sweat production (e.g., skin changes such as ichthyosis) or for children below one year of age. Local hyperthermia of about 1 °C within the head, 2 °C within the trunk, and about 3 °C within extremities is not likely to produce adverse effects. Increases in temperature greater than those just stated by a factor of two are at the limits of tolerance and may induce serious adverse reactions.

The increases in body temperature during MR procedures depend upon RF energy deposition and the rate of heat loss. Several models for computation of RF energy deposition in terms of SAR have been developed and measurements can be made in phantoms or animals to verify model predictions (see general review by Polk and Postow[38]). SAR alone provides information only about power deposition and thus is of limited value to the user, who is interested in resulting temperature increases. Under unrealistic "worst-case" conditions of no heat loss, temperature increases can be calculated from the SAR, the duration of exposure, and the specific heat (heat capacitance) of tissues using the formula,

$$\Delta T = \frac{SAR \cdot t}{4186 \cdot c},$$

where ΔT is the temperature increase in °C, t is the time in seconds, c is the specific heat in $kcal \cdot kg^{-1} \cdot °C^{-1}$, SAR is in W/kg, and 4186 is a conversion factor in J/kcal needed to obtain the proper dimensions of the equation. Assuming c for soft tissue as 0.83 $kcal \cdot kg^{-1} \cdot °C^{-1}$, a rule of thumb can be derived that 1-h exposure at 1 W/kg will result in an increase of about 1 °C. Alternatively, this can be restated that the same increase will occur if the total energy over the duration of exposure is 60 W · min/kg. These statements apply to SAR averaged over 1 kg. RF energy deposition is usually nonuniform and can result in hot spots or in the focusing of absorption over a small volume, resulting in local hyperthermia. Thus, models taking into account realistic RF energy deposition and heat dissipation within the body and heat exchange with the environment are necessary to predict thermal (temperature) effects. Such models are available[49] and are still being perfected. Computations were undertaken[50] of the temperature rise during imaging of the head at up to 3 W/kg averaged over its mass and no temperature rise was found of more than 1 °C in an unperfused region the size of an eye (approximated as a sphere). Similar SARs, or possible higher values, averaged over the exposed body part seem to be acceptable for the trunk, with the exception of persons with impaired blood flow and/or perspiration or on some medications. SAR considerations in relation to temperature increases are strictly dependent upon exposure parameters and equipment characteristics. Therefore, such considerations are more of interest to the designer and manufacturer to assure that acceptable temperatures are not exceeded.

The current FDA Guidance offers manufacturers the option of (i) adhering to a conservative whole-body SAR limit of 0.4 W/kg, the same as the ANSI C95.1 standard,[51] or (ii) demonstrating that the temperature increase in the body does not exceed the limits shown in the Appendix of this volume.

CONSIDERATIONS FOR FUTURE GUIDELINES AND STANDARDS

The future in MR technology seems to be one of an increasing pressure for larger magnetic fields, dB/dt, and RF power deposition. However, it is clear that this trend cannot continue indefinitely, both for reasons of safety and technical limitations.

For example, there are already several 4-T devices in clinical trials in the United States, but ordinary proton imaging devices are not likely to have much stronger fields because of the increasing importance of the chemical shift or cost considerations. It may be possible, however, for developments in the technology to actually take advantage of the chemical shift to produce images of specific chemical species, in which case fields higher than 4 T may be necessary. Imaging or spectroscopy of other nuclei may also require higher fields.

Higher static magnetic fields also mean higher frequencies for the RF fields, resulting in larger RF power deposition. At higher frequencies, phase differences in signals returning to the receiver coils may make imaging more difficult, but this may be manageable, at least up to 4 T.

Fast imaging procedures may also be important in the future, reducing the time required for a scan. These procedures usually involve higher values of $d\text{B}/dt$ from the gradient coils.

Clearly, it is important to set guidelines for MR that are safe, but which are not so restrictive that important diagnostic advances are unnecessarily inhibited. Determining the optimum trade-off is the task in several standards development efforts at the present time. Chief among these is that by IEC Subcommittee 62B, Working Group 21.[52] The FDA will probably wait until this new standard is completed before making major changes in its own guidance. The following considerations are some of the developments, mostly occurring since 1987, that have implications for the levels that are chosen for future guidelines and standards.

The threshold for biological effects seems most uncertain for static magnetic fields. Most of the concerns are theoretical in nature and actual clinical experience with the new 4-T systems may clarify just how much risk is involved in whole-body exposure to magnetic fields above 2 T. The clinical trials that are now under way should be well controlled and thorough with regard to possible adverse effects and the sponsors should recognize that the international community has a great interest in seeing the results of this research. Until the safety of levels above 2 T is demonstrated, which may occur before the IEC standard is finalized, the standard and guideline limits should probably not be raised above present levels.

Since 1987, there have been two important developments—one experimental and one theoretical—that affect our consideration of $d\text{B}/dt$ guidelines. Peripheral nerve stimulation has now been demonstrated in experimental imaging procedures using human volunteers.[53,54] Although some have suggested that the level of 20 T/s in the FDA and NRPB guidelines was quite conservative, the actual threshold levels for peripheral nerve stimulation have turned out to be slightly lower than the levels predicted in the theoretical studies by Reilly.[24,55] FIGURE 3 shows the theoretical threshold as a function of pulse width, and the experimental stimulation threshold data[53] are plotted as individual points.

The FDA guidance value was chosen to include a safety factor of about three with respect to the theoretical threshold. The actual safety factor now appears to be closer to two; thus, to avoid peripheral nerve stimulation, it will probably not be possible to relax the guideline levels very much, if at all.

The other consideration in setting the FDA guidance level for $d\text{B}/dt$ was that cardiac stimulation was thought to have a higher threshold than peripheral nerve stimulation. However, until recently, the cardiac stimulation problem had not been directly addressed for MR.

In a modeling study similar to the one that he did for peripheral nerve stimulation, Reilly[56,57] has now treated the case of cardiac stimulation. FIGURE 3 shows Reilly's threshold curves for both cardiac and peripheral nerve stimulation, assuming that the gradient field is parallel to the body. There are two curves for peripheral nerve, each representing a different value of the characteristic nerve response time constant. The figure shows that the threshold for peripheral nerve stimulation is, in fact, lower than for cardiac stimulation, except for pulse widths larger than 5 ms (frequencies less than 100 Hz). For pulses larger than 5 ms, there is very little difference between the two. However, it is unlikely that any MR systems will ever

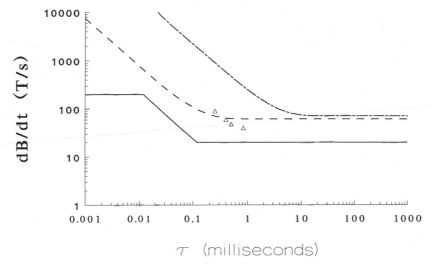

FIGURE 3. Thresholds and guidelines for dB/dt. Theoretical thresholds as a function of pulse width (τ) for peripheral nerve stimulation (PNS) (– –, PNS theoretical threshold;[56,57] △, experimental PNS data[53]), cardiac stimulation (CS) (– - –, CS theoretical data),[56,57] and FDA guidelines (—).

operate in this region. Hence, for any practical MR system, the conventional wisdom regarding peripheral nerve versus cardiac stimulation still appears to be true. The thresholds for cardiac fibrillation are estimated by Reilly to be at least a factor of five (and probably ten) higher than for cardiac stimulation.

Although peripheral nerve stimulation is probably not hazardous, it can be unpleasant to the patient and it may cause movement artifacts in the images. Therefore, it still seems appropriate to set the dB/dt limits at levels at least a factor of two below the threshold for peripheral nerve stimulation. This means that the present FDA guidance is unlikely to change for pulse widths longer than 120 μs.

The FDA guidance for RF power deposition allowed either (i) meeting a 0.4-W/kg SAR limit or (ii) providing valid scientific evidence that the SAR that is used does not cause temperature rises above specified limits. Many manufacturers have taken the latter approach to demonstrate safety. As a result, most 1.5-T systems in clinical usage in the United States have hardware or software controls on the SAR at levels above 0.4 W/kg, ranging from 1 to 2 W/kg.

Theoretical and clinical studies seem to indicate that a healthy person can handle up to 4 W/kg for up to an hour with less than a 1 °C temperature rise.[58,59] The difficulty for standards committees is that most patients undergoing MR scans are not healthy, although most have adequate thermoregulatory systems. For a small percentage of patients, their thermoregulatory systems are impaired to an extent that they may not be able to tolerate as much as 4 W/kg. The environmental conditions in the scan room also affect the tolerable limits on SAR. Most scan rooms meet the manufacturer's specifications (or are somewhat cooler than necessary), but not all do so at all times. Operators of MR systems generally have little appreciation for the potential risks to compromised patients of performing imaging sessions when room temperatures are elevated.

There seems to be no reason why the present FDA conservative SAR limit of 0.4 W/kg could not be relaxed in light of the recent clinical experience and modeling studies. However, there needs to be some provision in any new guidance or safety standards that protects the compromised patient.

The NRPB introduced a two-tiered system of limits on exposure in its 1984 MR Safety Guidance.[18] In this approach, there is a set of limits that should have an adequate margin of safety for the general population and another set of limits above which the system should not operate. This approach allows diagnostically important scans to be performed even when levels are above the first-tier limits, but also serves to warn the operator that proper supervision or patient screening is required.

The two-tiered approach to limits seems to have many advantages over the single safety limit for MR systems. It recognizes that MR systems, to provide the optimum trade-off between safety and effectiveness, must be capable of operating near the limits of patient safety. However, the variation in tolerance among patients would require limits that are too conservative for most patients under a single-limit approach to guidelines. The two-tiered approach is now being considered by the IEC MR working group and seems likely to be incorporated into future MR safety guidelines and standards.

REFERENCES AND NOTES

1. CZERSKI, P. & T. W. ATHEY. 1987. Safety of magnetic resonance *in vivo* diagnostic examinations: theoretical and clinical considerations. Center for Devices and Radiological Health Report (Rockville, Maryland).
2. The precise definitions of the three classes of devices may be found in the Medical Device Amendments of 1976, as further amended by the Safe Medical Device Act of 1990. Only a brief overview of the FDA's regulation of devices is intended here.
3. FDA. 1982 (February 25). Guidelines for evaluating electromagnetic risk for trials of clinical NMR systems. Bureau of Radiological Health Report.
4. FDA. 1988 (August 2). Guidance for content and review of a magnetic resonance diagnostic device 510(k) application: safety parameter action levels. Center for Devices and Radiological Health Report (Rockville, Maryland).
5. TENFORDE, T. S. 1983. Mechanisms for biological effects of magnetic fields. *In* Biological

Effects and Dosimetry of Static and ELF Electromagnetic Fields. M. Grandolfo, S. M. Michaelson & A. Rindi, Eds.: 71–92. Plenum. New York.

6. WIKSWO, J. P. & J. P. BARACH. 1980. An estimate of steady magnetic field strength required to influence nerve conduction. IEEE Trans. Biomed. Eng. **BME-27:** 722–723.

7. TENFORDE, T. S. 1983. Biological effects of stationary magnetic fields. *In* Biological Effects and Dosimetry of Static and ELF Electromagnetic Fields. M. Grandolfo, S. M. Michaelson & A. Rindi, Eds.: 92–128. Plenum. New York.

8. BEISCHER, D. E. & J. C. KNEPTON. 1966. The electroencephalogram of the squirrel monkey (*Saimiri sciureus*) in a very high magnetic field. Naval Aerospace Medical Institute Report (NASA), Order No. R-39 (Pensacola, Florida).

9. KHOLODOV, Y. A., M. M. ALEXANDROVSKAYA, S. N. DUKJANOVCE & N. S. UDAROVA. 1969. Investigations of the reactions of the mammalian brain to static magnetic fields. *In* Biological Effects of Magnetic Fields, Vol. 2. M. Barnothy, Ed.: 215–226. Plenum. New York.

10. VON KLITZIG, L., E. IHNEN & B. TERWEY. 1984. Statische 0.35-tesla Magnetfelder beeinflussen die akustisch evozierten Potentiale beim Menschen. Naturwissenschaften.

11. VON KLITZIG, L., H. J. SCHOPKA & H. WENDHAUSEN. 1986. Biological effects of static magnetic fields in animals and man. BGA-Schr. **3:** 86–88.

12. KOLIN, A. 1952. Improved apparatus and technique for electromagnetic determination of blood flow. Rev. Sci. Instrum. **23:** 235–240.

13. TOGAWA, T., O. OKAI & M. OSHIMA. 1967. Observation of blood flow EMF in externally applied strong magnetic fields by surface electrodes. Med. Biol. Eng. **5:** 169–170.

14. TENFORDE, T. S., C. T. GAFFEY & M. S. RAYBURN. 1985. Influence of stationary magnetic fields on ionic conduction processes in biological systems. Electromagnetic Compatibility 1985: Sixth Symposium and Technical Exhibition (5–7 March 1985, Zurich). Paper No. 37 G 2, p. 205–210.

15. MANSFIELD, P. & P. G. MORRIS. 1982. NMR imaging in biomedicine. *In* Advances in Magnetic Resonance (Suppl. 2). J. S. Waugh, Ed. Academic Press. New York.

16. KINOUCHI, Y., Y. KUBO, T. USHITA & T. S. TENFORDE. 1987. Analysis of magnetically induced potentials and currents around the ascending aorta. Bioelectromagnetics Society, Ninth Annual Meeting (21–25 June 1987, Portland, Oregon), Abstract p. 45.

17. NRPB (National Radiation Protection Board). 1981. Exposure to nuclear magnetic clinical resonance imaging. Radiography **47:** 258–260.

18. NRPB (National Radiation Protection Board). 1984. Ad hoc advisory group on NMR clinical imaging: revised guidance on acceptable limits of exposure during nuclear magnetic resonance clinical imaging. Br. J. Radiol. **56:** 974–977.

19. TENFORDE, T. S., C. T. GAFFEY, B. R. MOYER & T. F. BUDINGER. 1983. Cardiovascular alterations in *Macaca* monkeys exposed to stationary magnetic fields: experimental observations and theoretical analysis. Bioelectromagnetics **4:** 1–9.

20. WHO-UNEP-IRPA (World Health Organization–United Nations Environment Programme–International Radiation Protection Association). 1987. Environmental Health Criteria 69: Magnetic Fields. WHO. Geneva.

21. BERNHARDT, J. H. 1979. The direct influence of electromagnetic fields on nerve and muscle cells in man within the frequency range of 1 Hz and 30 MHz. Radiat. Environ. Biophys. **16:** 309–329.

22. BERNHARDT, J. H. 1985. Evaluation of human exposures to low frequency fields. *In* The Impact of Proposed Radiofrequency Radiation Standards on Military Operations. AGARD Lecture Series No. 138, JSBN92-835-1494-7, p. 8.1–8.18.

23. BERNHARDT, J. H. 1986. Assessment of experimentally observed bioeffects in view of their clinical relevance and the exposure at work places. *In* Proceedings of the Symposium on the Biological Effects of Static and Extremely Low Frequency Magnetic Fields. J. H. Bernhardt, Ed.: 157–168. MMV Medizin Verlag. Munich.

24. REILLY, J. P. 1987. Peripheral stimulation by pulsatile currents: applications to time-varying magnetic field exposure. Report No. MT 87-100 Prepared for the Center for Devices and Radiological Health (HFZ-133). FDA. Rockville, Maryland.

25. SILNY, J. 1986. The influence threshold of the time-varying magnetic field in the human organism. BGA-Schr. **3**(86): 105–112.

26. TENFORDE, T. S. & T. F. BUDINGER. 1986. Biological effects and physical safety aspects of NMR imaging and *in vivo* spectroscopy. *In* NMR in Medicine: The Instrumentation and Clinical Applications. S. R. Thomas & R. L. Dickson, Eds.: 493–548. Amer. Inst. Phys. New York.

27. BUDINGER, T. F. 1979. Thresholds for physiological effects due to RF and magnetic fields used in NMR imaging. IEEE Trans. Nucl. Sci. **NS-26:** 2821–2825.

28. BUDINGER, T. F. 1981. Nuclear magnetic resonance (NMR) *in vivo* studies: known thresholds for effects. J. Comput. Assist. Tomogr. **5:** 800–810.

29. McROBBIE, D. & M. A. FOSTER. 1985. Cardiac response to pulsed magnetic fields with regard to safety in NMR imaging. Phys. Med. Biol. **30:** 695–702.

30. McROBBIE, D. & M. A. FOSTER. 1984. Thresholds for biological effects of time-varying magnetic fields. Clin. Phys. Physiol. Meas. **5:** 67–78.

31. REILLY, J. P., V. T. FREEMAN & W. D. LARKIN. 1985. Sensory effects of transient electrical stimulation—evaluation with a neuroelectric model. IEEE Trans. Biomed. Eng. **BME-32:** 1001–1011.

32. REILLY, J. P. & R. H. BAUER. 1987. Application of neuroelectric model to electrocutaneous sensory sensitivity: parameter variation study. IEEE Trans. Biomed. Eng. **BME-34:** 752–754.

33. SAUNDERS, R. & H. SMITH. 1984. Safety aspects of NMR clinical imaging. Br. Med. Bull. **40:** 148–154.

34. SAUNDERS, R. & J. S. ORR. 1983. Biologic effects of NMR. *In* Nuclear Magnetic Resonance Imaging. C. L. Partain, A. E. James, F. D. Rollo & R. R. Price, Eds.: 383–396. Saunders. Philadelphia.

35. SILNY, J. 1984. Changes in VEP caused by strong magnetic fields. *In* Evoked Potentials. R. Nodar & C. Barber, Eds.: 272–279. Butterworths. London.

36. CZERSKI, P. 1986. The development of biomedical approaches and concepts in radiofrequency radiation protection. J. Microwave Power **21:** 9–23.

37. NCRP (National Council on Radiation Protection and Measurements). 1986. Biological effects and exposure criteria for radiofrequency electromagnetic fields. Report No. 86. NCRP. Bethesda, Maryland.

38. POLK, C. & E. POSTOW. 1986. Handbook of Biological Effects of Electromagnetic Fields. CRC Press. Boca Raton, Florida.

39. BARANSKI, S. & P. CZERSKI. 1976. Biological Effects of Microwaves. Dowden, Hutchinson, and Ross. Philadelphia.

40. SHIMADA, S. G. & J. T. STITT. 1983. Body temperature regulation during euthermia and hyperthermia. *In* Microwaves and Thermoregulation. E. R. Adair, Ed.: 139–159. Academic Press. New York.

41. HARDY, Y. O. & P. BARD. 1974. Body temperature regulation. *In* Medical Physiology (Thirteenth Edition). V. B. Mountcastle, Ed.: 1305–1342. Mosby. St. Louis, Missouri.

42. GUYTON, A. C. 1986. Textbook of Medical Physiology (Seventh Edition). Saunders. Philadelphia.

43. CHAPPUIS, P., P. PITTET & E. JEQUIER. 1976. Heat storage regulation in exercise during thermal transients. J. Appl. Physiol. **40:** 389–392.

44. DE LORGE, J. O. 1983. The thermal basis for disruption of operant behavior by microwaves in three animal species. *In* Microwaves and Thermoregulation. E. R. Adair, Ed.: 401–429. Academic Press. New York.

45. WAY, W. I., H. KRITIKOS & H. P. SCHWAN. 1981. Thermoregulatory physiologic responses in the human body exposed to microwave radiation. Bioelectromagnetics **2:** 341–356.

46. ACGIH (American Conference of Governmental Industrial Hygienists). 1985. Adopted threshold limit values—heat stress. *In* TLVs—Threshold Limit Values and Biological Exposure Indices for 1985–86, p. 68–74. ACGIH. Cincinnati, Ohio.

47. MICHAELSON, S. M. & H. P. SCHWAN. 1981. Factors governing the use of microwave/radiofrequency energies in cancer therapy. Adv. Radiat. Biol. **9:** 322–409.

48. GUY, A. W., J. C. LIN, P. O. KRAMAR & A. EMERY. 1975. Effect of 2450 MHz radiation on the rabbit eye. IEEE Trans. Microwave Theory Tech. **MTT-23:** 492–496.

49. ADAIR, E. R. & L. G. BERGLUND. 1986. On the thermoregulatory consequences of NMR imaging. Magn. Reson. Imag. **4:** 321–333.

50. ATHEY, T. W. 1989. A model of the temperature rise in the head due to magnetic resonance imaging procedures. Magn. Reson. Med. **9:** 177–184.

51. ANSI (American National Standards Institute). 1982. Safety levels with respect to human exposure to radio-frequency electromagnetic fields, 300 kHz to 100 GHz. Inst. Elec. Electronics Eng. New York.

52. IEC (International Electrotechnical Commission). 1992. Particular requirements for the safety of magnetic resonance systems for medical diagnosis. Subcommittee 62B, Working Group 21. Standard under Development. To be published.

53. COHEN, M. S., R. M. WEISSKOFF, R. R. RZEDZIAN & H. L. KANTOR. 1990. Sensory stimulation by time-varying magnetic fields. Magn. Reson. Med. **14:** 409–414.

54. BUDINGER, T. F., D. FISCHER, D. HENTSCHEL, H. REINFELDER & F. SCHMITT. 1990. Neural stimulation dB/dt thresholds for frequency and number of oscillations using sinusoidal magnetic gradient fields (abstract). Annual Meeting of the Society for Magnetic Resonance in Medicine.

55. REILLY, J. P. 1989. Peripheral nerve stimulation by induced electric currents: exposure to time-varying magnetic fields. Med. Biol. Eng. Comput. **23:** 101–110.

56. REILLY, J. P. 1989. Cardiac sensitivity to electrical stimulation. Report No. MT 89-100 Prepared for the Center for Devices and Radiological Health (HFZ-133). FDA. Rockville, Maryland.

57. REILLY, J. P. 1990. Peripheral nerve and cardiac excitation by time-varying magnetic fields: a comparison of thresholds. Report No. MT 90-100 Prepared for the Center for Devices and Radiological Health (HFZ-133). FDA. Rockville, Maryland.

58. ADAIR, E. R. & L. G. BERGLUND. 1989. Thermoregulatory consequences of cardiovascular impairment during NMR imaging in warm/humid environments. Magn. Reson. Imag. **7:** 25.

59. SHELLOCK, F. G., D. J. SCHAEFER & J. V. CRUES. 1990. Alterations in body and skin temperatures caused by MR imaging: is the recommended exposure for radiofrequency radiation too conservative? Br. J. Radiol. **62:** 904–909.

Session IV Summary

JOHN C. MONAHAN[a] AND JEFFREY C. WEINREB[b]

[a]Center for Devices and Radiological Health
Food and Drug Administration
Rockville, Maryland 20857

[b]Magnetic Resonance Imaging
New York University Medical Center
New York, New York 10016

Emanuel Kanal gave a physician's perspective on the major safety concerns of the clinical MRI environment. These include (1) effects of the static magnetic fields, (2) effects of the rapidly time-varying RF magnetic fields, (3) effects of the time-varying magnetic field gradients, and (4) claustrophobia. He described a number of potentially hazardous incidents that have occurred to patients in the environment of the clinical MR unit, including electrical and thermal burns (from surface coils, EKG leads, and pulse oximeters), as well as a variety of ferromagnetic objects that have been pulled into or onto the magnet. He stated that RF heating is a potential problem, especially in the elderly with compromised circulation and in infants, and that problems may be avoided by maintaining a flow of cool air because 75% of the body's heat is lost via radiation to the ambient air. Experimental subjects placed in 4-T magnets (which are not in clinical use at present) experienced vertigo, a metallic taste, and flashing lights. These sensations are not experienced with lower field strength clinical systems. E. Kanal made a plea for more study of the potential adverse effects of MRI, especially as newer techniques are introduced into the clinical arena. He also emphasized the critical importance of educating MRI physicians and technologists about the potential for these adverse effects.

Daniel Schaefer in his article on dosimetry discussed the effects of both gradient and radio-frequency (RF) fields. The safety of magnetic resonance (MR) imaging becomes more important as the technology evolves toward larger and faster gradients and toward the use of higher RF power levels. D. Schaefer, using a series of mathematical models, calculated the parameters of coil pairs and then related the derived values to experimental data on peripheral nerve and cardiac stimulation. He then examined the question of patient power absorption from RF fields during typical clinical scans and the potential temperature increases. Again, using mathematical models, he discussed whole-body and local specific absorption rates and the possibilities of adverse effects given the current understanding of thermal physiology. On the basis of these models, he proposed that a simple gradient safety standard could be based on the minimum flux required for cardiac stimulation. He also acknowledged the need for more experimental research with cardiac-compromised patients and their reaction to RF energy absorption.

Richard Olsen provided insight into the need for and the inherent difficulties in the development of personal dosimeters for MRI patients and staff. Current MR systems contain built-in safeguards, such as RF monitors and software checks, to prevent any overexposure to potentially hazardous RF fields. However, he stressed the need for an independent dosimeter system in the event of a failure or a bypassing of the safeguards. He then discussed the results of a study to determine localized SARs in a full-sized, muscle-equivalent human model exposed to realistic imaging protocols. A prototype muscle-equivalent dosimeter was also used to make additional SAR measurements on the human model. These measurements demonstrated that localized SARs were a relatively minor problem, but that MR scan time should be minimized to prevent thermal accumulation. R. Olsen concluded that the SARs developed by current generation MR instruments are sufficient to warrant the development of independent dosimeters.

In 1988, the Food and Drug Administration (FDA) reclassified MR devices from Class III (highest level of premarket regulation) to Class II (medium level of regulation). As part of the reclassification process, the FDA issued safety guidance for MR devices that they would have to meet in order to be considered Class II devices. T. Whit Athey presented a thorough summary of the FDA guidance and its underlying rationale. In addition, he provided a brief review of the general regulatory approach that the FDA takes for medical devices. Lastly, he presented the results of some recent studies that could impact future standards or guidance for MR instruments.

Thermal Responses in Human Subjects Exposed to Magnetic Resonance Imaging[a]

FRANK G. SHELLOCK

Division of Magnetic Resonance Imaging
Department of Radiology
Cedars-Sinai Medical Center
and
UCLA School of Medicine
Los Angeles, California 90048

INTRODUCTION

Magnetic resonance imaging (MRI) is an important diagnostic modality that requires exposing patients to three different types of electromagnetic radiation: a static magnetic field, gradient or time-varying magnetic fields, and radio-frequency (RF) electromagnetic fields. Each of these forms of electromagnetic radiation can cause significant biological effects if applied at sufficiently high exposure levels.[1-12]

The main biological effect of exposure to RF radiation is the production of heat that occurs due to resistive losses.[1-9] Therefore, the primary physiologic alterations associated with exposure to RF radiation are related to the thermogenic qualities of this electromagnetic field.[1,3-7,10]

Exposure to RF radiation may also cause athermal, field-specific alterations in biological systems that are produced without a significant increase in temperature.[11,12] This topic is somewhat controversial due to assertions concerning the role of electromagnetic fields in producing cancer and developmental abnormalities, along with the concomitant ramifications of such effects.[11,12] A recent report from the United States Environmental Protection Agency claimed that the existing evidence on this issue is sufficient to demonstrate a relationship between low level electromagnetic field exposures and the production of cancer.[13] To date, there have been no specific studies performed to study the potential athermal biological effects of RF radiation associated with MRI. However, those interested in a thorough review of this topic, particularly as it pertains to MRI, are referred to the extensive article written by Beers.[11]

Prior to 1985, there were no quantitative data available on thermoregulatory responses of human subjects exposed to RF radiation during MRI. In fact, there has been a general paucity of data on RF radiation–induced temperature changes in humans. Studies that have been performed in this area have examined thermal sensations or therapeutic applications of diathermy, usually involving only localized regions of the body.[2,8,9,14]

Although much work has been done with laboratory animals to determine thermoregulatory responses to heating from RF radiation,[2,8,9,15,16] these experiments

[a]This work was supported by PHS Grant No. 1 RO1 CA44014-03 awarded by the National Cancer Institute, National Institutes of Health.

do not apply to MRI because the pattern of RF absorption or the coupling of electromagnetic radiation to biologic tissues is highly dependent on the organism's size, anatomical factors, the duration of exposure, the sensitivity of the involved tissues, and a myriad of other variables.[2,8,9,15,16] Furthermore, there is no laboratory animal that sufficiently mimics or simulates the thermoregulatory system or responses of humans. For these reasons, results obtained in animal experiments cannot be simply "scaled" to human subjects.[8,15] Therefore, experiments performed on laboratory preparations may not be easily extrapolated nor are they directly applicable to human subjects for the clinical use of MRI.

Elaborate mathematic models have been devised to determine "worst-case" situations of how RF power is absorbed by human subjects during MRI.[17-19] A recognized major limitation of modeling, though, is that it is difficult to account for the numerous critical variables (i.e., age, drugs, cardiovascular disease, etc.) that affect the thermoregulatory function of human subjects, particularly in a patient population. More importantly, none of these models of thermal responses to RF radiation have ever been validated in human subjects during clinical MRI.

Due to the aforementioned considerations, it is imperative that studies pertaining specifically to MRI be conducted in a simulated setting or in the actual clinical setting in order to properly determine and characterize the thermal responses in human subjects.[4,7,20] Several investigations have been performed recently that have yielded extremely useful and important information about human thermal responses in human subjects exposed to MRI.[20-34] This article will review and discuss these specific studies as well as describe the various complicated factors involved in performing this type of research.

MRI AND THE ASSESSMENT OF SPECIFIC ABSORPTION RATE IN HUMAN SUBJECTS

Because one of the most apparent biological responses of exposure to MRI is the tissue heating that results from absorption of RF energy, investigators have typically quantified the RF exposure levels by the conventional means of determining the whole-body averaged specific absorption rate (SAR) (i.e., SAR is the mass normalized rate at which RF power is coupled to biologic tissue and is indicated in units of watts per kilogram, W/kg).[20-28,33,34] Measurements or estimates of SAR are not trivial, particularly in human subjects, and there are several methods of determining this parameter for the purpose of RF energy "dosimetry" during MRI.[20,28,34-38]

The SAR that is produced during MRI is a complex function of numerous variables including the frequency (which, in turn, is determined by the static magnetic field strength), the type of RF pulse used (i.e., 90° or 180°), the repetition time, the pulse width, the type of RF coil used (i.e., body coil or send/receive surface coil), the volume of tissue contained within the coil, the resistivity of the tissue, and the configuration of the anatomical region exposed, as well as other important factors.[1,3-7,37,38]

The efficiency and absorption pattern of RF energy are mainly determined by the physical dimensions of the tissue in relation to the incident wavelength.[2,8,9] Therefore, if the tissue size is large relative to the wavelength, energy is predominantly absorbed on the surface; if it is small relative to the wavelength, there is little absorption of RF power.[2,8,9] During MRI, tissue heating results primarily from magnetic induction with a negligible contribution from the electric fields,[37,38] so ohmic heating is greatest at the surface of the body and is minimal at the center of the body (FIGURE 1). Predictive calculations and measurements obtained in phantoms and in human subjects exposed to MRI support this pattern of temperature distribution.[2,8,9,37,38]

PHYSIOLOGICAL MEASUREMENTS OF THERMAL RESPONSES TO MRI IN HUMAN SUBJECTS

Obtaining physiologic measurements for evaluation of thermal responses within the harsh electromagnetic environment of MRI is not a simple task. The high

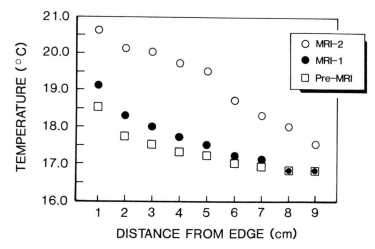

FIGURE 1. MRI was performed on a spherical, seedless watermelon (diameter, 24 cm) to study the depth of heating. Thermistor needles were inserted into the watermelon before (□) and after MRI performed with a 1.5-T/64-MHz MRI scanner using a quadrature body coil at whole-body averaged SARs of 1.0 W/kg (●) and 2.5 W/kg (○) for 30 min. Room temperature was 20.5 °C and relative humidity was 45%. The temperature plot shows that there is predominantly peripheral heating with relatively small temperature changes in the central part of the watermelon.

strength static magnetic fields can create missiles out of monitors that typically contain ferromagnetic components.[12,39,40] In addition, the static, gradient, and RF electromagnetic fields may adversely interfere with the proper operation of the monitoring equipment.[39,40] In turn, the monitors, themselves, may produce subtle or significant imaging artifacts that distort the MR images.[12,39,40] Therefore, monitors must be specially adapted or modified and then rigorously tested prior to use during MRI.

Currently, there are a variety of MRI-compatible monitors, as well as other patient support devices, that are commercially available.[39–42] Every physiologic parameter that is obtainable under normal circumstances in the critical care area or operating room may be recorded during MRI, including heart rate, oxygen saturation, end-tidal carbon dioxide, respiratory rate, blood pressure, and temperature.[39-42]

For assessment of thermal responses during MRI, volunteer subjects or patients have been routinely assessed continuously or semicontinuously with several different types of devices. For example, sublingual pocket temperature (note that there is a good relationship between sublingual pocket temperature and tympanic and esophageal temperatures[43]) is obtained immediately before and after MRI using a sensitive electronic thermometry system.[20,23,26] Skin temperatures are measured immediately before and after MRI procedures with a highly accurate infrared thermometer.[34,44] Body and skin temperatures measured at multiple sites are recorded before, during, and after MRI with a multichannel fluoroptic thermometry system that is unperturbed by electromagnetic radiation.[34,42] Heart rate, oxygen saturation, blood pressure, respiratory rate, and cutaneous blood flow, which are important physiologic variables that change in response to a thermal load, are also typically monitored during MRI to assess the thermoregulatory system of human subjects.[12,20-27,40] All of these parameters are obtained with MRI-compatible devices that have been extensively tested and demonstrated to provide accurate and sensitive data.

HUMAN THERMAL RESPONSES DURING MRI

Although the primary cause of tissue heating during MRI procedures is attributable solely to RF radiation, it should be noted that various reports have suggested that exposure to static magnetic fields used for MRI may also cause temperature changes.[45,46] The mechanism(s) responsible for such an effect remains unclear, but these publications have warranted investigations in human subjects to determine if there is any contribution of the static magnetic field to the temperature changes that may be observed during MRI. Therefore, studies were done[31,32] on body and skin temperatures in human subjects exposed to a 1.5-T static magnetic field. There were no statistically significant alterations observed in these recorded physiologic parameters.[31,32] Tenforde[47] examined this phenomenon as well in laboratory animals exposed to static magnetic fields as high as 7.55 T and also reported no effect. As far as the potential for production of heat by gradient magnetic fields is concerned, this is not believed to occur with conventional clinical MRI pulse sequences.[37,38]

The first study of human thermoregulatory responses during MRI was conducted by Schaefer et al.[25] and they investigated temperature changes and other physiologic alterations in volunteer subjects exposed to relatively high whole-body averaged SARs (i.e., approximately 4.0 W/kg). Their results indicated that there were no excessive temperature elevations or other untoward physiologic consequences related to this exposure to RF radiation.[25]

Several studies were subsequently conducted on volunteer subjects and patients undergoing clinical MRI procedures with the intent of obtaining information that would be applicable to the patient population typically encountered in the MRI setting.[20-28,30,33,34] The whole-body averaged SARs ranged from approximately 0.05 W/kg (i.e., for MRI procedures involving imaging with a send/receive head coil) to 4.0 W/kg (i.e., for MRI procedures involving the imaging of the spine or abdomen

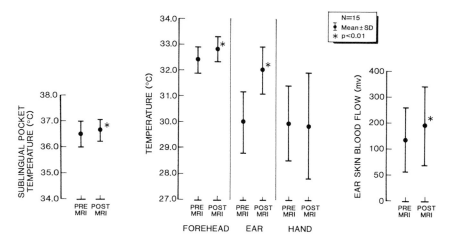

FIGURE 3. Sublingual pocket temperature, forehead skin temperature, ear skin temperature, hand skin temperature, and ear skin blood flow measured immediately before and after clinical MRI procedures involving the patient's head. There were statistically significant increases ($p < 0.01$) in sublingual pocket, forehead skin, and ear skin temperatures and in ear skin blood flow. (See reference 23.)

patients are scanned at whole-body averaged SARs higher than those previously evaluated (which is entirely possible; see last section in this article).

Dissipation of heat from the eye is a slow and inefficient process due to its relative lack of vascularization. Acute near-field exposures of RF radiation to the eyes or heads of laboratory animals have been demonstrated to be cataractogenic as a result

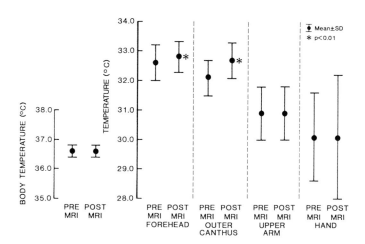

FIGURE 4. Average body (sublingual pocket) and skin temperatures measured immediately before and after MRI of the brain at 1.5 T/64 MHz using a head coil ($N = 35$). There were statistically significant increases in forehead skin and outer canthus skin temperatures. (See reference 26.)

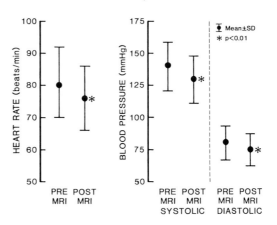

FIGURE 5. Average heart rate and systolic and diastolic blood pressures immediately before and after MRI of the brain at 1.5 T/64 MHz using a head coil ($N = 35$). There were statistically significant decreases in each of these measured parameters. (See reference 26.)

of the thermal disruption of ocular tissues if the exposure is of a sufficient intensity and duration.[56] An investigation conducted by Sacks et al.[57] revealed that there were no discernible effects on the eyes of rats produced by MRI at exposures that far exceeded typical clinical imaging levels. However, as previously indicated, it may not be acceptable to extrapolate these data to human subjects considering the coupling of RF radiation to the anatomy and the tissue volume of laboratory rat eyes compared to those of humans.

Corneal temperatures (corneal temperature is a representative site of the average temperature of the human eye[58]) have been measured in patients undergoing MRI of the brain using a send/receive head coil at local SARs up to 3.1 W/kg.[24] The largest corneal temperature change was 1.8 °C and the highest temperature measured was 34.4 °C. Because the temperature threshold for RF radiation–induced

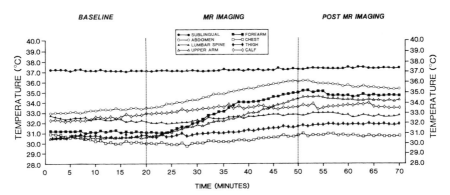

FIGURE 6. Sublingual and multiple skin temperatures measured at 1-min intervals with a fluoroptic thermometry system (Luxtron) before (baseline), during (MR imaging), and after (post–MR imaging) MRI performed at a whole-body averaged SAR of 2.8 W/kg. Note that there was little or no change in sublingual or body temperature, whereas there were slight to moderate changes in skin temperatures (depending on the site of measurement) during MRI. After MRI, some skin temperatures returned to the baseline level, whereas others remained elevated during the 20-min post-MRI evaluation period. (See reference 34.)

cataractogenesis in animal models has been demonstrated to be between 41 to 55 °C for acute near-field exposures, it does not appear that clinical MRI using a head coil has the potential to cause thermal damage in ocular tissue.[24] A more recent study[33] examined corneal temperatures in patients with suspected ocular pathology who underwent MRI using a special eye coil; again, there were no excessive corneal temperature elevations. The effect of MRI at higher SARs and the long-term effects of MRI on ocular tissues remain to be determined.

MRI AND "HOT SPOTS"

Theoretically, RF radiation "hot spots" caused by an uneven distribution of RF power may arise whenever current concentrations are produced in association with restrictive conductive patterns. There has been the suggestion that RF radiation "hot spots" may generate thermal "hot spots" under certain conditions during MRI. Because RF radiation is mainly absorbed by peripheral tissues, thermography has been used to study the heating pattern associated with MRI at high whole-body SARs.[22,30] This study demonstrated that there was no evidence of surface thermal "hot spots" related to MRI of human subjects. The thermoregulatory system apparently responds to the heat challenge by distributing the thermal load, producing a "smearing" effect of the surface temperatures (FIGURE 7). However, there is a possibility that internal thermal "hot spots" may develop during MRI. This issue is currently undergoing investigation in human subjects.

A report by Shuman et al.[35] indicated that there are significant temperature rises in internal organs produced by MRI. This study was conducted on anesthetized dogs and is unlikely to be pertinent to conscious adult human subjects because of the previously discussed factors related to the physical dimensions as well as due to the dissimilar thermoregulatory systems of these two species. Of note is that these data may have important implications for the use of MRI in pediatric patients because this patient population is typically sedated or anesthetized for MRI examinations and the physical dimensions of the dog are comparable to those of the pediatric population that frequently is examined by MRI.

FUTURE STUDIES OF THERMAL RESPONSES IN HUMANS DURING MRI

Recent advances in MRI have produced special pulse sequences (i.e., RARE, fast spin echo, etc.) that allow imaging to be performed five to ten times faster than previously possible.[59] This requires a substantial increase in RF power that is predicted, in some cases, to exceed a whole-body averaged SAR of 10 W/kg (D. J. Schaefer, personal communication). Both the clinical importance and the cost-effective use of MRI accomplished with these new pulse sequences are obvious. However, the safety of subjecting patients to RF energy at these potentially excessive levels is unknown. Therefore, studies are currently being designed and implemented to investigate human thermoregulatory responses to SARs that are even higher than those that have been studied in recent years.

In addition, there are now whole-body MRI scanners with a static magnetic field

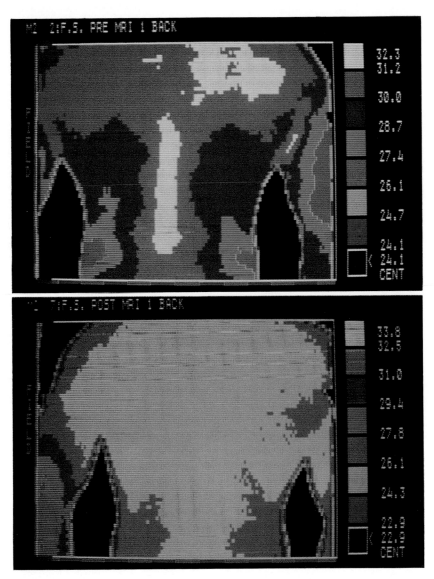

FIGURE 7. Thermographs obtained from the back of a human subject before (top) and after (bottom) a 45-min MRI procedure performed on the abdomen with a 1.5-T/64-MHz MRI scanner at a whole-body averaged SAR of 3.2 W/kg. There was no evidence of any surface "hot spots" or of excessive temperature elevations. The thermoregulatory system produced a "smearing" effect such that the increased surface temperatures after MRI were evenly distributed. (See references 22 and 30.)

strength of 4.0 T that are being used for a combination of imaging and spectroscopy on human subjects.[60,61] Imaging at 4.0 T uses approximately seven times as much RF energy as a 1.5-T MRI scanner.[61] Investigations evaluating thermal responses in human subjects will also need to be performed to assess the safety of these powerful MRI devices.

REFERENCES

1. PERSSON, B. R. R. & F. STAHLBERG. 1989. Health and Safety of Clinical NMR Examinations. CRC Press. Boca Raton, Florida.
2. MICHAELSON, S. M. & J. V. LIN. 1987. Biological Effects and Health Implications of Radiofrequency Radiation. Plenum. New York.
3. SHELLOCK, F. G. & J. V. CRUES. 1988. MRI: safety considerations in magnetic resonance imaging. MRI Decisions 2: 25–30.
4. SHELLOCK, F. G. 1989. Biological effects and safety aspects of magnetic resonance imaging. Magn. Reson. Q. 5: 243–261.
5. KANAL, E., F. G. SHELLOCK & L. TALAGALA. 1990. Safety considerations in MR imaging. Radiology 176: 593–606.
6. SHELLOCK, F. G. & J. V. CRUES. 1991. Biological effects and safety considerations of magnetic resonance imaging. In Magnetic Resonance Imaging Syllabus. American College of Radiology. In press.
7. SHELLOCK, F. G. 1990. MRI bioeffects and safety. In Magnetic Resonance Imaging of the Brain and Spine. S. Atlas, Ed. Raven Press. New York.
8. NCRP. 1986. Biological effects and exposure criteria for radiofrequency electromagnetic fields. Report No. 86. National Council on Radiation Protection and Measurements. Bethesda, Maryland.
9. GORDON, C. J. 1984. Thermal physiology. In Biological Effects of Radiofrequency Radiation, p. 4-1 to 4-28. EPA-600/8-83-026A.
10. EDELMAN, R. R., F. G. SHELLOCK & J. AHLADIS. 1990. Practical MRI for the technologist and imaging specialist. In Clinical Magnetic Resonance. R. R. Edelman & J. Hesselink, Eds. Saunders. Philadelphia.
11. BEERS, J. 1989. Biological effects of weak electromagnetic fields from 0 Hz to 200 MHz: a survey of the literature with special emphasis on possible magnetic resonance effects. Magn. Reson. Imag. 7: 309–331.
12. ADEY, W. R. 1981. Tissue interactions with nonionizing electromagnetic fields. Physiol. Rev. 61: 435–514.
13. SHULMAN, S. 1990. All aboard the bandwagon. Nature 346: 597.
14. COULTER, J. S. & S. L. OSBOURNE. 1936. Short wave diathermy in heating of human tissues. Arch. Phys. Ther. 17: 679–687.
15. GORDON, C. J. 1987. Normalizing the thermal effects of radiofrequency radiation: body mass versus total body surface area. Bioelectromagnetics 8: 111–118.
16. GORDON, C. J. 1988. Effect of radiofrequency radiation exposure on thermoregulation. ISI Atlas Sci. Plants Anim. 1: 245–250.
17. ATHEY, T. W. 1989. A model of the temperature rise in the head due to magnetic resonance imaging procedures. Magn. Reson. Med. 9: 177–184.
18. ADAIR, E. R. & L. G. BERGLUND. 1986. On the thermoregulatory consequences of NMR imaging. Magn. Reson. Imag. 4: 321–333.
19. ADAIR, E. R. & L. G. BERGLUND. 1989. Thermoregulatory consequences of cardiovascular impairment during NMR imaging in warm/humid environments. Magn. Reson. Imag. 7: 25–37.
20. SHELLOCK, F. G. & J. V. CRUES. 1987. Temperature, heart rate, and blood pressure changes associated with clinical MR imaging at 1.5 T. Radiology 163: 259–262.
21. KIDO, D. K., T. W. MORRIS, J. L. ERICKSON, D. B. PLEWES & J. H. SIMON. 1987. Physiologic changes during high field strength MR imaging. Am. J. Neuroradiol. 8: 263–266.

22. SHELLOCK, F. G., D. J. SCHAEFER, W. GRUNDFEST & J. V. CRUES. 1986. Thermal effects of high-field (1.5 tesla) magnetic resonance imaging of the spine: clinical experience above a specific absorption rate of 0.4 W/kg. Acta Radiol. Suppl. **369**: 514–516.

23. SHELLOCK, F. G., C. J. GORDON & D. J. SCHAEFER. 1986. Thermoregulatory responses to clinical magnetic resonance imaging of the head at 1.5 tesla: lack of evidence for direct effects on the hypothalamus. Acta Radiol. Suppl. **369**: 512–513.

24. SHELLOCK, F. G. & J. V. CRUES. 1988. Corneal temperature changes associated with high-field MR imaging using a head coil. Radiology **167**: 809–811.

25. SCHAEFER, D. J., B. J. BARBER, C. J. GORDON, J. ZIELONKA & J. HECKER. 1985. Thermal effects of magnetic resonance imaging. In Book of Abstracts, Soc. Magn. Reson. Med., Vol. 2: 925.

26. SHELLOCK, F. G. & J. V. CRUES. 1988. Temperature changes caused by clinical MR imaging of the brain at 1.5 tesla using a head coil. Am. J. Neuroradiol. **9**: 287–291.

27. SHELLOCK, F. G., B. ROTHMAN & D. SARTI. 1990. Heating of the scrotum by high-field-strength MR imaging. Am. J. Roentgenol. **154**: 1229–1232.

28. VOGL, T., K. KRIMMEL, A. FUCHS & J. LISSNER. 1988. Influence of magnetic resonance imaging on human body core and intravascular temperature. Med. Phys. **15**: 562–566.

29. CRUES, J. V., F. G. SHELLOCK & T. LEVY. 1986. Prevalence of high field MRI procedures requiring specific absorption rates below and above 0.4 W/kg: experience in 639 patients. In Book of Abstracts, Soc. Magn. Reson. Med., p. 1030–1031.

30. SCHAEFER, D. J., F. G. SHELLOCK, J. V, CRUES & C. J. GORDON. 1986. Infrared thermographic studies of human surface temperature in magnetic resonance imaging. In Proceedings of the Bioelectromagnetics Society, Eighth Annual Meeting, p. 68.

31. SHELLOCK, F. G., D. J. SCHAEFER & C. J. GORDON. 1986. Effect of a 1.5 T static magnetic field on body temperature of man. Magn. Reson. Med. **3**: 644–647.

32. SHELLOCK, F. G., D. J. SCHAEFER & J. V. CRUES. 1989. Effect of a 1.5 tesla static magnetic field on body and skin temperatures of man. Magn. Reson. Med. **10**: 371–375.

33. SHELLOCK, F. G., C. SCHATZ & D. BOYER. 1991. Increases in corneal temperature associated with MRI of the eye using a special ocular coil. J. MRI **1**(WIP suppl.): 27.

34. SHELLOCK, F. G., D. J. SCHAEFER & J. V. CRUES. 1989. Alterations in body and skin temperatures caused by MR imaging: Is the recommended exposure for radiofrequency radiation too conservative? Br. J. Radiol. **62**: 904–909.

35. SHUMAN, W. P., D. R. HAYNOR, A. W. GUY, G. E. WESBEY, D. J. SCHAEFER & A. A. MOSS. 1988. Superficial and deep-tissue increases in anesthetized dogs during exposure to high specific absorption rates in a 1.5-T MR imager. Radiology **167**: 551–554.

36. BARBER, B. J., D. J. SCHAEFER, C. J. GORDON, D. C. ZAWIEJA & J. HECKER. 1990. Thermal effects of MR imaging: worst-case studies in sheep. Am. J. Roentgenol. **155**: 1105–1110.

37. BOTTOMLEY, P. A., R. W. REDINGTON, W. A. EDELSTEIN & J. F. SCHENCK. 1985. Estimating radiofrequency power deposition in body NMR imaging. Magn. Reson. Med. **2**: 336–349.

38. BOTTOMLEY, P. A. & W. A. EDELSTEIN. 1981. Power deposition in whole body NMR imaging. Med. Phys. **8**: 510–512.

39. SHELLOCK, F. G. 1986. Monitoring during MRI—an evaluation of the effect of high-field MRI on various patient monitors. Med. Electron. **September**: 93–97.

40. HOLSHOUSER, B., D. B. HINSHAW & F. G. SHELLOCK. 1991. Sedation, anesthesia, and physiologic monitoring during MRI. In ARRS Categorical Course Syllabus: Spine and Body Magnetic Resonance Imaging. A. N. Hasso & D. D. Stark, Eds.: 9–15.

41. SHELLOCK, F. G. 1990. Monitoring sedated patients during MRI. Radiology **177**: 586 (letter).

42. WICKERSHEIM, K. A. & M. H. SUN. 1987. Fluoroptic thermometry. Med. Electron. **February**: 84–91.

43. HOUDAS, Y. & E. F. J. RING. 1982. Temperature distribution. In Human Body Temperature: Its Measurement and Distribution, p. 81–103. Plenum. New York.

44. SHELLOCK, F. G., S. A. RUBIN & C. E. EVEREST. 1986. Surface temperature measurement by IR. Med. Electron. **86**: 81–83.

45. SPERBER, D., R. OLDENBOURG & K. DRANSFELD. 1984. Magnetic field induced temperature change in mice. Naturwissenschaften **71**: 100–101.

46. GREMMEL, H., H. WENDHAUSEN & F. WUNSCH. 1983. Biologische Effeckte Statischer Magnetfelder bei NMR-Tomographic Am Menshen. Wiss. Mitt. Univ. Kiel Radiol. Klinik.
47. TENFORDE, T. S. 1986. Thermoregulation in rodents exposed to high intensity stationary magnetic fields. Bioelectromagnetics **7:** 341–346.
48. BURCH, G. E. & N. P. DePASQUALE. 1967. Hot Climates, Man and His Heart. Thomas. Springfield, Illinois.
49. JAUCHEM, J. R. 1985. Effects of drugs on thermal responses to microwaves. Gen. Pharmacol. **16:** 307–310.
50. ROWELL, L. B. 1983. Cardiovascular aspects of human thermoregulation. Circ. Res. **52:** 367–379.
51. SHELLOCK, F. G., J. K. DRURY, S. MEERBAUM & E. CORDAY. 1983. Possible hypothalamic thermostat increase produced by a calcium blocker. Clin. Res. **31:** 64A.
52. KENNY, W. L. 1985. Physiological correlates of heat intolerance. Sports Med. **2:** 279–286.
53. FOOD AND DRUG ADMINISTRATION. 1988. Magnetic resonance diagnostic device; panel recommendation and report on petitions for MR reclassification. Fed. Regist. **53:** 7575–7579.
54. BERMAN, E. 1984. Reproductive effects. *In* Biological Effects of Radiofrequency Radiation, p. 5-29 to 5-42. EPA-600/8-83-026A.
55. KURZ, K. R. & M. GOLDSTEIN. 1986. Scrotal temperature reflects intratesticular temperature and is lowered by shaving. J. Urol. **135:** 290–292.
56. ELDER, J. A. 1984. Special senses. *In* Biological Effects of Radiofrequency Radiation, p. 5-64 to 5-78. EPA-600/8-83-026A.
57. SACKS, E., B. V. WORGUL, G. R. MERRIAM & S. HILAL. 1986. The effects of nuclear magnetic resonance imaging on ocular tissues. Arch. Ophthalmol. **104:** 890–893.
58. MAPSTONE, R. 1968. Measurement of corneal temperature. Exp. Eye Res. **7:** 233–243.
59. HENNIG, J., A. NAUERTH & H. FRIEDBURG. 1986. RARE imaging: a fast imaging method for clinical MR. Magn. Reson. Med. **3:** 823–833.
60. REDINGTON, R. W., C. L. DUMOULIN, J. F. SCHENCK, P. B. ROEMER, S. P. SOUZA, O. M. MUELLER, D. R. EISNER, J. E. PIEL & W. A. EDELSTEIN. 1988. MR imaging and bioeffects in a whole body 4.0 tesla imaging system. *In* Book of Abstracts, Soc. Magn. Reson. Imag., Vol. 1: 20.
61. ORTENDAHL, D. A. 1988. Whole-body MR imaging and spectroscopy at 4 T: where do we go from here? Radiology **169:** 864–865.

Local and Global Thermoregulatory Responses to MRI Fields[a]

CHRISTOPHER J. GORDON

Neurotoxicology Division
Health Effects Research Laboratory
United States Environmental Protection Agency
Research Triangle Park, North Carolina 27711

INTRODUCTION

During magnetic resonance imaging (MRI) procedures, a subject is exposed to three novel environmental stimuli that have drawn attention over the past decade as potential health hazards:[1] (1) a relatively intense static magnetic field, (2) a time-varying magnetic field, and (3) a radio-frequency (RF) field. Thermoregulation is one of many physiological systems that can be affected by MRI, specifically by the RF radiation absorbed by the subject during MRI. Although there are some sparse, albeit controversial data on the possible effects of static magnetic fields on thermoregulation,[2] the major concern regarding potential health hazards of the MRI-induced thermal effects centers on the RF radiation absorbed by a subject during a scan.[1,3] The purpose of this report is to review the studies that have impacted on understanding the thermoregulatory effects of MRI with special emphasis on the problems of selecting appropriate animal models for assessing the potential risk of RF radiation exposure during MRI.

BASICS OF THE THERMOREGULATORY SYSTEM

Homeothermy refers to the ability to maintain a constant internal (i.e., core) body temperature over a relatively wide range of ambient temperatures (T_a) and under other conditions that may potentially change core temperature such as exercise and fever. Homeothermy is restricted primarily to most birds and mammals. The thermoregulatory system of homeotherms comprises several behavioral and autonomic motor outputs that function to achieve a balance between heat production and heat loss, thereby maintaining a constant core temperature (FIGURE 1).

The heat balance equation is useful to explain the fundamental properties of the thermoregulatory system:[4,5]

$$S = M - (K) - (C) - (E) - (R), \tag{1}$$

[a]This report has been reviewed by the Health Effects Research Laboratory, United States Environmental Protection Agency, and has been approved for publication. Mention of trade names or commercial products does not constitute endorsement or recommendation for use.

where

M = metabolic heat production (always +),
K = conductive heat transfer (+ for heat loss),
C = convective heat transfer (+ for heat loss),
E = evaporative heat transfer (+ for heat loss),
R = radiative heat transfer (+ for heat loss),
S = heat storage (+ for net increase).

At a comfortable T_a of 25 °C, radiation accounts for 67%, convection accounts for 10%, and evaporation accounts for 23% of the total heat loss. In a hot environment of 35 °C, dry heat loss is markedly attenuated because of the reduced temperature gradient of the skin and air; at this T_a, radiation accounts for 4%, convection

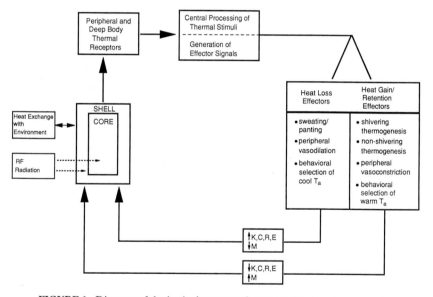

FIGURE 1. Diagram of the basic thermoregulatory mechanisms in mammals.

accounts for 6%, and evaporation accounts for 90% of the total heat loss.[6] When metabolic heat production is equal to the total rate of heat loss (i.e., K + C + E + R), then S = 0 and thermal homeostasis is achieved. When heat production exceeds heat loss, as would occur during heavy exercise or by exposure to a high T_a, then S > 0 and the subject becomes hyperthermic. When heat loss exceeds heat production, as would occur during exposure to acute cold stress, then S < 0 and the subject becomes hypothermic.

HEAT BALANCE DURING RF RADIATION EXPOSURE

One of the main aspects of exposure to RF radiation has been the concern over a hazardous elevation in body temperature. When a body is exposed to an RF radiation field, the electromagnetic energy absorbed causes agitation of polar molecules (principally water), resulting in the production of heat. The heat absorbed from RF radiation per unit of time is commonly expressed in terms of the specific absorption rate (SAR) in dimensions of W/kg and can be incorporated into the heat balance equation:

$$S = [M + SAR] - [K + C + E + R]. \tag{2}$$

Thus, if the total heat production, through elevations in M or SAR, exceeds the body's heat loss, then there will be an elevation in body temperature. Clearly, to maintain thermal homeostasis during RF radiation exposure, the subject must either reduce its metabolic rate or increase one or more of the avenues of heat loss.

The aforementioned discussion refers to the general effects of RF radiation on the core body temperature. Another concern of RF radiation as it pertains to MRI is the possibility of hazardous temperature elevations in local sites throughout the body. These "hot spots" can occur with uneven deposition of RF radiation; their formation is dependent on several crucial parameters including RF frequency, body morphology, and SAR.[7,8] A simplified version of equation 2 can be used to explain the etiology of hot spot formation in a particular tissue or organ that is not in contact with air:

$$S = [M + SAR] - [K + C]. \tag{3}$$

In this situation, there is no heat exchange by evaporation or radiation. The potential rise in tissue temperature then becomes proportional to its metabolic rate, SAR, and thermal conductance and inversely proportional to the blood flow:

$$\Delta \text{ tissue temperature} \propto \frac{M + SAR + \text{thermal conductance}}{\text{tissue blood flow}}. \tag{4}$$

Thus, well-vascularized tissues and organs are less susceptible to hot spot formation because the blood flow removes the RF heat load, thereby preventing a rise in temperature. Hot spots can also form peripherally; in this case, heat exchange with the air becomes a factor in governing the degree of temperature elevation.

ASSESSING THE THERMAL RISK OF MRI: PROBLEMS IN ANIMAL-TO-HUMAN EXTRAPOLATION

In the development of clinical MRI procedures, it was anticipated that subjects could be exposed to SARs as high as 4.0 W/kg for at least several minutes. Considering that this SAR was 10 times greater than the current guidelines for human exposure to RF radiation,[9] it was imperative that a risk assessment of the potential thermal effects of relatively high MRI scans be performed.

The standard approach in all biomedical research that evaluates potentially hazardous agents is appropriate experiments with an animal model. In the case of RF radiation, the search for an ideal animal model is hampered by the marked effect of body size on both the sensitivity to RF radiation exposure and the absorption of RF radiation at a given field strength. When body size is large relative to the wavelength of the RF radiation, the energy is absorbed mostly on the surface; when the subject is small in relation to the wavelength, there is inefficient absorption of the RF energy; the most efficient coupling of RF energy occurs when the body length is approximately one-half of the wavelength of the RF radiation. The condition of peak absorption is termed resonance and is most hazardous because there is deep and uneven absorption of the RF energy. During resonance, local SARs can be 10 to 20 times the value of the average SAR.[10] Not surprisingly, the resonant frequencies of experimental animals vary tremendously as a function of body mass[11] (FIGURE 2). MRI systems typically operate at an RF frequency of 65 MHz, which seems quite close to an adult human's resonant frequency. However, the data in FIGURE 2 are for far-field exposures with E-field polarization. Fortunately, in MRI, the quadrature arrangement of the coils results in a predominant peripheral deposition of the RF energy and the greatest amount of heating will be on the surface.[9]

The other problem in selecting animal models is the differential effect of body size on the sensitivity to RF radiation.[12] For example, in a general assessment of the SAR needed to affect an array of thermoregulatory variables in different species, a marked effect of body size on the SAR needed to affect a given variable is evident (TABLE 1). Small species such as the mouse and rat require relatively large SARs to activate a given thermoregulatory motor output compared to larger species. If higher SARs are required to activate thermoregulatory motor outputs in small species, it follows that the SARs needed to raise core body temperature will be inversely dependent on body mass. Our laboratory addressed this issue by exposing mouse,

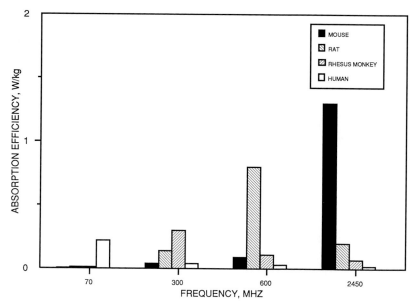

FIGURE 2. Relationship between body size and efficiency of absorption of RF radiation of models of various species. Note that the resonant frequency, or the frequency of maximum absorption efficiency, increases with decreasing body size. Absorption efficiency is equal to the SAR in W/kg per mW/cm² of incident power in the E-polarization. Data taken from Durney *et al.*[11]

TABLE 1. Selected Data on the Approximate Threshold SAR Needed to Activate Some Principal Thermoregulatory Effector Responses and Cause Significant Elevations (ΔT = 0.3–1.7 °C) in Core Temperature[a]

Species	T_a (°C)	Frequency (MHz)	SAR (W/kg)	Exposure Time (min)
Selection of Cool Ambient Temperature				
mouse	31.5	2450	5.3	60
hamster	30.2	2450	2.0	60
rat	5.0	2450	1.0	15
squirrel monkey	35.0	2450	1.1	10
Reduction in Metabolic Heat Production				
mouse	24	2450	10.0	30
rat	10	600	1.0	60
squirrel monkey	20	2450	0.9	10
Peripheral Vasodilation				
rat	20	600	2–6	90
rabbit	20	600	0.3	90
squirrel monkey	26	2450	1.5	10
rhesus monkey	20	225	2.1	120
Evaporative Heat Loss				
mouse	20	2450	29.0	90
squirrel monkey	33	2450	1.1	10
Elevation in Core Temperature				
mouse	20	2450	22.2	100
mouse	20	2450	57.1	90
hamster	22	2450	9.0	100
hamster	20	2450	17.4	90
rat	24	2450	4.2	60
rat	20	600	2.1	90
rabbit	20	600	1.4	90
squirrel monkey	23	2450	4.7	60
rhesus monkey	24	1290	4.1	480
rhesus monkey	24	225	1.2	120–240

[a]Taken from reference 13.

hamster, rat, and rabbit to near-resonant RF frequencies for 90 min while measuring core body temperature.[14] A double logarithmic plot of body mass and SAR needed to raise colonic temperature was inverse and linear (FIGURE 3). A major reason for the inverse relationship between body mass and thermal efficacy of SAR is that, as body mass increases, the surface area/body mass ratio decreases, which directly limits the ability of the animal to dissipate heat passively.[12,14] For example, the surface area/body mass ratio is 0.4 m²/kg for a mouse, 0.15 m²/kg for a rat, 0.07 m²/kg for a rabbit, and 0.025 m²/kg for a human.[15] To maintain thermal homeostasis, species with higher surface area/body mass ratios must generate proportionately higher amounts of heat per unit body mass. The higher surface area/body mass ratio also permits the same species to dissipate RF energy at much greater rates. Indeed, it has been suggested that expressing SAR in terms of surface area rather than body mass would allow for a better normalization of RF dose effects between species.[15] Thus, in selecting an

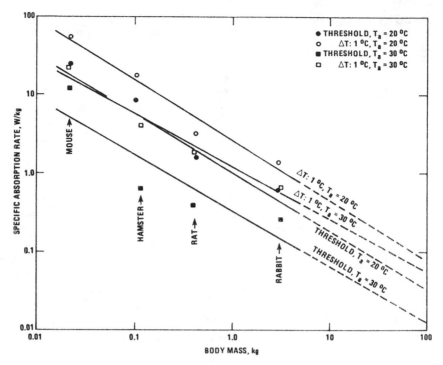

FIGURE 3. Relationship between body mass and thermal efficacy of RF radiation. Species were exposed to near-resonant RF radiation for 90 min at T_a values of 20 and 30 °C. Data points represent the SARs needed to elevate the species' core temperature by 1.0 °C. The SAR needed to raise the core temperature decreases with increasing body mass. Taken from reference 14.

experimental animal model to assess the thermal risk of high SAR MRI scans, it is clear that the body size of the animal will have to be equivalent to that of an adult human. If this is not possible, then appropriate scaling factors must be considered in extrapolating the observed effects in the experimental animal to the predicted effect in human subjects.

THERMOREGULATORY RESPONSES TO MRI

Experimental Animal Studies

To assess the thermal effects of MRI, the anesthetized, unshorn sheep was selected as an experimental animal model.[16] The sheep's body size approximates that of an adult human, but there are distinct differences in the thermoregulatory responses of the sheep and human. The sheep has a heavy insulative coat and pants to dissipate excess body heat. Humans subjected to typical MRI conditions would normally be lightly insulated and would increase skin blood flow and sweat to dissipate excess body heat. In spite of these differences in species, valuable information on the heating profile to relatively high SAR MRI scans can be collected in sheep.

Sheep were anesthetized, intubated, and fitted with thermocouples in various locations of the body including the jugular vein, colon, eye, and various sites on the skin. Both whole-body scans and head scans of 1.5 to 4 W/kg were used. Whole-body scans of 1.5 and 4 W/kg resulted in relatively rapid elevations in skin temperature and gradual elevations in core temperature (FIGURE 4). At the highest SAR of 4.0 W/kg, the rise in skin temperature was no more than 4 °C. Core temperature

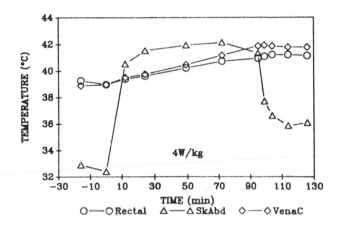

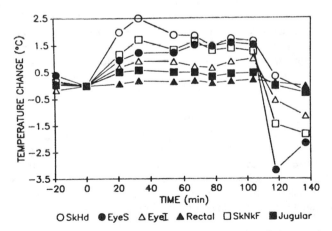

FIGURE 4. Time course of various skin and core temperatures of the anesthetized sheep during a 95-min, 4.0-W/kg whole-body MRI scan (upper graph) and a 105-min, 4.0-W/kg head MRI scan (lower graph). Terms: SkAbd = abdominal skin, VenaC = vena cava, SkHd = head skin, EyeS = eye surface, EyeI = internal eye, SkNkF = skin of neck, and Jugular = jugular vein. From Barber et al.[16]

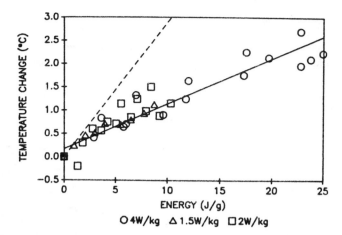

FIGURE 5. Relationship between the total energy absorption (i.e., W/kg × time of exposure) and the increase in core temperature of anesthetized sheep subjected to MRI at SARs of 1.5 to 4.0 W/kg. The dashed line shows the theoretical rise in temperature in the absence of heat loss. From Barber et al.[16]

increased by as much as 2.7 °C after 104 min of scanning at 4.0 W/kg. Overall, there was a linear relationship between the specific absorption (i.e., W/kg × time) and the rise in core temperature during whole-body scans of 1.5 to 4.0 W/kg (FIGURE 5).

A head scan in the anesthetized sheep of 4.0 W/kg led to abrupt elevations in the skin temperature of the head along with slight (1–2 °C) elevations in the temperature of the cornea and vitreous humor (FIGURE 4). Not surprisingly, core temperature elevations during a head scan were negligible, indicating little energy absorption in the body trunk. The temperature of the jugular vein, which drains blood from the brain, increased by 0.5 °C at the end of a 75-min, 4.0-W/kg head scan. This is indicative of substantial brain heating; however, there is no information on the actual changes in temperature of the CNS during MRI.

The experiments with sheep represent a possible worst-case scenario for high level MRI scans. The animals are anesthetized and intubated, thus eliminating the ability to pant to dissipate body heat. The fur of an unshorn sheep has an insulation value of approximately 7 clo (e.g., a light business suit has an insulative value of 1 clo). Thus, passive heat loss was tightly restricted in the sheep during MRI. Under these conditions, MRI scans of 4.0 W/kg had marked effects on the core and skin temperature; however, the elevations could not be considered as a health hazard. The temperature of the eye was also maintained within safe levels during high level whole-body and head scans. This is an important observation because there was concern over the possible cataractogenic effect of the RF radiation component, which has been demonstrated in several high energy RF studies.[17,18]

Human Studies

It would seem reasonable from the aforementioned results that a lightly insulated human subject could easily tolerate a 4.0-W/kg MRI scan. To test this hypothesis, a group of 11 adult volunteers were subjected to a 20-min, 4.0-W/kg whole-body scan while a variety of physiological variables including esophageal (i.e., core) temperature, various skin temperatures, metabolic rate, heart rate, blood pressure, and breathing rate were monitored.[19] As with the sheep study, the increase in skin temperature was markedly greater than that of core temperature (FIGURE 6). Overall, skin temperature near the isocenter of the scanner increased by as much as 3 °C, whereas core temperature increased an average of 0.3 °C after a 20-min scan. Heart rate and breathing rate were slightly elevated, whereas blood pressure measured 20 min before and 20 min after the termination of MRI was unchanged. Overall, the 20-min, 4.0-W/kg MRI procedure produced marked elevations in skin temperature and slight elevations in core temperature. Again, as with the sheep study, these temperature elevations are nowhere near those considered hazardous.

A variety of clinical investigations on the thermoregulatory effects of MRI have been performed by Shellock and colleagues. During whole-body scans at a T_a of 20–24 °C, slight ($\Delta T = 0.2$ °C), but significant elevations in core temperature were observed following exposure to SARs of 0.5 to 1.3 W/kg.[20] Significant elevations ($\Delta T = 0.4$ °C) in the temperature of the cornea were also noted following MRI. With a head scan at SARs ranging from 2.5 to 3.0 W/kg, the corneal temperature increased by only 0.5 °C with a range of 0 to 1.8 °C.[19] Average SARs in the head of 2.5 W/kg over a variety of exposure times resulted in slight, but significant elevations in the skin temperature of the forehead and outer canthus, but gave no change in the core temperature.[21] Interestingly, there were decreases in heart rate and blood pressure after MRI scans of the head; however, this may be attributed to the apprehension of the subjects rather than to specific effects of the MRI on these cardiovascular parameters. In another study, the time course of core and various skin temperatures was recorded in adult males exposed to SARs ranging from 2.8 to 4.0 W/kg (FIGURE 7). Skin blood flow above the umbilicus, which is in the area of

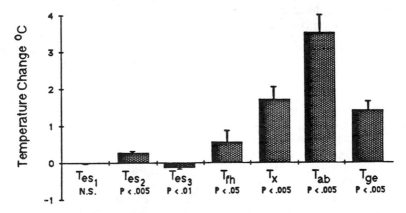

FIGURE 6. Change in esophageal (i.e., core; T_{es}) and various skin temperatures of 11 humans subjected to a 20-min whole-body MRI scan. Note larger elevations in the skin temperatures of the abdomen (T_{ab}) and xiphoid (T_x), which were closest to the isocenter of the body coil, compared to the temperatures of the forehead (T_{fh}) and genital area (T_{ge}). T_{es1}, T_{es2}, and T_{es3} represent the temperatures taken 20 min before MRI, immediately after MRI, and 20 min after the termination of MRI, respectively. From Schaefer.[19]

highest energy deposition during the whole-body scan, was measured noninvasively using laser-Doppler techniques. A 30-min scan resulted in a doubling of blood flow, marked elevations in skin temperature, and negligible elevations in core temperature.[22] Another area that is of concern is the potential heating of the scrotum during MRI. Impaired reproductive function and sterility can occur if heating of the scrotum is severe enough. An MRI scan with a mean SAR of 0.72 W/kg and an exposure time of 23 min led to an average increase in scrotal skin temperature of 1.5 °C with the largest increase equaling 3.0 °C.[23] Although these temperature elevations are not hazardous, it will be important in future studies to assure that testicular temperature does not exceed hazardous levels during MRI.

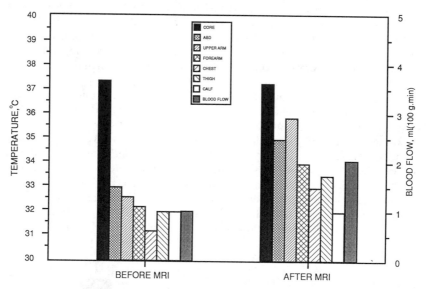

FIGURE 7. Effect of a whole-body MRI scan of 3.4 W/kg on cutaneous blood flow of the abdomen, core temperature, and skin temperature of various sites. Note that MRI resulted in a doubling of skin blood flow. From Shellock *et al.*[22]

Before the advent of MRI, little was known regarding the thermoregulatory response of humans when exposed to RF energy. The experimental and clinical MRI studies have provided a breadth of new data on the thermal effects of RF radiation. Whole-body SARs of <0.4 W/kg (i.e., the ANSI guideline) appear to have little effect on thermoregulation; SARs of 0.4 to 2.0 W/kg result in significant elevations in core and skin temperature; however, these temperature elevations are slight and appear to be quite safe. SARs of 4.0 W/kg result in 0.3 °C elevations in core temperature and up to 3.0 °C elevations in skin temperature depending on the location relative to the isocenter. Head scans also cause significant elevations in skin temperature, but it is important to note that little is known regarding the potential rise in brain temperature. This is of obvious importance because of the brain's high thermal sensitivity compared to other organs and tissues. However, modeling studies suggest that the rise in brain temperature during relatively high SAR scans would be negligible.[24]

Overall, the human thermoregulatory responses to MRI fall below the recommended exposure guidelines in the United States and United Kingdom. In the United States, the guidelines restrict core temperature from increasing over 1.0 °C and skin temperature from exceeding 40 °C. In the United Kingdom, the proposed guideline also limits the core temperature from increasing by 1.0 °C and prevents the local SAR in 0.1 kg of tissue from exceeding 10 W/kg in the head/trunk and 20 W/kg in the extremities. There are several unresolved issues in MRI safety that are relevant to the thermoregulatory response. Little is known of the response of patients with compromised thermoregulatory function including the very young and aged as well as those under complete anesthesia. A reduced ability to maintain thermal homeostasis in the very young and aged during heat and cold stress is well known. It is also likely that such populations would not thermoregulate as well as healthy adults during exposure to relatively high SAR scans. Superficial burning has been reported in anesthetized patients where cables had been laid too close to the skin. Although the present data suggest that there are no adverse effects, it should be emphasized that there is practically no information on the thermoregulatory capacity of the CNS during exposure to RF radiation. There is clearly a need to use both experimental and clinical approaches to understand the mechanisms of thermal homeostasis in the CNS during MRI.

REFERENCES

1. SHELLOCK, F. G. 1989. Biological effects and safety aspects of magnetic resonance imaging. Magn. Reson. Q. 5: 243–261.
2. SHELLOCK, F. G., D. J. SCHAEFER & J. V. CRUES. 1989. Exposure to a 1.5-T static magnetic field does not alter body and skin temperatures in man. Magn. Reson. Med. 11: 371–375.
3. SAUNDERS, R. D. & H. SMITH. 1984. Safety aspects of NMR clinical imaging. Br. Med. Bull. 40: 148–154.
4. GLOSSARY OF TERMS FOR THERMAL PHYSIOLOGY. 1987. Int. Union Physiol. Sci. Pflügers Arch. 410: 567–587.
5. GORDON, C. J. 1984. Effect of RF-radiation exposure on body temperature. In Biological Effects of Radiofrequency Radiation. J. A. Elder & D. F. Cahill, Eds.: 4-1 to 4-28. EPA-600/8-83-026F.
6. FOLK, G. E., JR. 1974. Textbook of Environmental Physiology. Lea & Febiger. Philadelphia.
7. GUY, A. W. 1971. Analysis of electromagnetic fields induced in biological tissues by thermographic studies on equivalent phantom models. IEEE Trans. Microwave Theory Tech. MTT-19: 205–214.
8. WEIL, C. M. & J. R. RABINOWITZ. 1984. RF-field interaction with biological systems. In Biological Effects of Radiofrequency Radiation. J. A. Elder & D. F. Cahill, Eds.: 3-6 to 3-24. EPA-600/8-83-026F.
9. ANSI. 1982. American National Standard safety levels with respect to human exposure to radio-frequency electromagnetic fields, 300 kHz–100 GHz (ANSI C95.1-1982). American National Standards Institute. New York.
10. GANDHI, O. P., J. CHEN & A. RIAZI. 1986. Currents induced in a human being for plane-wave exposure conditions (0–50 MHz) and for RF sealers. IEEE Trans. Biomed. Eng. BME-33: 757–767.
11. DURNEY, C. H., C. C. JOHNSON, P. W. BARBER et al. 1978. Radiofrequency Radiation

Dosimetry Handbook (Second Edition). USAF School Aerosp. Med. San Antonio, Texas.

12. GORDON, C. J. & J. H. FERGUSON. 1984. Scaling the physiological effects of exposure to radiofrequency electromagnetic radiation: consequences of body size. Int. J. Radiat. Biol. **46:** 387–397.

13. GORDON, C. J. 1988. Effect of radiofrequency radiation exposure on thermoregulation. ISI Atlas Sci. Anim. Plant Sci. **1:** 245–250.

14. GORDON, C. J., M. D. LONG & K. S. FEHLNER. 1986. Temperature regulation in the unrestrained rabbit during exposure to 600 MHz radiofrequency radiation. Int. J. Radiat. Biol. **49:** 987–997.

15. GORDON, C. J. 1987. Normalizing the thermal effects of radiofrequency radiation: body mass versus total body surface area. Bioelectromagnetics **8:** 111–118.

16. BARBER, B. J., D. J. SCHAEFER, C. J. GORDON, D. C. ZAWIEJA & J. HECKER. 1990. Thermal effects of MR imaging: worst-case studies on sheep. Am. J. Roentgenol. **153:** 1105–1110.

17. NCRP. 1986. Cataractogenesis. *In* Biological Effects and Exposure Criteria for Radiofrequency Electromagnetic Fields. Report No. 86, p. 191–206. National Council on Radiation Protection. Bethesda, Maryland.

18. SHELLOCK, F. G. & J. V. CRUES. 1988. Corneal temperature changes induced by high-field-strength MR imaging with a head coil. Radiology **167:** 809–811.

19. SCHAEFER, D. J. 1988. Safety aspects of magnetic resonance imaging. *In* Biomedical Magnetic Resonance Imaging: Principles, Methodology, and Applications. F. W. Wehrli *et al.*, Eds.: 553–578. VCH Pub. New York.

20. SHELLOCK, F. G., D. J. SCHAEFER, W. GRUNDFEST & J. V. CRUES. 1986. Thermal effects of high-field (1.5 tesla) magnetic resonance imaging of the spine: clinical experience above a specific absorption rate of 0.4 W/kg. Acta Radiol. Suppl. **369:** 514–516.

21. SHELLOCK, F. G. & J. V. CRUES. 1988. Temperature changes caused by MR imaging of the brain with a head coil. Am. J. Neuroradiol. **9:** 287–291.

22. SHELLOCK, F. G., D. J. SCHAEFER & J. V. CRUES. 1989. Alterations in body and skin temperatures caused by magnetic resonance imaging: is the recommended exposure for radiofrequency radiation too conservative? Br. J. Radiol. **62:** 904–909.

23. SHELLOCK, F. G., B. ROTHMAN & D. SARTI. 1990. Heating of the scrotum by high-field-strength MR imaging. Am. J. Roentgenol. **154:** 1229–1232.

24. ATHEY, W. T. 1989. A model of the temperature rise in the head due to magnetic resonance imaging procedures. Magn. Reson. Med. **9:** 177–184.

Health and Physiological Effects of Human Exposure to Whole-Body Four-Tesla Magnetic Fields during MRI

JOHN F. SCHENCK

General Electric Corporate Research and Development Center
Schenectady, New York 12301

INTRODUCTION

Three aspects of patient exposure to electromagnetic fields have been cause for concern since the introduction of magnetic resonance scanners: the radio-frequency transmitter fields, the time-dependent gradient fields, and the static field. Of course, other potential hazards, such as magnetic projectiles inadvertently introduced into the vicinity of the scanner or electric arcing of improperly wired components, also must be considered to assure patient safety. However, the three fields mentioned above are of special concern because they are intrinsic and essential features of the scanner operation and, on some level, each of them interacts with every component of the patient's body. From both the theoretical and the experimental standpoints, the safety aspects of the radio-frequency (rf) and gradient fields are more straightforward to deal with than are those of the static field. The reason is that, for rf and gradient fields, clear-cut end points for patient safety are known and accepted. These specifically are excessive tissue heating by the radio-frequency field and the inappropriate excitation of electrically excitable nerve, muscle, or myocardial tissue by the electric fields associated with the time-dependent gradients.

Although it seems reasonable that there also should be some limit to the ability of human tissues to withstand exposure to intense, static magnetic fields, it is not obvious what physical effect will establish this limit. Experience with the magnetic fields presently available has provided few clues about any ultimate limit to safe exposure for normal human subjects. The conjecture that there must exist an ultimate static magnetic field safety limit is reinforced by consideration of (i) the familiar and dramatic action of strong magnetic fields on magnetic materials such as iron and (ii) the devastating effects that even modest electric fields can produce in human tissues. Nonetheless, the mechanisms by which strong static magnetic fields will eventually be demonstrated to produce clear-cut tissue injury remain obscure.

Fortunately, the theoretical and experimental studies indicating that magnetic resonance imaging (MRI) would not be harmful to patients have been confirmed by the millions of scans safely performed in the last decade. However, the history of scanner development over this time period has involved the use of ever more intense fields of all three types in the attempt to achieve improved scanner performance. Therefore, there is a continuing practical as well as academic impetus for further understanding of the interaction between magnetic fields and human tissues.

Considering that the possibility of static magnetic field effects on human tissues had engaged many scientists and physicians of historical importance, such as

285

Paracelsus, Mesmer, Gilbert, Franklin, and Charcot, it is surprising that few serious scientific studies regarding this possibility were published until recently. The somewhat dubious use of "magnetotherapy" to treat disorders,[1] mostly with a psychosomatic overtone, such as hysteric paralysis and tarantism, finally led to a few skeptical reports[2-4] that denied the ability of the magnetic fields then available to produce measurable and repeatable responses in humans and other biological specimens. In recent decades, there have been many scientific reports of magnetic field–induced biological responses,[5-8] but many of these raise questions of (i) repeatability, (ii) the possibility of confounding factors, and (iii) the lack of dose-response information.[9,10] Several mechanisms of possible interactions between magnetic fields and human tissues are summarized in TABLE 1 and are discussed in more quantitative detail elsewhere.[11] At 4 T, these mechanisms all appear to be below the threshold for producing significant injury to normal human tissues.

This report summarizes data acquired from the exposure of volunteer subjects to an intense magnetic field, 4 T, which has only recently become available for whole-body human exposure. TABLE 1 provides quantitative estimates of some aspects of these interactions. Note that these are based on the parameters of the 4-T magnet; therefore, they include a substantial margin of safety for exposures to lower field strength magnets. In addition to the 4-T field strength, the crucial parameters for the magnet, as measured along its central axis, are the maximum field gradient, $\partial B/\partial z = 2.78$ T/m, and the maximum of the force product, $B(\partial B/\partial z) = 8.79$ T/m^2. This report also includes a discussion of the magnetic susceptibilities of human tissue components. This parameter is fundamental to the calculation of tissue responses to static fields.

SUMMARY OF HEALTH STUDIES

Until 1987, the strongest magnets available for whole-body MRI were the widely used 1.5-T units and a small number of 2-T machines. At that time, 4-T whole-body machines were installed in Schenectady, Erlangen,[42,43] and Hamburg. Presently, each one of these three machines has been moved to a clinical research site. One is at the National Institutes of Health (in Bethesda, Maryland) and the other two are at the University of Alabama and the University of Minnesota. Because the United States Food and Drug Administration has not approved the use of MRI scanners at field strengths above 2 T, the initial studies at Schenectady were done under a protocol approved by the Institutional Review Board of the Hospital of the University of Pennsylvania. This protocol required certain medical procedures (history and physical examinations, electrocardiograms, electroencephalograms, psychometric questionnaires, and standard blood tests) to be performed on the volunteers at the beginning of their exposure and after 12 months. As reported in more detail elsewhere,[44] the panel of 11 volunteers had recorded after one year a total exposure of 150 hours to the whole-body 4-T field. The individual exposures ranged from less than 1 hour to about 40 hours. The subjects were examined according to this protocol by an experienced industrial physician and no significant abnormalities in any of the volunteers were noted at the beginning or end of this period.

SUMMARY OF THE SENSORY STUDIES

Although no health abnormalities were noted, there were several instances of mild sensory effects attributed to the 4-T exposure. A questionnaire asking whether certain sensory effects had or had not been experienced was given to 8 volunteers who had experience at 4 T and to 22 additional volunteers who had experienced exposure at 1.5 T, but who had never been in stronger fields. Assuming that all differences between the responses of the two groups were caused only by the differences in the field strengths, statistically significant ($p < 0.05$) evidence was found for field-dependent sensations of vertigo, nausea, and metallic taste. No statistically significant evidence was found for a field-dependent incidence of headache, vomiting, tinnitus, balance difficulties, numbness, or hiccuping. Evidence was also found for magnetophosphenes[45] (transient visual sensations of flashing lights) associated with rapid movement of the eyes when the subject was in the magnet and the room was darkened. All the reported sensations at 4 T, at least in terms of clinical significance, were of a very mild degree and were absent or minimal if the subject was not required to move rapidly and extensively while inside the magnet.

A simple model can be proposed for the action of the magnetic field to produce sensations of vertigo and nausea. The sensation of angular rotation involves small deflections of the cupulas, structures located within the semicircular canals of the inner ear. This motion deforms sensory nerve cells and triggers nerve impulses to the brain.[46,47] Any motion of the head that changes the magnetic flux through one of the canals can be shown to produce a small magnetohydrodynamic (mhd) force on the orthogonal canals. A simple model gives the maximum value of the pressure drop across an orthogonal cupula when the head is rotated with an angular velocity, Ω, in a uniform magnetic field, B, as $P = ab\Omega B^2/\rho$ (a and b are the inner and outer radii of the toroidal canals of the membranous labyrinth and ρ is the electrical resistivity of the endolymphatic fluid). With $a = 1.5 \times 10^{-4}$ m, $b = 3 \times 10^{-3}$ m, $\rho = 0.5$ ohm-m, B = 4 T, and $\Omega = 10.5$ rad/s, $P = 1.5 \times 10^{-4}$ N/m^2. This is well above the threshold for the subjective sensation of rotation, 1.25×10^{-5} N/m^2. The brain receives information about the position and motion of the body from the vestibular and visual systems and from other sensory sources. According to the conflict hypothesis, nausea, the major component of motion sickness, is the consequence of discordant inputs from these sensory systems. The proposed mhd forces thus provide a plausible explanation of the mild nausea and vertigo sometimes found to accompany prolonged activity within the 4-T magnet. Alternative explanations for magnetic stimulation of the vestibular system include direct depolarization of the hair cell membranes by motion-induced currents and deflections of the cupulas caused by anisotropic susceptibility.

MAGNETIC SUSCEPTIBILITY

The magnetic susceptibility[48–50] of tissue components is fundamental to the analysis of the biological effects of magnetic fields. However, information on the magnetic susceptibilities of tissues and tissue components is sketchy and incomplete. Furthermore, much of what is available is difficult to use because of confusion over notation and units. This confusion arises, in part, because several closely related

TABLE 1. Potential Effects of Static Magnetic Fields on Human Tissue

Effect	Description	Assessment
Magnetic forces	Ferromagnetic materials and tissue components that are paramagnetic or less diamagnetic than water are drawn toward the regions of high fields; components more diamagnetic than water are driven toward low field regions.[12]	Human tissues apparently have no naturally occurring ferromagnetic components. However, such particles, introduced accidentally or iatrogenically, represent possible hazards. The tendency of magnetic forces to separate tissue components (based on susceptibility differences) is normally much smaller than that of gravitational forces (based on density differences).
Magnetic torques	Tissue components with permanent magnetic moments or anisotropic susceptibilities tend to rotate into alignment with the magnetic field.[12-25]	Alignment caused by anisotropy can be demonstrated *in vitro*, but *in vivo* it is probably prevented or reduced to insignificant levels by naturally occurring tissue forces.
Magnetostriction	Ferromagnetic materials change their size and shape slightly when they are exposed to static magnetic fields.[12-14]	These dimensional changes are very small even in ferromagnetic materials. Any effect in the nonferromagnetic materials that comprise human tissues will be very small compared to the normal effects of thermal expansion and mechanical stresses.
Equilibrium of chemical reactions	If the products of a chemical reaction have a different susceptibility than the reactants, the applied field will shift the reaction toward the more paramagnetic or less diamagnetic species.[26-32]	For the largest likely susceptibility differences, the free energy change in a reaction will be altered by about 1 J/mol at 4 T. This will have less effect on the equilibrium constant than a 0.01 °C temperature change.
Dynamics of chemical reactions	The likelihood of recombination of free radical pairs produced by the decomposition of certain organic molecules can be altered by the precession of the electron spins in an applied magnetic field.[33-38]	The field-induced change in reaction yields is usually rather small and has not been reported in biochemically significant reactions. This mechanism, however, deserves further consideration as a source of biologically significant magnetic field effects.

TABLE 1. Continued

Effect	Description	Assessment
Magnetoresistance and Hall effect	An applied magnetic field alters the path of charged current carriers such as ions and electrons. If the mean free path and the time between collisions are sufficiently long, the effective electrical resistivity is increased and transverse electric fields are generated (Hall effect).[39]	The activity of nerve and muscle is based on the currents associated with action potentials. The current carriers, however, are ions in solution with very short mean free paths (~ 1 Å) and short collision times ($\sim 10^{-12}$ s). Therefore, the magnetic field will have a negligible effect on these currents.
Flow and motion-induced currents	Ordinarily, the current density in tissue is given by $\vec{J} = \sigma\vec{E}$, where σ is the tissue conductivity and $\vec{E}$ is the electric field. In an applied magnetic field, an additional current, $\vec{J} = \sigma\vec{v} \times \vec{B}$, where $\vec{v}$ is the tissue velocity, is present. The maximum electric field induced external to the blood vessels is approximately $v\text{B}/2$. At 4 T, this is about 2 V/m and the corresponding current density is about 0.7 A/m².	These additional currents arise both from blood flow and from bulk motion of the body tissues through the field. This is the probable cause of the reported changes in the EKG and in the static field–induced magnetophosphenes. At 4 T, these effects are below excitation thresholds for most nerve and muscle cells,[40,41] but, in more intense fields, currents caused by blood flow may cause ectopic nerve and muscle excitation.
Magnetohydrodynamic (mhd) forces and pressures	Currents flowing in tissues experience a transverse body force proportional to $\vec{J} \times \vec{B}$. The resulting pressures and forces are transmitted to the tissues.	For the current densities present in tissues, these mhd forces are very small compared, for example, to the hemodynamic forces present in flowing blood. However, such forces operating in the inner ear are the likely cause of the sensations of vertigo and nausea sometimes reported by volunteers moving within the 4-T magnet.
Change in chemical concentrations	At equilibrium, the concentration of paramagnetic tissue components, such as oxygen and ferritin, will be increased in high field regions.	Over regions that are the size of cells, the effect is negligible. The equilibrium oxygen concentration at the center of the 4-T magnet is only 100 ppm above that outside the magnet.

quantities are referred to as susceptibilities and, in part, because two different sets of definitions for magnetization and susceptibility are in use. Because of several practical advantages, the mks (meter, kilogram, and second) system of units has become the system of choice for measuring and reporting electromagnetic field quantities. However, many physicists and almost all magnetochemists continue to use the older cgs (centimeter, gram, and second) system. Both systems use three fundamental magnetic field quantities:[51-53] the flux density, $\vec{B}$; the magnetic field strength, $\vec{H}$; and the magnetization, $\vec{M}$. However, the two systems define the relationships between these field quantities differently:

$$\vec{B} = \mu_0(\vec{H} + \vec{M}) \quad \text{(mks)}$$

$$\vec{B} = \vec{H} + 4\pi\vec{M} \quad \text{(cgs).}$$

Because of these differing definitions, more than a simple change of units is involved in converting between the two systems. For example, the susceptibility is defined by $M = \chi H$ in both systems and is dimensionless in both. Normally, the value of a

TABLE 2. Alternative Susceptibility Values for Water[a]

	MKS Units	CGS Units
Volume susceptibility χ	-9.03×10^{-6}	-0.719×10^{-6} emu/cm^3
Mass susceptibility $\chi_g = \chi/\rho$	-9.09×10^{-9} m^3/kg or -9.09×10^{-6} cm^3/g	-0.723×10^{-6} emu/g
Molar susceptibility $\chi_M = \dfrac{\chi(MW)}{\rho}$	-1.64×10^{-10} m^3/mole or -1.64×10^{-4} cm^3/mole	-1.30×10^{-5} emu/mole

[a] $\rho = 0.9933$ g/cm^3 = 993.3 kg/m^3 at 37 °C; MW = 18.015.

dimensionless quantity does not depend on the units used. However, because of the differing definitions, $\chi_{mks} = 4\pi\chi_{cgs}$.

A further complication results from the tradition in the cgs system of using a dimensional unit called the emu (for electromagnetic unit), which is formally equivalent to a cubic centimeter.[53] Even though χ_{cgs} is dimensionless, it is frequently reported using the redundant dimensional unit, emu/cm^3. The quantity defined as M/H is called the susceptibility or the volume susceptibility. Two related quantities are the mass susceptibility, $\chi_g = \chi/\rho$, and the molar susceptibility, $\chi_M = (MW)\chi/\rho$. Here, ρ is the mass density in g/cm^3 in the cgs system and in kg/m^3 in the mks system. By tradition, MW is the molecular weight with the implied unit of g/mol in both systems. Specifying densities in kg/m^3 sometimes leads to awkward numerical values and the density in the mks units may be specified in g/cm^3 as long as the correct conversion factors are used. Mass and molar susceptibilities are sometimes loosely reported as simply susceptibilities. Therefore, as illustrated in TABLE 2, six different quantities may conceivably be reported as the susceptibility of a given material. Good practice would dictate the abandonment of cgs units in favor of mks units, but, unfortunately, this procedure is not being followed in the magnetochemistry literature. Throughout the rest of this report, mks units will be used except for densities in g/cm^3 as indicated.

All atoms and molecules have the property of diamagnetism; that is, the orbits (or wave functions) of the electrons in the atoms or molecules of any material are modified by an applied field so as to produce, in each atom or molecule, a small magnetic moment directed oppositely to the applied field. This has the effect of reducing the total magnetic field within the material to a value slightly below that of the applied field (Lenz's law). Thus, for all materials, this effect provides a negative contribution to the magnetization and susceptibility.

The presence of ions, atoms, and molecules with unpaired spins provides a paramagnetic contribution to tissue susceptibility.[54] The transition elements are important examples. The transition elements known to be present in biological materials are iron (3–5 g), copper (70–120 mg), manganese (12 mg), nickel (10 mg), chromium (2 mg), cobalt (0.3 mg), vanadium (2 mg), molybdenum (13 mg), and tungsten. The numbers in parentheses give the total amount of the element expected in a 70-kg adult human.[55] These numbers, particularly for the less common elements, are very approximate. There is approximately 30 times more iron in the human body than all other transition elements combined. Iron is thus the major source of tissue paramagnetism. The additional sources of tissue paramagnetism include a few species that, because of peculiarities of their chemical bonding, have unpaired electron spins. The most physiologically important of these are oxygen, O_2, and nitric oxide, NO. Finally, tissues have in them, at small concentrations, some molecules in excited states and a variety of free radicals (short-lived, highly reactive chemical species) that have unpaired spins and associated magnetic moments.

A system with spin S has 2S+1 states that are labeled with the quantum number m_s. This quantity takes on integral or half-integral values ranging from $-S$ to S. Each of these states has a magnetic moment in the field direction of $g\mu_B m_s$, where $g = 2.0$ is the Landé factor and $\mu_B = eh/2m = 9.274 \times 10^{-24}$ J/T is the Bohr magneton. The energy of a magnetic dipole in a magnetic field is $U = -\overline{m} \cdot \overline{B} \equiv -g\mu_B m_s B$. The spacing between the energy levels is $g\mu_B B$. In thermal equilibrium, the probability of occupation of a given state is equal to $[\exp(-U/kT)]/Z$, where $Z = \sinh[(2S+1/2)x]/\sinh(x/2)$ is the partition function[56] and $x = B/B_e$. Note that $B_e = kT/g\mu_B$ is the field at which the magnetic energy difference between levels would be equal to the thermal energy, kT. At 37 °C, $B_e = 231$ T. The magnetic energy difference between adjacent energy states produced by a field of 4 T is less than the thermal energy by a factor of $231/4 \approx 58$. FIGURE 1 shows the energy level splitting for various values for S and B = 4 T at 37 °C. The figure also indicates the changes in the relative populations of the levels induced by a 4-T field. It is seen that, even at 4 T, only small changes in the occupation numbers are produced. This effect, though, is the basis of the paramagnetic contribution to the tissue susceptibility.

It is convenient to define $g\sqrt{S(S + 1)}$ as μ_{eff}, the effective number of Bohr magnetons per atom. With N as the concentration (particles/m^3), the paramagnetic contribution to the susceptibility is

$$\chi = \frac{N\mu_0\mu_{eff}^2\mu_B^2}{3kT}.$$

In biological applications, we are almost always interested in the susceptibility of a mixture, such as a solution of an iron compound in water, rather than that of a pure substance. If the material of interest contains n species with mass susceptibilities $\chi_g^{(i)}$,

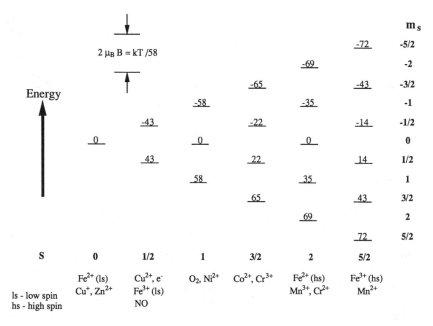

FIGURE 1. Energy levels for various spin states of paramagnetic ions and molecules at 4 T and 37 °C. The numbers give the equilibrium value for the change in occupation number assuming a total of 10,000 total atoms. For example, for S = ½ and at zero field, each of the two levels would be occupied by 5000 atoms. At 4 T, the number of atoms in the state with spin parallel to B would increase by 43. The number with spins antiparallel to B would decrease by 43. This diagram assumes that the spin-orbit coupling and the orbital angular momentum are negligible, leading to a g-value of 2.

molar susceptibilities $\chi_M^{(i)}$, mass concentrations ρ_i, and molar concentrations c_i, the total susceptibility is given by

$$\chi = \sum_{i=1}^{n} \rho_i \chi_g^{(i)} = \sum_{i=1}^{n} c_i \chi_M^{(i)}.$$

These formulas assume that the absolute value of χ is much less than 1, so the magnetizing field can be closely approximated by the applied field. This is always true in biological tissues that do not contain ferromagnetic components. Diamagnetic susceptibilities are essentially independent of temperature and paramagnetic susceptibilities are inversely proportional to temperature. At physiological temperatures, paramagnetism is much more powerful than diamagnetism on an atom by atom basis, but the low concentration of paramagnetic species indicates that the overall tissue susceptibility is normally diamagnetic.

MAGNETIC SUSCEPTIBILITY OF TISSUES

Water is the major chemical constituent of most tissues. It is diamagnetic and is the dominant factor in determining tissue susceptibility. Because it is itself the standard for experimental comparison, the susceptibility of water is not known with great certainty. A standard cgs value[52] for the mass susceptibility of water at 20 °C is -0.72145×10^{-6} emu/g. Precise measurements[57] have shown a slight, nearly linear, change in the mass susceptibility of water with temperature. Along with the density changes between 20 °C and 37 °C, this gives $\chi_{H_2O} = -9.03 \times 10^{-6}$ as the mks volume susceptibility of water at body temperature.

Few studies have been made on the susceptibilities of the lipid and protein constituents of cells. However, the susceptibilities of those diamagnetic tissue components that have been reported usually do not differ greatly from that of water. For example, the diamagnetic component of hemoglobin susceptibility[58] is -9.91×10^{-6}. As an example of a lipid, stearic acid (octadecanoic acid) has an anisotropic susceptibility[59,60] with an average value of -10.0×10^{-6}. There are very few published measurements available for hard tissues such as teeth, nails, bone, and calcifications. However, a recent publication[61] gives -8.7×10^{-6} as the susceptibility of cortical bone. Other diamagnetic tissue components, such as sodium, potassium, and chlorine, are present in too low a concentration to significantly affect tissue susceptibility. Consequently, it is likely that the diamagnetic susceptibilities of all soft tissue components are approximately equal to that of water, with a variation of approximately 10% to 20%.

The paramagnetic contribution from dissolved oxygen in body tissues is very small. Oxygen molecules have $S = 1$ and their concentration is proportional to the tissue oxygen partial pressure, p_{O_2}. At 37 °C and with a p_{O_2} of 760 mm of Hg (1 atmosphere), the equilibrium concentration of dissolved oxygen[62] in water is 1.09×10^{-3} mol/liter or 6.56×10^{-17} molecules/cm^3. At 37 °C, this gives a paramagnetic susceptibility due to dissolved O_2 of $5.82 \times 10^{-11} p_{O_2}$, where p_{O_2} is expressed in mm of Hg.

The reported values of body iron content[54,63] are variable, but a typical value for a normal adult human (70 kg) is a total body iron content of 3.7 grams distributed as 2500 mg in hemoglobin, 1000 mg in ferritin and hemosiderin, 130 mg in myoglobin, 80 mg in a labile pool possibly bound to membranes or to unknown proteins and chelating molecules, 8 mg in cytochromes and enzymes such as catalase, and 3 mg as transport iron bound to transferrin. A classical discovery[64,65] in biochemistry was the counterintuitive finding that, when oxygen molecules ($S = 1$) bind to the ferrous iron ($S = 2$) in hemoglobin or myoglobin, both molecules become diamagnetic ($S = 0$). Therefore, paramagnetic effects normally occur only in deoxyhemoglobin or deoxymyoglobin. If methemoglobin and/or metmyoglobin (which do not bind O_2) are present, there is a paramagnetic contribution from the ferric iron.

Depending on the circumstances, we may be interested in the effect of heme iron atoms on the susceptibility of individual molecules, of red blood cells, of whole blood, or of tissues. The hemoglobin molecule consists of four protein chains, each containing one iron atom (FIGURE 2). The total molecule has a molecular weight of 64,650, a density of 1.335 g/cm^3, and an approximate radius of 27 Å. The four iron atoms correspond to a density of 4.98×10^{19} particles/cm^3 and, with S = 2, they give a paramagnetic contribution to the susceptibility at 37 °C of 10.1×10^{-6}. Adding this to the diamagnetic susceptibility of the protein matrix, -9.91×10^{-6}, indicates that the overall deoxyhemoglobin molecule is just barely paramagnetic at body temperature with $\chi = 0.2 \times 10^{-6}$.

Within a red blood cell (rbc), the paramagnetism of deoxyhemoglobin molecules is diluted by intracellular water and other diamagnetic cellular components. The

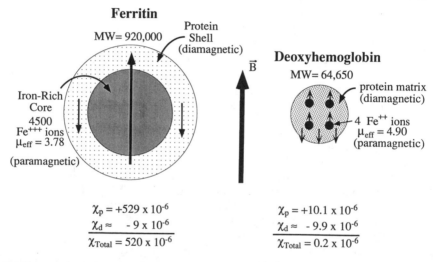

Ferritin

MW= 920,000

Protein Shell (diamagnetic)

$\vec{B}$

Deoxyhemoglobin

MW= 64,650

protein matrix (diamagnetic)

Iron-Rich Core
4500
Fe^{+++} ions
$\mu_{eff} = 3.78$

(paramagnetic)

4 Fe^{++} ions
$\mu_{eff} = 4.90$
(paramagnetic)

$\chi_p = +529 \times 10^{-6}$

$\underline{\chi_d \approx \quad -9 \times 10^{-6}}$

$\chi_{Total} = 520 \times 10^{-6}$

$\chi_p = +10.1 \times 10^{-6}$

$\underline{\chi_d \approx \quad -9.9 \times 10^{-6}}$

$\chi_{Total} = 0.2 \times 10^{-6}$

FIGURE 2. The major paramagnetic contribution to tissue susceptibility comes either from storage iron (ferritin and hemosiderin) or from heme iron in hemoglobin. Ferritin can have a high paramagnetic susceptibility because of the possibility of a large number of iron atoms in the mineral core. Each hemoglobin molecule has approximately 10,000 diamagnetic atoms and 4 paramagnetic iron atoms. At body temperature, these two contributions to the susceptibility of hemoglobin approximately cancel one another.

normal rbc[66] contains a total of 30.2 pg of hemoglobin in a volume of 90.1 cubic microns. This corresponds to a total of 280,000,000 hemoglobin molecules in each rbc. This dilution reduces the average iron concentration within the cell to 1.24×10^{19} atoms/cm^3 and gives 2.5×10^{-6} as the paramagnetic component of the susceptibility. Adding the diamagnetic component gives the overall susceptibility of the fully deoxygenated rbc as -6.52×10^{-6}. If the hematocrit (hct) is expressed as a decimal fraction, the paramagnetic contribution to the susceptibility of fully deoxygenated whole blood will be hct multiplied by 2.5×10^{-6}. For a normal value of hct = 0.45, this gives a paramagnetic contribution of 1.1×10^{-6} and a susceptibility for fully deoxygenated whole blood of -7.90×10^{-6}, which is only about 12% less diamagnetic than pure water. Thus, the paramagnetic effects of iron in blood are less substantial than sometimes assumed.

Ferritin is a storage form of iron[67-69] present in most tissues. The molecule (FIGURE 2) has a spherical mineral core that has the nominal chemical composition $(FeOOH)_8$-FeO-H_2PO_4 (MW = 879.7) and can contain as many as 4500 iron atoms that are in the Fe^{+++} state. The core is surrounded by a spherical protein shell. The core radius is approximately 40 Å and the shell's outer radius is approximately 62.5 Å. The protein shell has an MW = 480,000 and the fully loaded core has an MW = 440,000. Therefore, the molecular weight of the fully loaded molecule is 920,000. The iron atoms are sufficiently close to one another that there is a significant interaction between their magnetic dipole moments. Consequently, their spins do not behave completely independently. The interaction is antiferromagnetic, that is, it tends to produce antiparallel rather than parallel alignment of neighboring spins. At cryogenic temperatures, this leads to an antiferromagnetic ordered phase. It has been suggested that an ordered phase might be present even at body temperature. However, it appears that the iron is paramagnetic at body temperature,[68] although the interaction reduces μ_{eff} to 3.78 rather than 5.92, which would be expected from completely independent spins with S = 5/2. The iron concentration in the core is 1.68×10^{22} atoms/cm³ and this gives a paramagnetic $\chi = 2020 \times 10^{-6}$ at body temperature. Adding a value of -9×10^{-6} as a rough estimate of the core diamagnetism gives $\chi_{core} = 2011 \times 10^{-6}$. Using the same estimate for the diamagnetism of the protein shell gives $\chi = 520 \times 10^{-6}$ for the entire molecule. Hemosiderin is usually regarded as a degraded form of ferritin that consists of the ferritin mineralized cores intermingled with a partially digested protein matrix. Physically and chemically, it is much less thoroughly characterized than ferritin. We assume that the susceptibility of the iron in hemosiderin is equal to that of the iron in ferritin. The concentration of storage iron (ferritin plus hemosiderin) is normally specified as mg of iron/g of wet tissue. Calling this concentration c_i and taking ρ as the tissue density (g/cm³), the iron concentration, N, in particles/m³ is given by $(10^3)c_i\rho N_0/MW$, where MW = 55.847 is the molecular weight of iron and N_0 is Avogadro's number. This gives $N = (1.08 \times 10^{25})c_i\rho$ iron atoms/m³. With $\mu_{eff} = 3.78$, $\chi = (1.30 \times 10^{-6})c_i\rho$ is the paramagnetic contribution from storage iron to the tissue susceptibility. For the normal liver,[70,71] c_i is approximately 0.21 mg/g and ρ is 1.05 g/cm³ (FIGURE 3). An expression that accounts for the contribution of dissolved oxygen and storage iron to the susceptibility of soft tissues is[72-74]

$$\chi_{tissue} = \chi_{H_2O} + (5.82 \times 10^{-11})p_{O_2} + (1.30 \times 10^{-6})c_i\rho.$$

The blood content varies from tissue to tissue[75] and its contribution to the susceptibility will depend on the hematocrit and the level of oxygen saturation. It is clear that the susceptibility of all the soft tissues is very small in magnitude and, except in cases of extreme iron overload, it is diamagnetic. In fact, tissue susceptibility is ordinarily not much different from that of water. Estimates for the susceptibility of tissue components can be used to compare the magnetic forces on tissue components with the gravitational forces that tissues are continually exposed to (FIGURE 4).

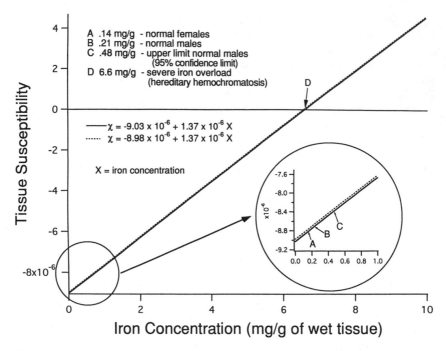

FIGURE 3. The calculated susceptibility for liver tissue shows that, under normal conditions, the susceptibility even in this iron-rich organ varies only in a narrow range near that of water. The effect of dissolved oxygen, even at an unphysiologically high p_{O_2} of 760 mm of Hg, is negligible (dashed line). Only under conditions of severe iron overload will the liver become weakly paramagnetic.

DISCUSSION

Several possible physiological effects of strong static magnetic fields have been considered. In all cases, a strong argument can be made that the potential hazards of these effects up to field strengths of 4 T are well below thresholds set by the stability of human tissues with regard to routine stresses and strains encountered in daily life. Of course, there are many physiological and biochemical processes that are not now understood thoroughly and, hence, it is not possible to exclude the possibility of field-induced pathology coming from some unsuspected source. Therefore, these arguments should not produce complacency about magnetic field exposure. However, they do provide (i) a basis for understanding the fact that harmful effects are not normally observed during human exposure to strong fields and (ii) a basis for explaining those low level sensory effects that appear to be present at 4 T. Special consideration continues to be necessary when using very strong fields to image patients with special medical situations: for example, patients with magnetically sensitive foreign bodies such as pacemakers, pregnant patients, and, possibly, patients known to be especially vulnerable to cardiac dysrhythmias.

Very many experimental observations of biological effects of static magnetic fields have been reported. However, only a few, such as magnetotactic bacteria and the *in vitro* alignment of particles with anisotropic susceptibility, can be considered as incontrovertible. It appears that additional effects involving the migratory behavior of some birds and fishes[76] may be approaching this level of certainty. Apart from apparently harmless effects associated with susceptibility, changes in the electrocardiogram,[77] and the NMR signal itself, the other proposed effects of static magnetic fields on human tissues have an aspect of uncertainty about them. These effects require additional experimental confirmation and theoretical explanation before they can be accepted as unchallenged biological and physical facts.

The apparent safety of human exposure to static fields as strong as 4 T is difficult to reconcile with recent proposals of field-induced pathology produced by slowly changing (100 Hz or less) magnetic fields at the milligauss (10^{-7} T) level. For the most part, the arguments presented earlier for purely static magnetic fields do not need to be modified when considering slowly changing magnetic fields. However, it must be remembered that all time-dependent magnetic fields are accompanied by electric fields and these have not been considered in this article. It would also seem that the magnetic field effects on the dynamics of some chemical reactions should be given a more thorough analysis as a possible source of biological effects.

It has been argued that the presence of sensory effects at high field strengths is a cause for concern because the existence of even low level effects in tissues that are part of a sensory apparatus may imply additional and possibly harmful effects in other tissues that do not happen to be part of a sensory monitoring system. This argument can be at least partially countered by noting that the sensory tissues involved—the retina, the taste buds, and the hair cells of the inner ear—are renowned for the extreme level of their sensitivity to low energy stimuli and all of

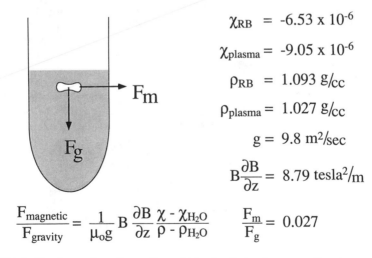

$$\chi_{RB} = -6.53 \times 10^{-6}$$

$$\chi_{plasma} = -9.05 \times 10^{-6}$$

$$\rho_{RB} = 1.093 \text{ g/cc}$$

$$\rho_{plasma} = 1.027 \text{ g/cc}$$

$$g = 9.8 \text{ m}^2/\text{sec}$$

$$B\frac{\partial B}{\partial z} = 8.79 \text{ tesla}^2/\text{m}$$

$$\frac{F_{magnetic}}{F_{gravity}} = \frac{1}{\mu_0 g} B \frac{\partial B}{\partial z} \frac{\chi - \chi_{H_2O}}{\rho - \rho_{H_2O}} \qquad \frac{F_m}{F_g} = 0.027$$

FIGURE 4. The force of gravity on the red blood cells *in vitro* causes the phenomenon of erythrocyte sedimentation. This rate is approximately 5 mm/h in normal individuals. Even in the 4-T magnet, the maximum magnetic force on deoxygenated red cells would be much smaller than the force of gravity. *In vivo*, these effects are overwhelmed by the continual mixing and agitation produced by hemodynamic forces. The magnetic force, of course, will be in the direction of the maximum increase in the magnitude of the magnetic field.

them are sensitive to excitations (photon fluxes, chemical concentrations, and angular accelerations) that are many orders of magnitude below those that are known to cause tissue injury.

It is interesting to speculate on the ultimate limits of static magnetic field exposure for normal, healthy subjects. The sensory effects reported at 4 T are expected to increase as B^2. It has been suggested that the development of a 10-T whole-body scanner is a next logical step in this research area. A subject who moves rapidly while inside such a magnet may experience quite strong sensations of vertigo, magnetophosphenes, and metallic tastes. Because of individual variations, it is likely that some subjects will find these effects distinctly uncomfortable, whereas others may not even notice them. However, by minimizing patient motion while inside the bore and by using proper patient selection, such field strengths will probably be readily tolerated by the majority of subjects.

What then will be the ultimate limit of tolerance to intense static magnetic fields for the healthiest and most adventurous humans? For fields in the 100–200 T range, there will be a significant alteration in the population of the various spin states in iron atoms, oxygen molecules, and free radicals. The rates of many chemical reactions such as oxygen binding to hemoglobin and those of the electron transport chain of the mitochondria could be affected in a dangerous fashion. However, before this level is reached, perhaps between 25 and 50 T, the flow-induced electric fields surrounding blood vessels would exceed the threshold for nerve and muscle stimulation. It seems likely that no human could expect to safely and routinely tolerate field exposure above this level. If this effect really does occur, it will likely be observed using small mammals in small bore, high field magnets long before whole-body human exposure to such fields becomes possible.

The experimental test of these speculations is probably in the distant future. In the meantime, it is interesting to recall that at one time there was widespread use of magnetotherapy. This was a technique in which a physician would place magnets on or near patients for the purpose of curing various diseases. A century ago,[3] A. E. Kennelly (codiscoverer of the ionosphere) and F. Peterson, perplexed that there was no scientific study of the physiological basis of this therapy, borrowed from Thomas Edison the largest magnet then available. After studying a dog and a young boy and performing other experiments with this (marginally) whole-body 0.15-T magnet, they summarized their work in a way that remains thought-provoking today:[3]

> The ordinary magnets used in medicine have purely suggestive or psychic effect and would in all probability be quite as useful if made of wood. While we have demonstrated conclusively the above facts, we do not deny the possibility of there being invented some day magnets enormously more powerful than any yet known to us, which may produce effects upon the nervous system perceptible to some of the sensory organs, for magnetism is certainly a remarkable force, and we find it very difficult to understand why it seems to have no influence whatever upon the human body and its wonderfully delicate neuroelectric mechanism.

ACKNOWLEDGMENTS

It is a pleasure to acknowledge the discussions and assistance from many colleagues and the assistance in the preparation of this manuscript from J. A. Agresta, M. Henry, and R. E. Argersinger.

REFERENCES

1. BARTHOLOW, R. 1887. Medical Electricity (Third Edition). Lea & Febiger. Philadelphia.
2. HERMANN, L. 1888. Hat das magnetische Feld direkte physiologische Wirkungen? Pflügers Arch. Gesamte Physiol. Menschen Tiere **43:** 217–234.
3. PETERSON, F. & A. E. KENNELLY. 1892. Some physiological experiments with magnets at the Edison Laboratory. N.Y. Med. J. **56:** 729–734.
4. DRINKER, C. K. & R. M. THOMSON. 1921. Does the magnetic field constitute an industrial hazard? J. Ind. Hyg. **3:** 117–129.
5. BARNOTHY, M. F., Ed. 1964. Biological Effects of Magnetic Fields. Plenum. New York.
6. BARNOTHY, M. F., Ed. 1969. Biological Effects of Magnetic Fields, Vol. 2. Plenum. New York.
7. TENFORDE, T. S., Ed. 1978. Magnetic Field Effects on Biological Systems. Plenum. New York.
8. MARET, G., J. KIEPENHEUER & N. BOCCARA, Eds. 1986. Biophysical Effects of Steady Magnetic Fields. Springer-Verlag. Berlin/New York.
9. BUDINGER, T. F. & C. CULLANDER. 1984. Health effects of *in vivo* nuclear magnetic resonance. *In* Biomedical Magnetic Resonance. T. L. James & A. Margulis, Eds. Radiology Research and Education Foundation. San Francisco.
10. SAUNDERS, R. D. & H. SMITH. 1984. Safety aspects of NMR clinical imaging. Br. Med. Bull. **40:** 148–154.
11. SCHENCK, J. F. 1991. Quantitative estimates of magnetic field effects on biological tissues. In preparation.
12. STRATTON, M. A. 1941. Electromagnetic Theory. McGraw–Hill. New York.
13. CHIKAZUMI, S. & S. H. CHARAP. 1964. Physics of Magnetism. Wiley. New York.
14. CHEN, C-W. 1977. Magnetism and Metallurgy of Soft Magnetic Materials. North-Holland. Amsterdam. (Reprinted 1985. Dover. New York.)
15. HONG, F. T., D. MAUZERALL & A. MAURO. 1971. Magnetic anisotropy and the orientation of retinal rods in a homogeneous magnetic field. Proc. Natl. Acad. Sci. U.S.A. **68:** 1283–1285.
16. GEACINTOV, N. E., F. VAN NOSTRAND, J. F. BECKER & J. B. TINKEL. 1972. Magnetic field orientation of photosynthetic systems. Biochim. Biophys. Acta **267:** 65–79.
17. HONG, F. T. 1977. Photoelectric and magneto-orientation effects in pigmented biological membranes. J. Colloid Interface Sci. **58:** 471–497.
18. MARET, G., M. V. SCHICKFUS, A. MAYER & K. DRANSFELD. 1975. Orientation of nucleic acids in high magnetic fields. Phys. Rev. Lett. **35:** 397–400.
19. TORBET, J., J-M. FREYSSINET & G. HUDRY-CLERGEON. 1981. Oriented fibrin gels formed by polymerization in strong magnetic fields. Nature **289:** 91–93.
20. WORCESTER, D. C. 1978. Structural origins of diamagnetic anisotropy in proteins. Proc. Natl. Acad. Sci. U.S.A. **75:** 5475–5477.
21. MURAYAMA, M. 1966. Molecular mechanism of red cell "sickling". Science **153:** 145–149.
22. MURAYAMA, M. 1965. Orientation of sickled erythrocytes in a magnetic field. Nature **206:** 420–422.
23. BRODY, A. S., M. P. SORETTE, C. A. GOODING, J. LISTERUD, M. R. CLARK, W. C. MENTZER, R. C. BRASCH & T. L. JAMES. 1985. Induced alignment of flowing sickle erythrocytes in a magnetic field: a preliminary report. Invest. Radiol. **20:** 560–566.
24. BRODY, A. S., S. H. EMBURY, W. C. MENTZER, M. L. WINKLER & C. A. GOODING. 1988. Preservation of sickle cell blood flow patterns during MR imaging: an *in vivo* study. Am. J. Roentgenol. **151:** 139–141.
25. MANKAD, V. N., J. P. WILLIAMS, M. D. HARPEN, E. MANCI, G. LONGENECKER, R. B. MOORE, A. SHAH, Y. M. YANG & B. G. BROGDON. 1990. Magnetic resonance imaging of bone marrow in sickle cell disease: clinical, hematologic, and pathologic correlations. Blood **75:** 274–283.
26. ATKINS, P. 1976. Magnetic field effects. Chem. Br. **12:** 214–218.
27. ATKINS, P. W. & T. P. LAMBERT. 1976. The effect of a magnetic field on chemical reactions. Annu. Rep. Prog. Chem. **A72:** 67–88.
28. HABERDITZL, W. 1967. Enzyme activity in high magnetic fields. Nature **213:** 72–73.
29. MALING, J. E., M. WEISSBLUTH & E. E. JACOBS. 1965. Enzyme-substrate reactions in high magnetic fields. Biophys. J. **5:** 767–776.

30. RABINOVITCH, B., J. E. MALING & M. WEISSBLUTH. 1967. Enzyme-substrate reactions in very high magnetic fields—I. Biophys. J. **7:** 187–204.
31. RABINOVITCH, B., J. E. MALING & M. WEISSBLUTH. 1967. Enzyme-substrate reactions in very high magnetic fields—II. Biophys. J. **7:** 319–327.
32. KOMOLOVA, G. S., G. D. ERYGIN, T. B. VASILEVA & I. A. EGOROV. 1972. Effect of high strength constant magnetic field on enzymatic hydrolysis of nucleic acids. Dokl. Akad. Nauk SSSR Ser. Biol. **204:** 995–997.
33. MCLAUGHLAN, K. A. 1981. The effects of magnetic fields on chemical reactions. Sci. Prog. (Oxford) **67:** 509–529.
34. BROCKLEHURST, B. 1976. Spin correlation in the geminate recombination of radical ions in hydrocarbons. Part I—Theory of the magnetic field effect. J. Chem. Soc. Faraday Trans. 2 **72:** 1864–1869.
35. OZEKI, S. & H. UCHIYAMA. 1988. Magnetoadsorption of NO on iron oxides. J. Phys. Chem. **92:** 6485–6486.
36. TURRO, N. J. 1983. Influence of nuclear spin on chemical reactions: magnetic isotope and magnetic field effects (a review). Proc. Natl. Acad. Sci. U.S.A. **80:** 609–621.
37. GOULD, I. R., N. J. TURRO & M. B. ZIMMT. 1984. Magnetic field and magnetic isotope effects on the products of organic reactions. In Advances in Physical Organic Chemistry, Vol. 20. V. Gold & D. Bethel, Eds. Academic Press. New York.
38. STEINER, U. E. & T. ULRICH. 1989. Magnetic field effects in chemical kinetics and related phenomena. Chem. Rev. **89:** 51–147.
39. KITTEL, C. 1963. Quantum Theory of Solids. Wiley. New York.
40. WINFREY, A. T. 1990. The electrical thresholds of ventricular myocardium. J. Cardiovasc. Physiol. **1:** 393–410.
41. REILLY, J. P. 1989. Peripheral nerve stimulation by induced electric currents: exposure to time-varying magnetic fields. Med. Biol. Eng. Comput. **27:** 101–110.
42. BARFUSS, H., H. FISCHER, D. HENTSCHEL, R. LADEBECK & J. VETTER. 1988. Whole-body MR imaging and spectroscopy with a 4-T system. Radiology **169:** 811–816.
43. BARFUSS, H., H. FISCHER, D. HENTSCHEL, R. LADEBECK, A. OPPELT, R. WITTIG, W. DUERR & R. OPPELT. 1990. In vivo magnetic resonance imaging and spectroscopy with a 4 T whole-body magnet. NMR Biomed. **3:** 31–45.
44. SCHENCK, J. F., C. L. DUMOULIN, R. W. REDINGTON, H. Y. KRESSEL, R. T. ELLIOTT & I. L. MCDOUGALL. 1991. In preparation.
45. LÖVSUND, P., A. ÖBERG, S. E. G. NILSSON & T. REUTER. 1980. Magnetophosphenes: a quantitative analysis of thresholds. Med. Biol. Eng. Comput. **18:** 326–334.
46. OMAN, C. M. & L. R. YOUNG. 1972. The physiological range of pressure difference and cupula deflections in the human semicircular canal. Acta Oto-Laryngol. (Stockholm) **74:** 324–331.
47. OMAN, C. M., E. N. MARCUS & I. S. CURTHOYS. 1987. The influence of semicircular canal morphology on endolymph flow dynamics. Acta Oto-Laryngol. (Stockholm) **103:** 1–13.
48. SENFTLE, F. E. & W. P. HAMBRIGHT. 1969. Magnetic susceptibility of biological materials. In Biological Effects of Magnetic Fields, Vol. 2. M. F. Barnothy, Ed.: 261–306. Plenum. New York.
49. GUPTA, R. R. 1986. Diamagnetic susceptibility. In Landolt-Börnstein Numerical Data and Functional Relationships in Science and Technology. New Series, Vol. 16. K-H. Hellwege & A. M. Hellwege, Eds. Springer-Verlag. Berlin/New York.
50. VAN VLECK, J. H. 1932. The Theory of Electric and Magnetic Susceptibilities. Oxford University Press. London/New York.
51. QUICKENDEN, T. I. & R. C. MARSHALL. 1972. Magnetochemistry in SI units. J. Chem. Educ. **49:** 114–116.
52. BATES, L. F. 1961. Modern Magnetism (Fourth Edition). Cambridge University Press. London/New York.
53. CARLIN, R. L. 1986. Magnetochemistry. Springer-Verlag. Berlin/New York.
54. COTTON, F. A. & G. WILKINSON. 1988. Advanced Inorganic Chemistry (Fifth Edition). Wiley. New York.
55. OTSUKA, S. 1988. Introduction. In Metalloproteins: Chemical Properties and Biological Effects. S. Otsuka & T. Yamanaka, Eds. Kodansha. Tokyo.

56. PATHRIA, R. K. 1972. Statistical Mechanics. Pergamon. Elmsford, New York.
57. PHILO, J. S. & W. M. FAIRBANK. 1980. Temperature dependence of the diamagnetism of water. J. Chem. Phys. **72:** 4429–4433.
58. PHILO, J. S., U. DREYER & T. M. SCHUSTER. 1984. Diamagnetism of human apo-, oxy-, and (carbonmonoxy)-hemoglobin. Biochemistry **23:** 865–872.
59. LONSDALE, K. 1939. Diamagnetic anisotropy of conjugated compounds. J. Chem. Soc. **1:** 364–368.
60. LONSDALE, K. 1939. Diamagnetic anisotropy of organic molecules. Proc. R. Soc. London **A171:** 541–568.
61. SAMANAWEERA, T. S., G. H. GLOVER, T. O. BINFORD & J. R. ADLER. 1991. Correction and quantification of MR susceptibility distortion applied to stereotaxic surgery. *In* Society of Magnetic Resonance in Medicine Tenth Annual Meeting, Book of Abstracts, p. 1225.
62. TRUESDALE, G. A., A. L. DOWNING & G. F. LOWDEN. 1955. The solubility of oxygen in pure water and sea-water. J. Appl. Chem. **5:** 53–62.
63. WILLIAMS, W. J., E. BUETLER, A. J. ERSLEV & R. W. RUNDLES. 1977. Hematology (Second Edition). McGraw–Hill. New York.
64. PAULING, L. & C. D. CORYELL. 1936. The magnetic properties and structure of hemoglobin, oxyhemoglobin, and carbonmonoxyhemoglobin. Proc. Natl. Acad. Sci. U.S.A. **22:** 210–216.
65. SERAFINI, A. 1989. Linus Pauling: A Man and His Science. Paragon House. New York.
66. DICKERSON, R. E. & I. GEIS. 1983. Hemoglobin: Structure, Function, Evolution, and Pathology. Benjamin. New York.
67. HARRISON, P. M., P. J. ARTYMIUK, G. C. FORD, O. M. LAWSON, J. M. A. SMITH & J. L. WHITE. 1989. Ferritin: function and structural design of an iron-storage protein. *In* Biomineralization: Chemical and Biochemical Perspectives. S. Mann, J. Webb & R. Williams, Eds. Verlag Chemie. Weinheim, Germany.
68. MICHAELIS, L., C. D. CORYELL & S. GRANICK. 1943. The magnetic properties of ferritin and some other colloidal ferric compounds. J. Biol. Chem. **148:** 463–480.
69. FRANKEL, R. B. & R. P. BLAKEMORE, Eds. 1991. Iron Biominerals. Plenum. New York.
70. SENFTLE, F. E. & A. THORPE. 1961. Magnetic susceptibility of normal liver and transplantable hepatoma tissue. Nature **190:** 410–413.
71. OVERMOYER, B. A., C. E. MCLAREN & G. M. BRITTENHAM. 1987. Uniformity of liver density and nonheme (storage) iron distribution. Arch. Pathol. Lab. Med. **111:** 549–554.
72. BRITTENHAM, G. M., D. E. FARRELL, J. W. HARRIS, E. S. FELDMAN, E. H. DANISH, W. A. MUIR, J. H. TRIPP & E. M. BELLON. 1982. Magnetic-susceptibility of human iron stores. N. Engl. J. Med. **307:** 1671–1675.
73. BAUMAN, J. H. & J. W. HARRIS. 1967. Estimation of hepatic iron stores by *in vivo* measurement of magnetic susceptibility. J. Lab. Clin. Med. **70:** 246–257.
74. BRITTENHAM, G. M., P. E. ZANZUCCHI, D. E. FARRELL, J. H. TRIPP, W. A. MUIR & J. W. HARRIS. 1980. Non-invasive *in vivo* measurement of human iron overload by magnetic susceptibility studies. Trans. Assoc. Am. Physicians **93:** 156–163.
75. SNYDER, W. S., M. J. COOK, E. S. NASSET, L. R. KARHAUSEN, G. P. HOWELLS & I. H. TIPTON. 1975. Report of the Task Group on Reference Man. International Commission on Radiological Protection Publication No. 23. Pergamon. Elmsford, New York.
76. SAKAKI, Y., T. MOTOMIYA, M. KATO & M. OGURA. 1990. Possible mechanism of biomagnetic sense organ extracted from sockeye salmon. IEEE Trans. Magn. **26:** 1554–1556.
77. TENFORDE, T. S., C. T. GAFFEY, R. P. LIBURDY & L. LEVY. 1985. Biological effects of magnetic fields. *In* Annual Report of the Biology and Medicine Divisions, Lawrence Berkeley Laboratory (LBL-20345), p. 60–67.

Safety of Patients with Medical Devices during Application of Magnetic Resonance Methods

GERALD M. POHOST,[a,b] GERALD G. BLACKWELL,[a] AND
FRANK G. SHELLOCK[c]

[a]Division of Cardiovascular Disease
[b]Center for NMR Research and Development
University of Alabama at Birmingham
Birmingham, Alabama 35294

[c]Section of Magnetic Resonance Imaging
Department of Diagnostic Radiology
Cedars-Sinai Medical Center
and
UCLA School of Medicine
Los Angeles, California 90048

INTRODUCTION

Although clinically applicable magnetic resonance methods are generally regarded as noninvasive, safe, and effective diagnostic modalities with none of the hazards associated with approaches based on ionizing radiation, there are potential hazards. Among the most important potential hazards to patients are those related to implanted or attached medical devices, which are so commonly encountered in modern clinical practice.[1-8] Devices such as cardiac pacemakers, surgical vascular clips, and heart valves are among the most frequently encountered. These devices can be considered to be in three different categories: (a) metallic implants or foreign bodies; (b) magnetically, electrically, mechanically, or radio-frequency activated devices; and (c) externally located devices. The hazards associated with MR procedures in patients with implanted devices or other objects are related to movement or dislodgment, possible electric current induction, heating, malfunction, or artifact production and resultant misinterpretation. The purpose of this report is to provide a review of the implanted or attached medical devices that may be associated with morbidity or even mortality in patients undergoing magnetic resonance imaging procedures.

TABLE 1 presents a summary of the risks associated with a variety of commonly encountered devices or objects. Assessment of risk in individuals with a possible ferromagnetic implant, object, or device should include (1) careful history check for previous implant surgery or penetrating wounds, (2) careful physical examination to look for surgical scars, and (3) planar radiograph of a region in question.

METALLIC IMPLANTS OR FOREIGN BODIES

One of the greatest potential risks to individuals undergoing a magnetic resonance study is that associated with ferromagnetic metallic implants or foreign bodies. At the present time, there have been well over 40 publications that have examined the ferromagnetic properties of numerous metallic implants and foreign bodies. Needless to say, a substantial percentage of patients are at risk for magnetic resonance imaging or spectroscopy due to the presence of these ferromagnetic objects. Alternatively, some of these objects will present little or no risk to the subject under investigation. A variety of factors influence risk for magnetic resonance diagnostic procedures in patients with surgically implanted or accidentally encountered ferromagnetic objects (TABLE 2).

It is essential to know prior to exposure to a magnetic resonance procedure if there is any possibility that the patient has a ferromagnetic object and, if so, the location of that object because certain locations must be considered dangerous, whereas others do not pose a risk or hazard. For example, if the object is located near important vascular, neural, or other soft tissues where movement or dislodgment could lead to morbidity or mortality, magnetic resonance procedures should be avoided.

An acceptable approach for screening for metallic objects was developed with respect to the eye. Williams *et al.*[9] demonstrated that metallic fragments as small as $0.1 \times 0.1 \times 0.1$ mm within the orbit were detectable by standard plain X rays. A series of metallic fragments of various sizes from $0.1 \times 0.1 \times 0.1$ to $3.0 \times 1.0 \times 1.0$ mm were examined to determine if they were displaced within the eyes of laboratory animals during exposure within an MR system ($B_0 = 2.0$ T). Only the largest fragment ($3.0 \times 1.0 \times 1.0$ mm) was found to move in a circular way without causing any discernible clinical damage. Thus, this study suggests that the use of a plain X-ray examination is an acceptable technique for determining if an intraocular metallic fragment represents a potential hazard. A report from the Society for Magnetic Resonance Imaging suggests that each imaging site "should develop a standardized policy for screening patients with suspected metallic foreign bodies; the policy should include guidelines as to which patients require radiographic and/or CT examinations and the specific radiographic or CT technique(s) to be used."[7]

Various implantable devices and objects that have been studied are indicated in TABLE 3. These include vascular clips and clamps, intravascular devices, prosthetic heart valves, and ocular and otologic implants. Among the most dangerous implantable objects when subjected to a magnetic resonance procedure is the ferromagnetic aneurysm clip.[10] *In vitro* and laboratory animal studies have demonstrated the hazard of subjecting ferromagnetic aneurysm clips to static magnetic fields[1] because they can be displaced, damaging adjacent cerebral tissue, or they can even be extracted, resulting in morbidity or mortality. Thus, patients known to have or suspected of having such clips must not be examined using magnetic resonance procedures unless the clip is definitely nonmagnetic. In addition, certain carotid artery clamps have been shown to be deflected by the magnetic field in a 1.5-T system.[11] However, in general, most carotid artery vascular clamps have been imaged by magnetic resonance systems with field strengths up to 0.6 T without problem. Metallic intravascu-

TABLE 1. Hazard Potential of Devices or Objects with MR Procedures[a]

Device or Object	n	Hazard Potential	Comments
Internal			
Aneurysm & hemostatic clips	26	4	Nonferromagnetic clips are safe (grade 0). No morbidity or mortality reported to date with aneurysm or hemostatic clips.
Carotid artery clamps	5	1 or 4	The Poppen-Blaylock clamp is unsafe (grade 4).
Intravascular coils, stents & filters	14	0	These devices are usually firmly incorporated into the vessel wall and are unlikely to be dislodged.
Prosthetic heart valves	29	0–4	Starr-Edwards mitral prostheses < model 6000 may be unsafe (grade 3). This is especially true with paravalvular leak or dehiscence (grade 4).
Vascular access ports	33	0–3	Electronically controlled infusion pumps can be damaged and MR methods are contraindicated in patients with such systems (grade 3).
Ocular implants	12	3	The Fatio eyelid spring and the retinal tack made from martensitic stainless steel may be unsafe at 1.5 T.
Ocular foreign body		3	Two reports of a ferrous foreign body penetrating the eye and resulting in eye injury.
Otologic implants:			
cochlear	3	2	Activated by magnetic field. Can be damaged. One implant reported to be severely damaged.
others		1	McGee piston prosthesis (platinum and 17Cr-4Ni model) is unsafe (grade 3).
Orthopedic implants	15	0	Heating has not been a significant problem.
Dental devices & materials	16	1	Devices that are magnetically activated present a potential problem.
Penile implants	9	0–2	Only one, the Dacomed Omniphase, demonstrated significant deflection force at 1.5 T. No experience with MR exposure.
Contraceptive diaphragm		0	Although strongly attracted, it has presented no discomfort in practice. Large artifacts can obscure diagnostic information.
Bullets and pellets		0–4	Shrapnel produces artifacts. Unsafe if located near a vital structure.

TABLE 1. Continued

Device or Object	Hazard Potential	Comments
Pacemakers	4	Causes asynchronous pacing. Can cause cessation of pacing or rapid pacing. Pacemakers should be considered to be a contraindication to MR procedures; two patients with pacemakers have died during MRI.
Defibrillators/cardioverters	4	MR contraindicated with these devices.
Neurostimulators	3	Report of one device that was severely damaged.
External Swan-Ganz thermodilution catheter	2–3	Swan-Ganz thermodilution wires melted at skin entry site.
Pulse oximeter Pulse plethysmography ECG wires and leads	3	Over 75 incidents of burns reported, 6 with third-degree burns. Includes report of severe third-degree chest burns where ECG cables crossed and came into contact with patient's chest. Pulse oximeter third-degree burns of finger have been reported.
External prostheses (nose, teeth, ears, braces)	2	Prostheses held in place with magnets could have subcutaneous magnets damaged, requiring replacement.
Hearing aids	1	Hearing aids have been irreversibly damaged.
Halo vests	1	Conductive, nonferromagnetic vest reported to show arcing without morbidity.

[a]Hazard potential: 0 = none; 1 = mild risk, can cause mild discomfort; 2 = mid to moderate risk and discomfort; 3 = can cause severe morbidity, but not usually life-threatening; 4 = life-threatening risk; n = number of devices reported in the literature.

TABLE 2. Risk Factors for Ferromagnetic Objects in Patients Undergoing MR Procedures

Static and gradient magnetic field strength
Degree of ferromagnetism
Mass of object
Geometry of object
Location of object
Orientation of object
Mobility of object
Duration of time that the object has been in place

TABLE 3. Objects and Devices Studied

Aneurysm and hemostatic clips
Carotid artery clamps
Dental materials
Prosthetic heart valves
Intravascular devices (stents, filters, etc.)
Vascular access ports
Ocular implants
Cochlear and other otologic implants
Orthopedic implants
Contraceptive diaphragms and IUDs
Penile implants
Bullets, pellets, and shrapnel
Miscellaneous

lar stents, filters, and coils can also be ferromagnetic. These devices typically become firmly incorporated into the vessel wall after several weeks and, therefore, it is unlikely that any of them would become dislodged by magnetic forces during magnetic resonance procedures.[12] Only a very few of more than 30 implantable vascular access ports have been shown to be deflected by static magnetic fields and these deflection forces are relatively insignificant.[13] Thus, magnetic resonance procedures can be performed safely in patients with one of these types of implants.

Moreover, in the category of intravascular or extravascular objects, heart valves are an important subset. Deflection forces associated with heart valves are relatively minor and, therefore, these pose no hazard. The possible exception to this is the Starr-Edwards mitral valve prosthesis with a series number less than 6000.[14] This type of valve was used between 1960 and 1964 and is uncommonly encountered today. Soulen and colleagues suggest that MR studies should not be performed in patients with this prosthesis in magnets with fields greater than 0.35 T if there is the possibility of dehiscence or a paravalvular leak.[14]

There are several other commonly encountered implantable or attached objects that may be ferromagnetic. For example, the majority of a number of dental devices and materials have exhibited measurable deflection forces.[15] However, only those few that are magnetically activated represent a potential problem.

MAGNETICALLY, ELECTRICALLY, RADIO-FREQUENCY, OR MECHANICALLY ACTIVATED DEVICES

The FDA requires clear labeling of MR systems to indicate contraindication in patients with electrically, magnetically, radio-frequency, or mechanically activated devices because the electromagnetic field of the MR system could interfere with the operation of these devices.

Cardiac pacemakers are commonly encountered implanted devices, especially in the older population. The majority of pacemakers are complex externally programmable devices that use a radio-frequency transmitter to change their pacing parameters. Stimulation rate (for ventricle and/or atrium), electric current output, duration and configuration of the electrical pulse, and time delay between atrial and ventricular pulses are some of the parameters that can be externally reprogrammed. In addition, many pacemaker pulse generators are converted from an impulse sensitive or synchronous mode to a fixed rate or asynchronous mode using an externally applied magnet. The magnet activates a reed switch and the device produces stimulating pulses at a fixed rate. The rate is related to the residual battery power and provides a means to evaluate the state of the battery.

Thus, exposure to strong external magnetic or electromagnetic fields could lead to the following: conversion of a demand pulse generator from the synchronous to the asynchronous mode, damage to the fragile reed switch, reprogramming of the pacemaker parameters, induced currents in the electrode wires, or displacement of the pulse generator.[16] It should be noted that the behavior of a cardiac pacemaker pulse generator near or within an MR device is related to the intrinsic properties of that pulse generator and to the parameters of the MR system. For example, advanced dual-chamber programmable demand pacemakers from *in vitro* and *in vivo* experience suggest that ultrafast atrial rates of up to 800/min or total inhibition of the pacemaker may occur and lead to devastating consequences. Both the continuation of pacing and the ultrafast rhythms are not related to the static magnetic field, but they only occur during actual imaging.[17]

Most pulse generators contain magnetically activated reed switches that are used to convert pulse generators from a synchronous mode into an asynchronous mode. These fragile-appearing reed switches have not been reported to be substantially damaged by exposure to magnetic resonance devices. Undoubtedly, the reed switch will be activated and the patient will be paced asynchronously due to the static magnetic field. Generally, asynchronous pacing is safe; however, in patients with unstable cardiac conditions such as acute myocardial infarction or unstable angina pectoris, there is substantial risk for ventricular fibrillation. It is the sensitivity of the reed switch of some pacemakers that has determined the "safety boundary" for magnetic resonance devices as being 5 gauss. Although most reed switches will be activated only by fields in considerable excess of 5 gauss, patients as well as others (i.e., visitors, health-care workers, etc.) with pacemakers and other magnetically sensitive devices should be kept outside of regions where the magnetic field is in excess of 5 gauss (5.0×10^{-4} T). The only two reported deaths related to magnetic resonance imaging have occurred in patients with pacemakers. In one case, the patient had no escape ventricular rhythm and the patient apparently died due to asystole. The second patient developed ventricular fibrillation during the imaging procedure that was not recognized immediately because ECG monitoring was not used.

TABLE 4 lists other implantable electronic devices. Patients with implantable

TABLE 4. Devices Activated Magnetically, Electrically, Mechanically, or with Radio Frequency

Cardiac pacemakers
Implantable defibrillators
Implantable infusion pumps
Neurostimulators
Cochlear implants
Bone growth stimulators

defibrillators/cardioverters should not be subjected to magnetic resonance procedures. The risk includes triggering the device, which has the potential to induce ventricular fibrillation, and damaging the device, which will inhibit or eliminate the possibility of its functioning to defibrillate or cardiovert. Also, there is a risk of induced current in the lead wire. Implantable infusion pumps sometimes contain an electronic feedback mechanism to allow the infusion rate to change. For example, in diabetics with insulin pumps, an electronic method to control the pump as a function of blood glucose levels is present. Magnetic resonance procedures could alter the infusion rate or damage the pump and, accordingly, they are contraindicated in such patients. The presence of a neurostimulator should also be a contraindication to magnetic resonance procedures. One such stimulator has been reported to be badly damaged and nonfunctional after a magnetic resonance procedure. The same is true of cochlear implants, which are sensitive to static magnetic fields and are also electronically and/or magnetically activated.[18] Cochlear implants have been reported to be damaged after exposure to magnetic resonance imaging.

EXTERNALLY LOCATED DEVICES

Many individuals who are in need of magnetic resonance procedures will have external or attached devices. These include intravenous lines, thermodilution catheters, pulse oximeters, pulse plethysmographs, monitoring electrodes, ECG cables, hearing aids, halo vests (for cervical spine fixation),[19] and various types of limb or cosmetic prostheses. Untoward effects have been reported in patients subjected to magnetic resonance procedures with such devices present.[20,21] For example, a Swan-Ganz thermodilution catheter has been reported to demonstrate melting at the site of introduction of the catheter into the patient, suggesting a radio-frequency heating phenomenon.[22] Up to 75 incidents have been reported of burns developed at the site of a pulse oximeter, pulse plethysmograph, or monitoring electrode. In several patients, third-degree burns have been noted.[23] For example, in an infant being monitored with a pulse oximeter, third-degree burns involving the finger used for monitoring were noted. Similar observations have been made in adult patients. Another important problem is that of burns sustained by patient contact with ECG monitoring wires. One patient developed third-degree burns of his chest while being imaged in the area where the ECG electrode wires inappropriately crossed one another.[22]

Another problem with magnetically or electronically activated devices is damage to these devices. Hearing aids can be electronically destroyed by exposure to magnetic resonance procedures. In addition, certain prostheses used in plastic surgery are held in place using magnets. Such magnets can be demagnetized or irreparably damaged in the MR system. Newly developed dental prostheses frequently use magnets to hold teeth in place and there are other types of orthodontic prostheses that also use magnets. In these cases as well, these prostheses may require replacement in patients subjected to magnetic resonance procedures.

Halo vests generally used for spine fixation after cervical spine trauma are composed of metallic materials that can produce mild to severe artifacts. If the vest contains ferromagnetic components, there exists the possibility of movement or dislodgment, a potential hazard in such patients. Even in those patients in which the vest contains no ferromagnetic components, but only conductive materials, there is a theoretical hazard of inducing an electrical current because the vest contains a closed loop conductor. There has been a report of arcing in such a vest during magnetic resonance imaging. A halo vest was recently developed with little ferromagnetic or conductive potential. Such a device was evaluated as an alternative to more traditional vests and permits MR imaging.[19] This device was found to be safe with no artifacts generated on the resultant MR images.

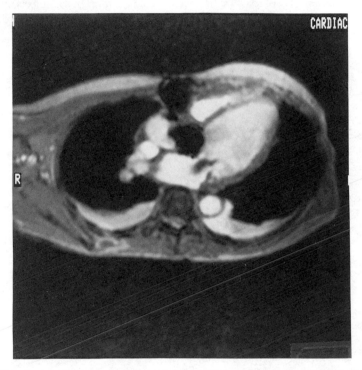

FIGURE 1. Long-axis image of the heart in a patient with a Medtronic-Hall tilting disk prosthesis in the aortic position. An artifact is well seen in the midst of the heart, obscuring the upper septum and a portion of the left atrium. In addition, the stainless steel wire suture material used to close the sternal incision can be observed as another signal void artifact anterior to the valve. Other findings of interest include a small amount of mitral regurgitation and bilateral pleural effusions.

IMAGING ARTIFACTS AND MISINTERPRETATION

One of the most bothersome effects of ferromagnetic objects is their propensity to generate bothersome artifacts considerably larger than the size of the object. Such artifacts can obscure or confound diagnostic information. An illustrative example of this problem occurred in 1980 when an NMR scientist who worked in our laboratory at the Massachusetts General Hospital volunteered to be among the first persons to undergo MR imaging.

The system consisted of a 0.15-T four-ring resistive magnet with an aperture of 50 cm. In one tomographic cut, there was a circular defect located in the skull that looked like a lytic bone lesion from a metastatic tumor. Every person who saw the study was quite concerned and it was difficult to tell our colleague that he could have a terminal disease. Finally, he was apprised of the situation and he had a plane film of his head. This film showed the culprit: a 2-mm metallic fragment, shrapnel from an encounter in Vietnam.

A wide variety of artifacts have been reported.[20] Ferromagnetic objects affect the image by disrupting the local magnetic field. The degree of image disruption depends

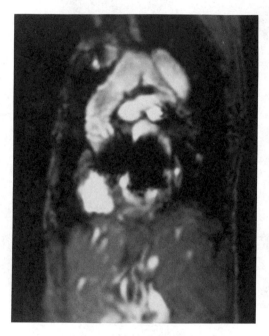

FIGURE 2. Large signal void artifact created by two prosthetic cardiac valves in a patient with Marfan's syndrome and an aortic dissection. The valves are located in the aortic and mitral positions. The large area of signal void markedly reduces the diagnostic power of this imaging study.

upon the shape and orientation of the object in addition to its magnetic susceptibility. Typical artifacts appear as areas of signal void (FIGURES 1 and 2). Other image artifacts can be observed in association with objects that are conductors, but that are nonmagnetic due to resultant eddy currents. Other unusual artifacts have been observed in patients with tattooed eyeliner and certain types of eye makeup made from ferrous materials.

CONCLUSIONS

A major risk associated with the clinical application of MR procedures (imaging or spectroscopy) is related to the presence of implanted or external ferromagnetic devices or objects. MR exposure can lead to significant deflection of a ferromagnetic object or to malfunction of an electronic device. In conductive materials, heating can lead to burns or to melting of the device. If the patient's life depends on the device (such as with a pacemaker), malfunction can be lethal. Thus, good clinical evaluation including careful history and screening, physical examination, and plain X ray, if needed, can minimize the risk of MR procedures. In addition, knowledge of the characteristics of the object will help define risk and will allow determination of the patient's risk-benefit ratio for the MR procedure. Under certain conditions, even if there is some risk, the physician may decide to cautiously proceed with the MR procedure if the information to be acquired is essential. Conversely, an alternative and potentially less effective approach may be selected.

REFERENCES

1. NEW, P. F. J., B. R. ROSEN, T. J. BRADY, F. S. BUONANNO, J. P. KISTLER, C. T. BURT, W. S. HINSHAW, J. H. NEWHOUSE, G. M. POHOST & J. M. TAVERAS. 1983. Potential hazards and artifacts of ferromagnetic and nonferromagnetic surgical and dental materials and devices in nuclear magnetic resonance imaging. Radiology **147**: 139–148.
2. SHELLOCK, F. G. & J. V. CRUES. 1988. High-field strength MR imaging and metallic biomedical implants: an *ex vivo* evaluation of deflection forces. Am. J. Roentgenol. **151**: 389–392.
3. SHELLOCK, F. G. 1988. MR imaging of metallic implants and materials: a compilation of the literature. Am. J. Roentgenol. **151**: 811–814.
4. SHELLOCK, F. G. 1989. Biological effects and safety aspects of magnetic resonance imaging. Magn. Reson. Q. **5**: 243–261.
5. TEITELBAUM, G. P., C. A. YEE, D. D. VAN-HORN, H. S. KIM & P. M. COLLETTI. 1990. Metallic ballistic fragments: MR imaging safety and artifacts. Radiology **175**: 855–859.
6. KANAL, E., F. G. SHELLOCK & L. TALAGALA. 1990. Safety considerations in MR imaging. Radiology **176**: 593–606.
7. SHELLOCK, F. G. & E. KANAL. 1991. SMRI safety committee policies: policies, guidelines, and recommendations for MR imaging safety and patient management. J. MRI **1**: 97–101.
8. SHELLOCK, F. G. & J. S. CURTIS. 1991 (August). MR imaging and biomedical implants, materials, and devices: an updated review. Radiology. In press.
9. WILLIAMS, S., D. H. CHAR, W. P. DILLON, N. LINCOFF & M. MOSELEY. 1988. Ferrous intraocular foreign bodies and magnetic resonance imaging. Am. J. Ophthalmol. **105**: 398–401.
10. ROMNER, B., M. OLSSON, B. LJUNGGREN, S. HOLTÅS, H. SÄVELAND, L. BRANDT & B. PERSSON. 1989. Magnetic resonance imaging and aneurysm clips: magnetic properties and image artifacts. J. Neurosurg. **70**: 426–431.
11. TEITELBAUM, G. P., M. C. W. LIN, A. T. WATANABE, J. F. NORFRAY, T. I. YOUNG & W. G. BRADLEY. 1990. Ferromagnetism and MR imaging: safety of carotid vascular clamps. Am. J. Neuroradiol. **11**: 267–272.
12. LIEBMAN, C. E., R. N. MESSERSMITH, D. N. LEVIN & C. T. LU. 1988. MR imaging of the inferior vena caval filter: safety and artifacts. Am. J. Roentgenol. **150**: 1174–1176.
13. SHELLOCK, F. G. & T. MEEKS. 1991. *Ex vivo* evaluation of ferromagnetism and artifacts for implantable vascular access ports exposed to a 1.5 T MR scanner. J. MRI. In press.
14. SOULEN, R. L., T. F. BUDINGER & C. HIGGINS. 1985. Magnetic resonance imaging of prosthetic heart valves. Radiology **154**: 705–707.
15. SHELLOCK, F. G. 1989. *Ex vivo* assessment of deflection forces and artifacts associated with high-field strength MRI of "mini-magnet" dental prosthesis. Magn. Reson. Imag. **7**(suppl. I): 38.
16. ERLEBACHER, J. A., P. T. CAHILL, F. PANNIZZO & R. J. R. KNOWLES. 1984. Effects of

magnetic resonance imagers on external and implantable pulse generators. PACE **7:** 720–727.

17. ERLEBACHER, J. A., P. T. CAHILL, F. PANNIZZO & R. J. R. KNOWLES. 1986. Effect of magnetic resonance imaging on DDD pacemakers. Am. J. Cardiol. **57:** 437–440.
18. SHELLOCK, F. G. & C. J. SCHATZ. 1991. Metallic otologic implants: *in vitro* assessment of ferromagnetism at 1.5 T. Am. J. Neuroradiol. **12:** 279–281.
19. SHELLOCK, F. G. & G. SLIMP. 1990. Halo vests for cervical spine fixation during MR imaging. Am. J. Roentgenol. **154:** 631–632.
20. PUSEY, E., R. B. LUFKIN, R. K. J. BROWN *et al.* 1986. Magnetic resonance imaging artifacts: mechanism and clinical significance. Radiographics **6:** 891–911.
21. ECRI. 1988 (May 27). A new MRI complication? *In* Health Devices Alert, p. 1.
22. KANAL, E. & F. G. SHELLOCK. 1990. Burns associated with clinical MR examinations. Radiology **175:** 585.
23. SHELLOCK, F. G. & G. SLIMP. 1989. Severe burn of the finger caused by using a pulse oximeter during MR imaging. Am. J. Roentgenol. **153:** 1105.

The Design of RF Systems for Patient Safety

JEFFREY R. FITZSIMMONS

Department of Radiology
University of Florida
Gainesville, Florida 32610

The concern over surface absorption rates (SAR) due to radio-frequency (RF) power deposition is well motivated for modern high power MRI systems.[1] High field (1.5-T) systems typically have 15-kW power amplifiers that are capable of delivering average SARs well above the FDA limits. In addition, there are other aspects of these high power environments that pose safety problems for the patient. Any wires in the bore of the magnet may build up very high voltages along their length and may become sources of high voltage breakdown near the patient's body. Moreover, the presence of surface coils in the bore presents further potential for high local SARs. Energy from the transmitter coil can be transferred quite effectively to the surface coil, concentrating the flux over a small region of interest. In response to these problems, a number of engineering solutions have been proposed and implemented by various manufacturers. What we will do here is to explore each of these problems in turn and discuss what may be done to preclude or minimize the potential for excessive RF energy deposition in the patient.

RF POWER OUTPUT AND SAR

As stated earlier, the power amplifier is capable of generating very large RF fields within the bore of the magnet that may easily exceed the SAR limits set by the FDA. Depending on the MRI system design, it may be very easy or impossible to violate these limits. Our concern here is that the system be designed in such a way that the operator may not easily or mistakenly expose the patient to excessive RF energy.

The early MRI systems did not have to concern themselves with power deposition because it was easy to show that, at low fields and with low RF power amplifiers (5 kW or less), it was not possible to exceed the FDA guidelines with the available pulse techniques. Therefore, they could proceed to tune the RF power output over some predetermined range and thereby determine the 90° pulse. The 180° pulse could then be calculated either by the same algorithm or from the already determined 90° pulse and the RF power level could be set accordingly (this type of system is shown in FIGURE 1a).

With modern high field systems (1–4 T), it became necessary to at least estimate the SAR before patient scanning so that the decision could be made about whether the FDA guidelines were going to be exceeded. Some current systems use a look-up table (LUT) based on previously determined values; thus, when the operator inputs the patient's weight and the sequence type, the system can estimate the SAR within some limits. This average SAR is then presented on the operator screen and data acquisition is allowed to proceed as long as the estimated SAR is within the guidelines (FIGURE 1b). Unfortunately, this type of algorithm does not preclude excessive exposure. It would be easy to make the mistake of inputting the wrong patient weight (say, 200 pounds instead of 20 pounds). The system would then calculate the average SAR based on a large person instead of the pediatric case at

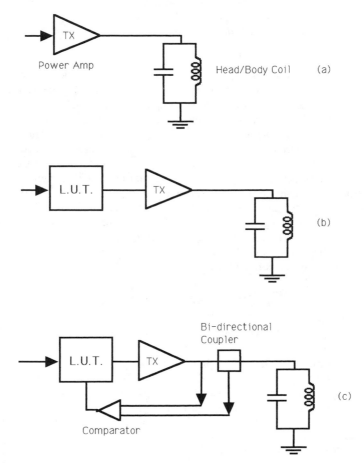

FIGURE 1. Block diagram of transmitter control methods: (a) direct drive of an RF coil without feedback; (b) use of a look-up table (LUT) for storage of power levels appropriate for body mass; (c) use of an LUT for power level with feedback from a bidirectional coupler.

hand. The tip-angle tuning procedure would, of course, adjust the 90° pulse appropriately to the load at hand; however, because the body mass would be wrong, the system might allow a much higher duty cycle before the calculated SAR limit was reached.

An alternative way to address this problem would be to make use of the inherently available information regarding patient body mass. The body coil (or head coil) is sensitive to loading. Large loads cause large impedance changes that may be corrected for by either retuning the coil or, in the case of fixed tuned coils, increasing the power output. For systems that tune each coil to the load, the degree of impedance mismatch may be used to estimate the patient's body mass. Another LUT could be used to store these data. This information could then be compared to the data supplied by the operator to determine if the two sources are in agreement. If both agree within some predefined range, then the data acquisition phase should proceed. In the case of MRI systems that do not tune coils, the same information is available in a different form. An impedance mismatch still exists when a large load is placed in the coil so that power will be reflected back to the driving source. A bidirectional coupler may be employed to measure the amount of reflected power and this can in turn be used to estimate the patient's body mass (FIGURE 1c). In addition, the power level arrived at for a 90° pulse will be an index of body mass in an untuned system because the transmitter must make up for the mismatch by adding power. Therefore, we again have a method of checking the data input by the operator to see if it is within some range. When these sources of data are out of range, the system should not be permitted to continue with data acquisition. The operator should be advised that the FDA limits would be exceeded. An instruction to change the duty cycle by adjusting some pulse parameter would be appropriate (TR or the number of slices, for example). An added advantage of output power monitoring is that the duty cycle can be monitored at the hardware level so that the transmitter can be shut down immediately when the limits are exceeded.

Finally, it should not be an easy matter for the operator to override the SAR limits that are installed in the system at manufacture. It can be found on typical MRI systems that a simple keystroke is all that is needed to go beyond the established limits, thus making such limits irrelevant. The system designer should look carefully at how these limits are implemented on each system so as to assure that the patient will not be exposed inadvertently to high levels of RF energy.

HIGH VOLTAGE EFFECTS

In addition to excessive levels of RF, we must also be concerned about local effects that may occur even when operating well within the FDA guidelines. A recent survey on incidents related to MRI use revealed that a number of patients received first- and second-degree burns from surface coil and EKG leads that were exposed and near the patient's skin.[2] Any piece of wire in the magnet bore that is a sizable portion of a wavelength may absorb a considerable amount of energy from the transmitting coil. As a consequence, large voltages may build up on the surface of the wire with no path for discharge except free space (FIGURE 2).

If the wire happens to be poorly insulated or partly exposed and it is laying on the patient's chest or arm, the voltage present may discharge through space into the skin, causing significant local burns. This problem may be further aggravated by coiling up wire in the bore and placing the coil on top of the patient. In any case, because the surface coil is only grounded at the preamplifier input, there is no way to discharge the voltages safely. Therefore, the manufacturer must be extra careful to provide substantial insulation along the length of any wires that enter the bore of the magnet.

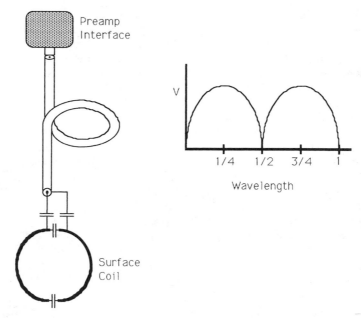

FIGURE 2. Example of a typical preamp to surface coil lead with a plot of voltage versus wavelength. Voltage may build up along the surface coil lead depending on its length and geometric configuration.

In addition, any junctions or connectors must be further insulated to guard against this type of shock and burn hazard.

LOCAL SAR EFFECTS

There is one more problem that has been a consequence of using receive-only surface coils inside of the whole-body transmitter coils. The energy generated by the high power transmitter may be coupled very effectively to any surface coil in the bore, resulting in a flux concentration over the region of the surface coil.[3] Unless the surface coil is properly decoupled from the transmitting coil, there will be high circulating currents in the surface coil that will result in an SAR that is far in excess of the calculated average SAR from the transmitter coil alone. In experiments done in our laboratory, significant temperature increases were achieved over small sample sizes in as little as 10 minutes of exposure to a high duty cycle pulse sequence (FIGURE 3). We used an inversion spin-echo pulse sequence with a TR of 50 milliseconds, a TI of 6 milliseconds, and a TE of 20 milliseconds. With a 50-ohm load attached to the coil, we obtained a temperature rise of 4 °C in 10 minutes. With no load attached to the coil, we measured a 9 °C temperature rise in 10 minutes.

There are several ways to minimize the problem of local heating due to surface coils. The general tactic has been to decouple the surface coil during the transmit pulse period. This serves several purposes simultaneously. First, it eliminates any added tip-angle variation that would otherwise distort the image. Second, such decoupling will also minimize the voltage presented to the preamplifier circuit that could otherwise destroy the first stage in the amplifier. Finally, the same circuitry will eliminate the potential hazard of high local SAR to the patient.

There are many ways to effect such decoupling; however, the most popular and easiest to implement is one using some diode gating scheme. The diode suppression circuits come in two varieties. The first is a passive decoupling method that was first introduced by Flugen[4] on the early Technicare systems. As these systems pioneered MRI development, they were the first to use separate transmit and receive coils and thus faced the decoupling problem. This method is shown in FIGURE 4a. Basically, a pair of crossed diodes are used in series with a small inductor. When the transmitter fires, the large voltage induced in the surface coil quickly forward-biases the diodes, putting them in a low resistance mode. This small resistance is in series with an inductor that has been chosen to change the resonant frequency of the tuned circuit by a significant degree (several megahertz at least). The result is that very little current is allowed to flow in the tuned circuit and, consequently, very little additional flux concentration results. This circuit is quite effective and will produce excellent suppression if the diodes are chosen carefully. The second method for achieving suppression is to use PIN diodes and to actively drive them into conduction during the transmission period.[5] This requires an external source of power that can be

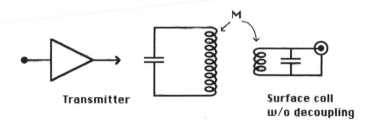

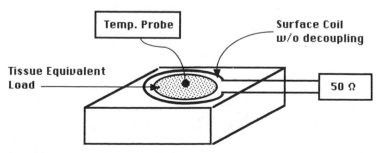

FIGURE 3. RF heating experiment. The top panel shows the coupling mechanism from the transmitter power amplifier through the body coil coupled to the surface coil. The bottom panel shows the heating phantom placed under the surface coil with a saline solution and temperature sensing probe.

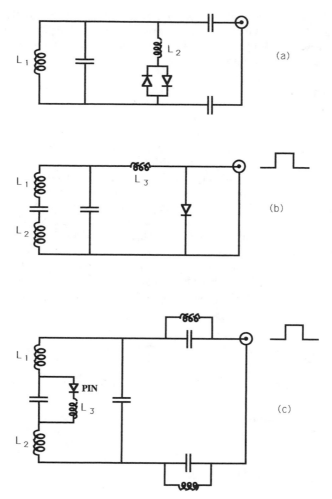

FIGURE 4. Decoupling methods: (a) passive decoupling with crossed diodes to effect a frequency shift; (b) active decoupling using a PIN diode at the terminal end of the surface coil matching circuit; (c) active decoupling using a PIN diode at a break point along the surface coil and with RF chokes to conduct the dc drive for the PIN diode.

delivered down the same coaxial line that connects the RF coil to the preamplifier (active suppression methods shown in FIGURES 4b and 4c). This technique of using the transmission line for dc and RF at the same time has been used for years in the television preamplifier field. An advantage to this approach is that it achieves the minimum diode on resistance because it does not depend on the coupled transmitter voltage to activate it. However, in practice, the results achieved are very similar to the passively activated suppression network. In both cases, the diode low on resistance must be applied in such a way that the currents in the tuned inductor are minimized.

There are advantages and disadvantages to both methods of decoupling. The passive network may fail, leaving the coil completely coupled to the transmitter coil. This limitation can be addressed by adding a few RF chokes to the circuit and sending a test current down the coax. If the diodes are there and are working properly, they will conduct accordingly and the acquisition may proceed. If the diodes fail the test, the system can generate an error message for the operator to replace the coil. With the PIN diode arrangement, we are essentially testing the diode during every acquisition. However, the cable ground may break (a common problem with surface coils) and then there will again be no protection. If the current to the diode is being monitored by the computer, this condition can be detected and reported to the operator. Finally, some manufacturers have chosen to insert a fuse into the surface coil circuit that does not activate unless everything else has failed. This fuse can be chosen so that it will open at a given threshold of RF power

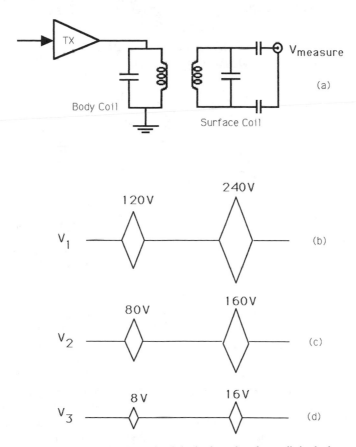

FIGURE 5. Decoupling test: (a) schematic of the body and surface coils in the bore of a 1.5-T (64-MHz) system; (b) voltage measurements made at the surface coil with no decoupling method present; (c) voltage measurements made with a 50-ohm load present at the surface coil terminals; (d) voltage measurements made with a 50-ohm load and with diode decoupling present.

deposition.[6] If the design is effective, we can expect results similar to those given in FIGURE 5. Here, a tuned surface coil was inserted into a 1.5-T system and a typical spin-echo sequence was executed. The large voltage shown as V_1 is the measured result with no suppression circuit on the surface coil. The voltage V_2 is the result of loading the surface coil with a 50-ohm load, but still without suppression. The voltage V_3 is measured with both a 50-ohm load and diode suppression. As can readily be appreciated, the voltages present in the nonsuppressed condition are quite high as compared to the relatively small voltage present when the circuit is decoupled and loaded properly.

Given the aforementioned methods, we need only be concerned about the type of diode that is used to accomplish suppression. The requirements are several, including high frequency performance, low junction capacitance, low on resistance, and (finally) nonmagnetic materials. There are a wide range of diodes available; however, the specification of nonmagnetic materials reduces the field considerably. We have

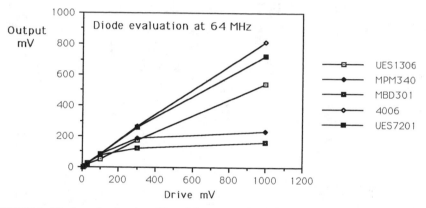

FIGURE 6. Diode evaluation data. Plot of the suppression efficiency of several types of diodes at 64 MHz with a drive source of 0–1 V coupled through to a tuned circuit and matched to 50 ohms.

investigated a number of diodes by building a simple test set as an analogue of the transmitter coil/surface coil situation. A signal generator is used to drive a primary coil while the secondary coil is closely coupled to the primary. The diode suppression network is inserted in the tuned circuit secondary just as it would be on a typical surface coil. An RF millivoltmeter is attached to the output of the secondary coil so that the signal suppression efficiency can be directly measured. The results for some typical diodes are shown in FIGURE 6. It should be apparent from these data that the diodes that turn on at lower drive voltages would be preferable to those with higher thresholds. Holding this output voltage to only 200 mV will assure that very little energy is added to the local SAR. It should also be pointed out that this test is somewhat unfair for those PIN diodes in the group that would normally require external current to put them in the low resistance mode.

SUMMARY AND CONCLUSIONS

The design of MRI systems has become a very complex challenge covering many fields, including physics, chemistry, engineering, and computer science. We could consider the entire system software as a source of patient safety; however, here, we have only addressed the hardware aspects of the RF system. We have seen that the design engineer must take considerable care to assure that the powerful RF transmitters used in these systems are interlocked with proper output power monitoring. Hardware power monitoring as well as software algorithms may be involved in limiting the SAR to the patient. However, as much as possible, the system should be designed at the hardware level to limit power output (duty cycle) as well as to assure that the calculated SAR is based on measured variables (patient loading of the RF coil). The possibility of patient burns resulting from poorly insulated leads should be minimized by heavily insulating any wires that lay on or near the patient. Finally, the potential for increased SAR due to surface coil coupling should be minimized by passive as well as active decoupling circuits. The implementation of the suggested designs should bring the reported safety-related RF incidents to an absolute minimum. The safety record of MRI has been excellent to date; however, there is still room for minimizing risk to the patient.

REFERENCES

1. BUDINGER, T. F. 1979. Threshold for physiological effects due to RF and magnetic fields used in NMR imaging. IEEE Trans. Nucl. Sci. NS-26: 2821–2825.
2. KANAL, E. & F. G. SHELLOCK. 1990. Burns associated with clinical MR examinations (letter). Radiology 175: 585.
3. BOESIGER, P., R. BUCHLI, M. SANER & D. MEIER. 1987. Increased rf power absorption in human tissue due to coupling between body coil and surface coil. Abstr. Annu. Meet. Soc. Magn. Reson. Med. (17–25 August 1987, New York).
4. FLUGEN, D. C. 1987 (March 10). Radiofrequency coils for NMR imaging. United States Patent No. 4,649,348.
5. EDELSTEIN, B. 1986 (October 28). Nuclear magnetic resonance imaging antenna subsystem having a plurality of non-orthogonal surface coils. United States Patent No. 4,620,155.
6. HEDGES, L. K. 1989. A fuse for magnetic resonance imaging probes. Magn. Reson. Med. 9: 278–281.

Development of Contrast Media for Magnetic Resonance Imaging

H. A. GOLDSTEIN, J. R. WIGGINS, AND F. KASHANIAN

Berlex Laboratories
Wayne, New Jersey 07470

INTRODUCTION

When it was first introduced, magnetic resonance imaging (MRI) was acclaimed to have several important advantages over computed tomography (CT). Among them, it provides tomographic images in any imaging plane, whereas CT is limited to the transaxial plane; it does not require the use of ionizing radiation; and it provides excellent images without the use of contrast media. Indeed, the absence of ionizing radiation and the apparent lack of a need for contrast material make the use of MR imaging an extremely safe procedure. However, similar claims for image quality and a lack of need for contrast agents were also made for CT when it was first introduced. In practice, contrast-enhanced CT has become an important addition to the radiological repertoire; a similar appreciation of the uses of contrast in MRI is now growing.[1] As with CT, the use of contrast agents may increase the efficacy of MRI at the cost of making the procedure minimally invasive and in some instances increasing the total imaging time required.

Although unenhanced MRI is an extremely safe procedure, adverse experiences have been reported.[2] Claustrophobia in patients predisposed to this condition and intolerance of the noise associated with the cycling of the magnet are two of the most common adverse experiences; tissue damage caused by torquing of embedded shrapnel and injuries due to projectiles attracted to the magnet are unusual, but important problems to be considered. Contraindications to MRI have also become known, including aneurysm clips, cardiac pacemakers, and cochlear implants.[3]

By way of background, it should be noted that the basic principle of MRI is the differential signal arising from differences in the spin-lattice (T1) and spin-spin (T2) relaxation times of specific protons in different physiological pools of water and tissue molecules (e.g., fat) when exposed to a magnetic gradient. Because hydrogen is the most abundant element, clinical MRI is based on the magnetic resonance properties of hydrogen. Resonance occurs when radio-frequency is applied at the Larmor frequency; when this radio-frequency is applied perpendicular to the main magnetic field, the effect is to rotate the magnetization away from its resting state. T1 values are strongly dependent on the frequency and increase with increasing free water content. T2 is more dependent on chemical structure, but is affected less by frequency or water content than is T1.

Contrast agents for other imaging modalities are direct-acting agents. Iodinated agents directly absorb X rays; the decay of radioactive tracers used in nuclear medicine is detected by specific detectors. Contrast agents for MRI act only indirectly; these agents alter the magnetic resonance properties of their surrounding environment and it is this change that is detected by the instrument. In clinical MRI,

322

contrast agents alter the relaxation properties of protons in selected regions of tissue water and thus increase the difference in signal between adjacent tissues. Any agent that alters the resonance of hydrogen has the potential to be used as a contrast agent in MRI; these include paramagnetic, diamagnetic, ferromagnetic, and superparamagnetic molecules. Paramagnetic agents are those that have one or more unpaired electrons and thus have a magnetic moment. The magnetic moment is increased when paramagnetic agents are placed in a magnetic field, as the unpaired electrons line up with the field. When the field is removed, these electrons gradually relax to their baseline state; in the process of this relaxation, some of the additional magnetic moment is transferred to adjacent protons, altering their resonance properties. To the extent that T1 relaxation is affected more than T2, this additional magnetic moment makes these protons appear brighter on an MR image. (At higher concentrations of the contrast agent, T2 may be affected more than T1 and thus the enhanced regions will appear less bright in the presence of the contrast agent.[4]) Diamagnetic agents, such as kaolin, have essentially zero magnetic moment because all the electrons in the molecule are paired and are generally too weak to alter relaxation rates. Ferromagnetic agents retain some magnetization after removal of the magnetic field. Superparamagnetic agents behave like ferromagnetic agents, but do not retain magnetization after removal of the magnetic field. Superparamagnetic agents, such as iron oxide, have such a strong magnetic moment that the T2 relaxation is primarily affected. Superparamagnetic agents thus give rise to negative enhancement.

Most of the agents in clinical use or undergoing clinical trials are based on the rare earth element, gadolinium, which with its seven unpaired electrons is theoretically the most relaxive paramagnetic ion. However, because free gadolinium, like all of the rare earths, is toxic, it must be sequestered by a chelating agent in order to be clinically useful. The chelating agent must itself be nontoxic.

The efficacy of transition metal chelates depends in part on the accessibility of water molecules to the outer coordination sphere of the metal; hence, the nature of the chelate affects efficacy. In addition, because both T1- and T2-weighted images are enhanced in a dose-dependent manner, contrast enhancement with paramagnetic agents is not a simple linear relationship. Contrast enhancement with paramagnetic agents is clearly biphasic; higher doses may be less effective in contrast enhancement, as mentioned earlier (FIGURE 1).

MR imaging is relatively young as a clinically important diagnostic method and it is not surprising that the use of contrast agents in MRI has become important only recently. Although there are a number of agents currently undergoing clinical trials, there is presently only one contrast agent, gadopentetate dimeglumine, marketed for use with MRI in the United States. Gadopentetate dimeglumine (Magnevist® Injection, Berlex Laboratories, Wayne, New Jersey) is currently indicated for use in adults and children (two years and older) for MRI of the brain and spine. The purpose of this review is to discuss the safety and efficacy of contrast agents in MRI using gadopentetate dimeglumine for illustration because this is the agent for which there is the greatest clinical experience and the most published information.

The clinical development of MR contrast agents, as for all other drugs in the United States, can be divided into four distinct stages. Safety and efficacy are estimated in (1) studies in animals, including toxicology, and in other preclinical models and (2) extensive clinical trials in humans [including Phase 1, which investigates safety, pharmacokinetics, and (in some cases) efficacy in normal subjects or patients; Phase 2, in which the emphasis is on the determination of safety and efficacy in patients; and Phase 3, in which additional information on safety and efficacy in specific indications is gathered].[5] Additional information comes from (3) postmarketing clinical studies (Phase 4 studies) and (4) postmarketing surveillance, which relies on voluntary (spontaneous) reporting of adverse experiences, and formal pharmacoepidemiologic studies.

PRECLINICAL STUDIES

For gadopentetate dimeglumine, studies in animals demonstrated the potential utility of contrast agents in MRI. Doses of 0.01 mmol/kg to 1.0 mmol/kg body weight were administered to anesthetized rats, rabbits, and a baboon. Gadopentetate

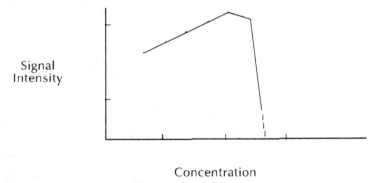

FIGURE 1. Effect of the concentration of paramagnetic MR contrast agents on image intensity. Redrawn from reference 4.

dimeglumine clearly enhanced the contrast between normal and pathologic tissue in the brain in a dose-dependent manner, facilitating the detection of tumors and infarcts by MRI.[6]

Because of the toxicity of free gadolinium, it is also important to show that the chelated gadolinium complex is stable in the body. Gadopentetate has a thermodynamic stability constant of 22.1 and a conditional stability constant at pH 7.4 of 17.7; thus, the chelate is chemically very stable. Additional studies in the rat have shown that gadopentetate has the same clearance as does ^{99m}TcDTPA.[7] Other studies have shown that less than 0.3% of the injected dose of radiolabeled gadopentetate remains in the body after seven days.[6,8] Together, these data suggest that the gadolinium-DTPA complex is quite stable under physiologic conditions.

Studies in anesthetized dogs showed that the administration of the usual imaging dose (0.1 mmol/kg) of gadopentetate dimeglumine had no effect on blood pressure when injected either within ten seconds or over one minute.[9] Similarly, the administration of a much higher dose (0.5 mmol/kg) administered over one minute also had no effect on blood pressure. However, a transient decrease in blood pressure (21 mmHg) was seen when this higher dose was administered rapidly, a decrease that returned to control values within one minute after injection.

The safety of contrast agents is frequently defined by comparing its effective imaging dose (as determined clinically) with its acute lethal dose in animals. The intravenous LD_{50} of gadopentetate dimeglumine in mice and rats ranges from about 5 mmol/kg to about 15 mmol/kg, providing a "Safety Index" of approximately 50 to 150 for the usual effective dose (0.1 mmol/kg). For comparison, the "Safety Index" for iodinated X-ray contrast agents ranges from about 6 for ionic agents to approximately 15 for nonionic agents.[10]

CLINICAL STUDIES

Preliminary trials of intravenous gadopentetate dimeglumine in normal volunteers have utilized doses of gadopentetate dimeglumine from 0.005 to 0.25 mmol/kg. In normal volunteers, gadopentetate has a volume of distribution of about 250 mL/kg, an elimination half-life of 1.58 hours, and a plasma clearance of 1.76 mL/min · kg.[11] These data are consistent with an agent that is distributed in extracellular water and that is cleared completely by the kidney.

Both the safety and efficacy of gadopentetate dimeglumine have been demonstrated in numerous reports.[12–22] In clinical trials,[12,13] efficacy was assessed by a number of parameters, including evaluating contrast score, the facilitation of visualization of lesions, and the number of lesions observed. In all these studies, each patient received a single intravenous injection of 0.1 mmol/kg of gadopentetate dimeglumine; the majority of these studies were open-label in design, with the patient serving as his or her own control. Contrast score was a rating of conspicuity, using a four-point rating scale ranging from 0 (no contrast) to 3 (excellent contrast). In some studies, intensity scores were used to provide a relative measure of the pre- and post-gadopentetate signal intensity in identical regions of interest; a reference standard of gadopentetate dimeglumine was placed by the patient's head. In addition, randomly selected films were also read in a blinded fashion both before and after the addition of gadopentetate dimeglumine.

In the majority of patients examined, film contrast scores increased for T1-weighted images when preinjection results were compared to postinjection results. In addition, the investigator's diagnostic ability was improved or facilitated after the injection of gadopentetate dimeglumine in a majority of the patients. For example, in one placebo-controlled double-blind study published by Russell and colleagues,[12] 88 patients with cerebral lesions underwent MRI: 57 patients received gadopentetate dimeglumine, 26 patients received saline, and data from 5 patients were not valid. Nine of 17 patients for whom a diagnosis could not be made prior to the administration of gadopentetate dimeglumine could be diagnosed after the injection of the paramagnetic agent. By comparison, none of the 5 patients for whom a diagnosis could not be made prior to administration of placebo could be diagnosed after injection of placebo.

In rare cases, contrast enhancement can result in a loss of information. This happens when enhancement of a relatively dark lesion increases the intensity of the lesion to that of the surrounding tissue (i.e., the signal becomes isointense). A similar loss of information can in theory be seen when higher doses are used; higher doses will increase the image intensity of the background, potentially leading to a loss of difference in image intensity between the lesion and surrounding tissue.[13]

For MR imaging, particularly brain imaging, the absence of contrast enhancement may also provide useful clinical information.[14] Because gadopentetate dimeglumine makes brain lesions more visible, the absence of contrast enhancement has been used to confirm the absence of significant lesions involving the blood-brain barrier.

Most of the clinical experience to date with gadopentetate dimeglumine has centered on imaging of the brain and spine. However, these are not the only anatomical regions that may benefit from contrast-enhanced imaging. Preliminary work has been reported using gadopentetate dimeglumine for enhancement of many other anatomical regions, including breast, liver, kidney, lung, etc.[23-31]

Biodistribution is an important determinant of the efficacy of an MR contrast agent. The intravenous formulation of gadopentetate dimeglumine distributes in extracellular water and is excluded by the intact blood-brain barrier. For brain imaging, the appearance of gadopentetate within the brain itself identifies regions of breakdowns of the blood-brain barrier. In the spine, the addition of contrast allows one to discriminate scar tissue (which becomes brighter with gadopentetate) from herniated disk material (which enhances only much more slowly).[32]

The extracellular distribution of gadopentetate dimeglumine defines its efficacy and, therefore, its efficacy in certain indications may be limited. Animal studies have been reported for MR contrast agents that remain entirely within the vascular bed;[33] such agents may provide a better view of tissue perfusion than do agents such as gadopentetate that distribute in extracellular water. Tissues such as liver tissues, which are highly vascularized and have a large extracellular space, present special challenges for MR contrast; gadopentetate has been used successfully to enhance hepatic tumors, but the efficacy is very dependent on the imaging protocol used.

Gadopentetate dimeglumine and other agents such as superparamagnetic iron oxide and perfluorooctylbromide are currently being evaluated for oral use, specifically to mark the bowel.[34] Such formulations are essentially not absorbed and so remain within the gastrointestinal tract; their utility lies in identifying bowel loops and in allowing the differential diagnosis between bowel and pathology.

The safety of intravenous gadopentetate dimeglumine has been reported in over 1000 adult patients in the United States.[35] Safety was assessed by monitoring of adverse experiences for up to 48 hours after injection, by a battery of laboratory tests before and after injection, and by physical examinations, including vital signs and neurological examinations, before and after injection.

Overall, one or more adverse experiences were reported in a total of 213 adult patients (of 1068, 19.9%). Adverse experiences were rated on a three-point scale (mild, moderate, severe) and their relationship to the study drug was assessed by the investigator on a five-point scale (not related, remotely, possibly, probably, definitely related). Adverse experiences reported by more than one patient are summarized in TABLE 1. It is seen that 134 (12.5%) patients had one or more adverse experiences that were characterized by the investigator as remotely, possibly, or probably related to the administration of gadopentetate dimeglumine; none was characterized as definitely related. Of these, seven adverse experiences were judged to be both severe in intensity and related to the administration of gadopentetate dimeglumine (TABLE 2). Overall, most of the adverse experiences were mild in severity, transient, and not troublesome.

The safety of gadopentetate dimeglumine was also assessed by comparing

TABLE 1. Most Common Adverse Experiences in Adult Patients Referred for MR Imaging of the Brain and Spine[a]

Adverse Experience	No. Total ($N = 1068$)	Percent
headache	69	6.5
injection site coldness and/or localized coldness	38	3.6
nausea	20	1.9
paresthesia	11	1.0
dizziness	10	0.9
vomiting	9	0.8
localized pain	8	0.7
hypertension	7	0.7
localized warmth	6	0.6
anxiety	5	0.5
injection site pain	5	0.5
rash	5	0.5
vasodilatation	5	0.5
localized burning	4	0.4
diarrhea	4	0.4
fever	4	0.4
injection site burning	4	0.4
injection site reaction	4	0.4
injection site warmth	4	0.4
pain	4	0.4
hypotension	3	0.3
grand mal convulsion	3	0.3
back pain	3	0.3
sweating	3	0.3
taste abnormality	3	0.3
cough	2	0.2
drowsiness	2	0.2
dry mouth	2	0.2
gastrointestinal distress	2	0.2
pallor	2	0.2
stiffness	2	0.2
tachycardia	2	0.2
throat irritation	2	0.2
tiredness	2	0.2
weakness	2	0.2

[a]From reference 35.

precontrast and postcontrast physical examinations (including neurological examinations) and batteries of laboratory tests. Physical examinations were unremarkable. Neurologic evaluations were performed in 713 patients before and after the administration of gadopentetate dimeglumine. Even though many patients had abnormal neurological findings based on underlying disorders, concurrent illness, or concomi-

TABLE 2. Adverse Experiences Rated Severe by Investigators and Related to Administration of Gadopentetate Dimeglumine[a]

Adverse Experience	Treatment-related Reactions ($N = 1068$)	Percent
headache	3	0.3
nausea	2	0.2
vomiting	1	0.1
agitation	1	0.1

[a]From reference 35.

tant medication, no drug-related changes were noted after the administration of gadopentetate dimeglumine. Laboratory changes were generally limited to transient increases in serum iron and, to a lesser extent, serum bilirubin, which appeared 2–4 hours after dosing and which usually returned to baseline within 24–48 hours (TABLE 3).

In most studies of the brain and spine, gadopentetate dimeglumine is administered at a rate of 10 mL/min. However, in some imaging procedures, it may be desirable to administer the drug at a faster rate. One study was undertaken specifically to investigate the effects of the rate of administration of gadopentetate dimeglumine on blood pressure.[36] In this study, after injection of gadopentetate dimeglumine at a bolus rate (10 mL/15 s), there were no clinically significant changes or trends in the blood pressure or heart rate. The results obtained after gadopentetate dimeglumine injection were not statistically significantly different from the results obtained after placebo injection. No adverse experiences or clinically significant changes in laboratory evaluations were noted.

POSTMARKETING DATA

The clinical trials with gadopentetate dimeglumine showed that this MR contrast agent was safe and effective. However, it is generally recognized that rare adverse

TABLE 3. Serum Iron Levels[a]

	No. of Patients	Mean	Standard Deviation	Minimum	Maximum
Male Patients					
baseline	415	85.6	38.3	4	328
2–4 h	349	120.6	57.9	11	341
24 h	396	93.2	52.2	13	366
48 h	108	83.9	38.9	8	196
Female Patients					
baseline	304	78.2	35.2	3	211
2–4 h	270	103.0	49.2	13	328
24 h	283	84.1	46.7	9	291
48 h	64	79.6	41.2	18	233

[a]Levels are in micrograms per deciliter. Baseline levels are preinjection. Times are postinjection. From reference 35.

experiences probably will not be discovered in the clinical development process, but rather will emerge only in the postmarketing period, when large numbers of patients are exposed to the drug.[37] The search for rare adverse experiences has led to the development of postmarketing studies and especially to postmarketing surveillance methods.

In general, data collected in the postmarketing period are less stringently controlled than data collected during clinical trials. Postmarketing studies and surveys utilize standardized protocols and data collection forms, but the numbers of patients involved preclude the detailed monitoring of patient records associated with premarket trials, except in cases of serious and unexpected adverse experiences. Spontaneous postmarketing surveillance is uncontrolled and depends entirely on the voluntary reporting of adverse experiences. Moreover, federal regulations require that all adverse experiences be included in postmarketing surveillance reports without assessment of the relationship to the drug (21CFR§314.80). Such spontaneous adverse experience reporting in the postmarketing phase probably underestimates the overall incidence of adverse experiences.

To date, approximately 2.2 million patients have received gadopentetate dimeglumine for MRI in the United States; gadopentetate dimeglumine is also marketed in several other countries (including Japan and Germany). A postmarketing survey did not reveal any unexpected adverse experiences.[38] Postmarketing surveillance has also shown that the nature of adverse experiences is similar to that reported during the premarket trials. Serious adverse experience reports have been very rare.[2]

CONCLUSIONS

Gadopentetate dimeglumine has shown that MRI as a diagnostic modality can benefit from contrast enhancement and that the risk-benefit ratio is quite favorable. The future is likely to bring additional contrast media for MRI. Some of these agents, particularly those designed for more targeted imaging, may further improve image enhancement for selected indications. The original claim that MR images are so good that contrast is not needed has been set aside; the considerations in contrast-enhanced MR now lie in determining which imaging procedures can most benefit from the addition of contrast to MRI.

REFERENCES

1. KIEFFER, S. A. 1990. Gadopentetate dimeglumine: observations on the clinical research process. Radiology **174:** 7–8.
2. KANAL, E., F. G. SHELLOCK & L. TALAGALA. 1990. Safety considerations in MR imaging. Radiology **176:** 593–606.
3. EDELMAN, R. R., F. G. SHELLOCK & J. AHLADIS. 1990. Practical MRI for the technologist and imaging specialist. *In* Clinical Magnetic Resonance Imaging. R. R. Edelman, J. R. Hesselink, J. Newhouse & D. J. Sartoris, Eds.: 39–72. Saunders. Philadelphia.
4. RUNGE, V. M., J. A. CLANTON, W. A. HERZER, S. J. GIBBS, A. C. PRICE, C. L. PARTAIN & A. E. JAMES, JR. 1984. Intravascular contrast agents suitable for magnetic resonance imaging. Radiology **153:** 171–176.
5. FINKEL, M. J. 1977. General Considerations for the Clinical Evaluation of Drugs HEW (FDA 77-3040). U.S. Govt. Printing Office. Washington, District of Columbia.

6. WEINMANN, H-J., R. C. BRASCH, W-R. PRESS & G. E. WESBEY. 1984. Characteristics of gadolinium-DTPA complex: a potential NMR contrast agent. Am. J. Roentgenol. 142: 619–624.

7. WEDEKING, P., S. EATON, D. G. COVELL, S. NAIR, M. F. TWEEDLE & W. C. ECKELMAN. 1990. Pharmacokinetic analysis of blood distribution of intravenously administered ^{153}Gd-labeled Gd(DTPA)$_2$- and ^{99m}Tc(DTPA) in rats. Magn. Reson. Imag. 8: 567–575.

8. WEDEKING, P. & M. TWEEDLE. 1988. Comparison of the biodistribution of ^{153}Gd-labeled Gd(DTPA)$_2$-, Gd(DOTA)-, and Gd(acetate)$_n$ in mice. Int. J. Radiat. Appl. Instrum. B15: 395–402.

9. SULLIVAN, M. E., H. A. GOLDSTEIN, K. J. SANSONE, S. A. STONER, W. L. HOLYOAK & J. R. WIGGINS. 1990. Hemodynamic effects of Gd-DTPA administered via rapid bolus or slow infusion: a study in dogs. Am. J. Neuroradiol. 11: 537–540.

10. SOVAK, M. 1987. New developments in radiographic contrast media. In Contrast Media: Biologic Effects and Clinical Application. Volume 1. Z. Parvez, R. Moncada & M. Sovak, Eds.: 28–45. CRC Press. Boca Raton, Florida.

11. WEINMANN, H-J., M. LANIADO & W. MUTZEL. 1984. Pharmacokinetics of GdDTPA/dimeglumine after intravenous injection into healthy volunteers. Physiol. Chem. Phys. Med. NMR 16: 167–172.

12. RUSSELL, E. J., T. F. SCHAIBLE, W. DILLON, B. DRAYER, J. LIPUMA, A. MANCUSO, K. MARAVILLA & H. A. GOLDSTEIN. 1989. Multicenter double-blind placebo-controlled study of gadopentetate dimeglumine as an MR contrast agent: evaluation in patients with cerebral lesions. Am. J. Neuroradiol. 10: 53–63.

13. SZE, G., G. K. STIMAC, C. BARTLETT, W. P. DILLON, V. M. HAUGHTON, W. ORRISON, F. KASHANIAN & H. A. GOLDSTEIN. 1990. Multicenter study of gadopentetate dimeglumine as an MR contrast agent: evaluation in patients with spinal tumors. Am. J. Neuroradiol. 11: 967–974.

14. ELSTER, A. D., D. M. MOODY, M. R. BALL & D. W. LASTER. 1989. Is Gd-DTPA required for routine cranial MR imaging? Radiology 173: 231–238.

15. HEALY, M. E., J. R. HESSELINK, G. A. PRESS & M. S. MIDDLETON. 1987. Increased detection of intracranial metastases with intravenous Gd-DTPA. Radiology 165: 619–624.

16. HESSELINK, J. R., M. E. HEALY, G. A. PRESS & F. J. BRAHME. 1988. Benefits of Gd-DTPA for MR imaging of intracranial abnormalities. J. Comput. Assist. Tomogr. 12: 266–274.

17. PETERMAN, S. B., R. E. STEINER, G. M. BYDDER, D. J. THOMAS, J. S. TOBIAS & J. R. YOUNG. 1985. Nuclear magnetic resonance imaging (NMRI) of brain stem tumors. Neuroradiology 27: 202–207.

18. RUNGE, V. M. & D. Y. GELBLUM. 1990. The role of gadolinium-diethylenetriaminepentaacetic acid in the evaluation of the central nervous system. Magn. Reson. Q. 6: 85–107.

19. BIRD, C. R., B. P. DRAYER, M. MEDINA, H. L. REKATE, R. A. FLOM & J. A. HODAK. 1988. Gd-DTPA-enhanced MR imaging in pediatric patients after brain tumor resection. Radiology 169: 123–126.

20. COHEN, B. H., E. BURY, R. J. PACKER, L. N. SUTTON, L. T. BILANIUK & R. A. ZIMMERMAN. 1989. Gadolinium-DTPA-enhanced magnetic resonance imaging in childhood brain tumors. Neurology 39: 1178–1183.

21. PARTAIN, C. L., T. A. POWERS, M. P. FREEMAN et al. 1988. Gadolinium-enhanced MRI in pediatric patients with masses in the brain and spinal cord. Magn. Reson. Imag. 6: 122 (abstract).

22. POWERS, T. A., C. L. PARTAIN, R. M. KESSLER, M. W. FREEMAN, R. H. ROBERTSON, S. H. WYATT & H. T. WHELAN. 1988. Central nervous system lesions in pediatric patients: Gd-DTPA-enhanced MR imaging. Radiology 169: 723–726.

23. CRAWFORD, S. C., H. R. HARNSBERGER, R. B. LUFKIN & W. N. HANAFEE. 1989. The role of gadolinium-DTPA in the evaluation of extracranial head and neck mass lesions. Radiol. Clin. North Am. 27: 219–242.

24. CHOYKE, P. L., J. A. FRANK, M. E. GIRTON, S. W. INSCOE, M. J. CARVLIN, J. BLACK, H. A. AUSTIN & A. DWYER. 1989. Dynamic Gd-DTPA-enhanced MR imaging of the kidney: experimental results. Radiology 170: 713–720.

25. CARR, D. H. 1985. Paramagnetic contrast media for magnetic resonance imaging of the mediastinum and lungs. J. Thorac. Imag. **1:** 74–78.
26. DANIELS, D., L. CZERVIONKE, K. POJUNAS, G. A. MEYER, S. J. MILLEN, A. L. WILLIAMS & V. M. HAUGHTON. 1987. Facial nerve enhancement in MR imaging. Am. J. Neuroradiol. **8:** 605–607.
27. GLAZER, G. 1988. MR imaging of the liver, kidneys, and adrenal glands. Radiology **166:** 303–312.
28. HEYWANG, S., D. HAHN, H. SCHMIDT, I. KRISCHKE, W. EIERMANN, R. BASSERMAN & J. LISSNER. 1986. MR imaging of the breast using gadolinium-DTPA. J. Comput. Assist. Tomogr. **10**(2): 199–204.
29. KAISER, W. & E. ZEITLER. 1989. MR imaging of the breast: fast imaging sequences with and without Gd-DTPA. Radiology **170:** 681–686.
30. PETTIGREW, R., L. AVRUCH, W. DANNELS, J. COUMANS & M. BERNARDINO. 1986. Fast-field-echo MR imaging with Gd-DTPA: physiologic evaluation of the kidney and liver. Radiology **160:** 561–563.
31. REVEL, D., R. BRASCH, H. PAAJANEN, W. ROSENAU, W. GRODD, B. ENGELSTAD, P. FOX & J. WINKELHAKE. 1986. Gd-DTPA contrast enhancement and tissue differentiation in MR imaging of experimental breast carcinoma. Radiology **158:** 319–323.
32. HUEFTLE, M. G., M. T. MODIC, J. S. ROSS, T. J. MASARYK, J. R. CARTER, R. G. WILBER, H. H. BOHLMAN, P. M. STEINBERG & R. B. DELAMARTER. 1988. Lumbar spine: postoperative MR imaging with Gd-DTPA. Radiology **167:** 817–824.
33. WOLFE, C. L., M. E. MOSELEY, M. G. WIKSTRON, R. E. SIEVERS, M. F. WENDLAND, J. W. DUPON, W. E. FINKBEINER, M. J. LIPTON, W. W. PARMLEY & R. C. BRASCH. 1989. Assessment on myocardial salvage after ischemia and reperfusion using magnetic resonance imaging and spectroscopy. Circulation **80:** 969–982.
34. HAHN, P. F. 1991. Gastrointestinal contrast agents. Am. J. Roentgenol. **156:** 252–254.
35. GOLDSTEIN, H. A., F. K. KASHANIAN, R. F. BLUMETTI, W. L. HOLYOAK, F. P. HUGO & D. M. BLUMENFIELD. 1990. Safety assessment of gadopentetate dimeglumine in U.S. clinical trials. Radiology **174:** 17–23.
36. KASHANIAN, F. K., H. A. GOLDSTEIN, R. F. BLUMETTI, W. L. HOLYOAK, F. P. HUGO & M. DOLKER. 1990. Rapid bolus injection of gadopentetate dimeglumine: absence of side effects in normal volunteers. Am. J. Neuroradiol. **11:** 853–856.
37. NIES, A. S. 1990. Principles of therapeutics. In Goodman and Gilman's Pharmacological Basis of Therapeutics (Eighth Edition). A. G. Gilman, T. W. Rall, A. S. Nies & P. Taylor, Eds.: 62–83. Pergamon. Elmsford, New York.
38. LAFLORE, J., H. GOLDSTEIN, R. ROGAN, T. KEELAN & A. EWELL. 1989. A prospective evaluation of adverse experiences following the administration of Magnevist® (gadopentetate dimeglumine) injection. Soc. Magn. Reson. Med., p. 1067 (abstract).

Clinical Indications for MRI

DAVID D. STARK

Department of Radiology
Massachusetts General Hospital
Boston, Massachusetts 02114

INTRODUCTION

Ten years ago, most clinicians and radiologists saw no advantages of MRI over CT and other established imaging technologies. It soon became apparent, however, that MRI was a superior technique for imaging degenerative, ischemic, and neoplastic disorders of the brain. With the clinical development of multislice 2DFT methods, application to routine clinical practice was possible and the dissemination of MRI was well under way by 1983.

The introduction of surface coils in 1984 opened new opportunities in imaging the spine and started a second wave of enthusiasm for widespread utilization of MRI. In 1986, it was recognized that high resolution surface coil imaging techniques developed for the spine could be applied to imaging of the knee. This started a third wave of applications in the joints and other areas of the musculoskeletal system.

Most recently, gradient echo and high speed imaging techniques have matured to a point where clinically relevant MR angiography and body MRI are feasible. Although these techniques do not enjoy the broad popularity of musculoskeletal MRI, it is clear that another decade of technical innovation and clinical development has begun.

It now seems likely that, by the turn of the century, magnetic resonance will become the dominant technology used in diagnostic imaging. This review will briefly summarize the established and anticipated indications of MRI in the major organ systems.

ORGAN SYSTEM APPLICATION

Central Nervous System

MRI is now the procedure of choice for all congenital, traumatic, hereditary, vascular, infectious, autoimmune, metabolic, and neoplastic disorders of the central nervous system. For selected indications, such as acute trauma or where agitation or sedation presents problems, it may be better logistically to perform plain radiography, angiography, or CT scanning. For the evaluation of suspected acute subarachnoid hemorrhage, CT scanning is still more sensitive than MRI. Fractures of the temporal bone or skull base and many bony destructive lesions may also be better visualized within section CT than with MR. Nevertheless, in many of these conditions, the multiplanar format of MR may be a dominant advantage.

The cervical, thoracic, and lumbar spine are now preferentially imaged by MR, largely replacing myelography, CT, and CT myelography. The major remaining indication for CT of the spine is thin-section CT scanning of the cervical spine to examine the bony cortex in cases of acute trauma or degenerative foraminal stenoses.

Musculoskeletal System

The physical examination remains the best test for diseases of the joints including trauma, degeneration, and other arthritic processes. Plain radiographs are efficient and sensitive in the evaluation of bony dislocation, fracture, tumor, or infection. Cross-sectional imaging with CT has a limited role in evaluating complex bony trauma. CT adds relatively little to the assessment of tumors due to poor contrast with soft tissues and artifacts from dense cortical bone.

When the physical examination or plain radiography suggests a serious abnormality, MRI is the procedure of choice for further evaluation of the entire range of musculoskeletal disorders. MRI has largely replaced arthrography and offers additional information about tendons, ligaments, and muscles not previously available. MR shows excellent contrast between tumor, fat, and muscle and has become an indispensable tool in planning surgery on soft tissue regions of the musculoskeletal system.

Body Imaging

Cross-sectional imaging of the neck, chest, abdomen, and pelvis is demanding because the terrain is vast and a large number of organs and potential diseases are encompassed. Skeletal surveys can be accomplished simply by the use of plain radiographs. Simple surveys of the abdomen or pelvis can be achieved inexpensively with ultrasound; however, limited visualization due to intervening bowel gas or bone is a frequent occurrence that limits diagnostic ultrasound examinations.

CT scanning, despite its expense, is established as the preferred test for body imaging. CT has the advantage of providing fast (2 s) sequential image sections that can be repeated if patient motion degrades a single slice. CT produces excellent anatomic definition as the organs of interest are contrasted against fat, bone, and air.

The major limitation of CT is poor contrast between pathology and adjacent normal tissue. For example, the contrast between liver metastases and normal liver tissue is notoriously poor on CT. MRI has the same advantages of CT as a cross-sectional imaging modality and offers additional soft tissue contrast. MR image contrast can be varied to detect individual diseases. Slice geometry can be matched to the demands of individual anatomic structures.

At the present time, indications for MRI in the body are limited by the availability of machine time. Few machines in routine clinical practice as of 1991 have the high speed and short echo time capabilities required for efficient body MRI.

CONTRAINDICATIONS

The safety of MRI is one of its great advantages over competing technologies. The absence of ionizing radiation is also attractive. Despite some uncertainties about the risks of exposure to radio-frequency (RF) electromagnetic energy, time-varying magnetic fields, and large static magnetic fields, very few known hazards have been defined. RF heating may occur with certain research techniques or pulse sequences not necessary for established diagnostic applications. Time-varying magnetic fields may produce hazardous electrical currents in the body, but again only with gradient systems operated well beyond the range established as routine for clinical work. Similarly, there are no known hazards, although there is no way to exclude unknown hazards, from exposure to static field strengths above 2 T, the limit for generally available commercial technology.

The major hazards of MRI, such as claustrophobia and missile injuries, are related to the magnet design and the static magnetic fields. These hazards exist independent of the anatomic area under study. Exposure to RF or time-varying magnetic field gradients is, of course, concentrated to those parts of the body within the RF or gradient coil.

In summary, the hazards of MRI are minimal or, at worst, undefined for the imaging conditions practiced in a routine clinical environment. The hazards discussed in great detail elsewhere in this volume are often unrelated to the specific imaging protocol or organ under study. They are associated with the development of advanced technology that will expose the patient to larger static and time-varying magnetic fields.

SUMMARY

Safety considerations for MRI will continue to require careful attention and detailed scientific investigation. As new insights are gained into the hazards of time-varying electromagnetic and static magnetic fields, more sophisticated assessment of the true risk will be possible. At the present time, for established clinical indications, the risk of a mismanagement of disease appears to outweigh the minimal or unknown risks of MRI.

Other than the mechanical hazards of implanted or external metallic or electrical devices, MRI seems to be an extraordinarily safe and compatible environment for patients undergoing evaluation of suspected diseases.

Session V Summary

ROBERT S. BALABAN

Laboratory of Cardiac Energetics
National Heart, Lung, and Blood Institute
Bethesda, Maryland 20892

Magnetic resonance imaging (MRI) and spectroscopy (MRS) are noninvasive techniques used for evaluating the structure and function of the body. However, the noninvasive nature of MRI is limited to surgical exposure because the body is intimately exposed to large magnetic and electrical fields during these procedures. This section has been devoted to the evaluation of patient safety during exposure to these electromagnetic fields.

One of the most obvious safety issues in the MRI/MRS exam is RF radiation–induced heating. Numerous models have been proposed to predict the local and whole-body thermal responses to RF energy, but most of these models have proved to be inadequate due to the complex geometry and physiology of the body. Thus, direct measurements of thermal heating in the body under a variety of RF deposition schemes are necessary to evaluate this problem and to hopefully develop more appropriate models. As discussed by F. G. Shellock and C. J. Gordon, whole-body specific absorption rates (SAR) on the order of 4.0 W/kg resulted in temperature elevations below the known thresholds for adverse physiological effects. Hence, it appears that this level of whole-body SAR is acceptable in the MR exam. However, much more work must be performed to evaluate the maximum threshold of the whole body; the effects of different pathologies, or even anesthesia, on this threshold; and the effects of local heating generated by the more popular use of surface coils in MRS and MRI exams.

Another concern is the construction of the MR exam coils, which are used to transmit the RF energy and receive the MR signal from the subject. Once properly calibrated, the instrument can control the amount of energy applied to the patient, but it cannot control the RF distribution inside the magnet. This requires proper design and construction of RF coils and other conductive devices that are placed inside the magnet. These issues are discussed by J. R. Fitzsimmons and include the proper insulation of RF coils, the distribution of the parallel capacitance of the coil to prevent large voltages and dielectric coupling to the patient, and hardware (i.e., fuses) and software controls to limit RF energy and detect open or inappropriate circuits. Extreme care must be taken to assure that this coil is not serving as a concentrator of RF energy from the body coil to small regions of the body, especially in MRS studies where custom, homebuilt, surface coils are usually used. It is highly recommended that active detuning of these coils be used and that an active test confirming this detuning be incorporated into the protection circuits.

Another obvious safety issue in the MR exam is the presence of foreign ferromagnetic objects in or around the body that could become projectiles or be moved internally in the body in a strong magnetic field. These objects are of two basic classes: (1) those that are accidentally placed in the body via old injuries (internal) or by not properly screening a patient or attendant in the magnet (i.e., scissors in pocket) and (2) medical devices that provide a useful service to the patient. In our own experience, we have found that active screening of patients and personnel is the best method of avoiding magnetic foreign objects in the magnet, coupled with routine inspections of the MR scan room for inappropriate objects that may have entered the room on "off-hours". We use a hand-held detector on all personnel upon entering the scan room. The hand-held device is superior to the whole-body screen because it provides information on the topology of the detected magnetic objects. This is advantageous because the warning for a belt buckle, which could be ignored, will not be confused by a pair of scissors in a shirt pocket as would occur with a whole-body scanner. G. M. Pohost and colleagues discussed both the effects of medical devices on the patient in a magnetic field as well as the MRI scan. In addition, the effect of the magnetic field on the performance of medical devices, most notably pacemakers, was discussed. Several devices have been found to be contraindicated for MR studies. These included Poppen-Blaylock carotid artery clamps, pacemakers, some bullets and pellets, and defibrillators/cardioverters. These dangers indicate that a good clinical evaluation, physical exam, and history, as well as a plain X-ray film, if needed, should be employed before any MR exam. The issue of ferromagnetic implanted medical devices should be further investigated with regard to good medical practice. If the medical device, for example, a vascular clip, could be equally effective made from nonmagnetic materials as from magnetic materials, it only seems reasonable that the nonmagnetic materials should be used. This follows from the simple reasoning that it may be possible to limit the extent of medical evaluation that a given patient can have (i.e., MRI) at a later date by implanting a magnetic device.

The most invasive aspect of MR exams, with the exception of an inserted coil for prostate or vaginal exams, is the use of injected contrast agents used for a variety of purposes including blood flow, blood-brain barrier assessment, and viability. These agents are complex chelates of paramagnetic or supermagnetic elements that are suitable for injection. The evaluation of these agents with regard to safety is similar to any injected contrast or pharmaceutical. H. A. Goldstein and colleagues reviewed this procedure and provided details on gadopentetate dimeglumine, which is the only approved contrast agent available at this time.

At present, 1.5 to 2 tesla static magnetic fields have been approved by the FDA for human studies. The use of higher magnetic fields is still under investigation with numerous 3-T and 4-T sites beginning operation around the world. J. F. Schenck described his experiences with patients and normal volunteers with a 4-T whole-body magnet. No health abnormalities have been found in these studies. However, significant sensory side effects attributed to the high magnetic field have been described. These include vertigo, nausea, and a metallic taste in the mouth. Effects were only noted during the study and no effect was severe enough to terminate the study. It has been suggested that many of these sensory effects may be due to local electrical currents set up in the ear and mouth. Thus, the initial experiences at 4 T indicate that no significant medical effects are apparent and that only minor sensory effects are present. However, before the effects of these high fields can be ignored, a further study with a larger population sample and in different pathologies should be performed. It would also be of interest to establish the "medical" threshold for static magnetic fields. Animal studies up to 8 to 11 T seem to indicate no significant effects. However, these studies have not been systematically performed.

In summary, there are significant risks associated with the MR exam, most notably RF-induced heating and foreign metal objects or medical devices. However, with proper patient screening, with appropriate information on RF heating and magnetic field gradient effects, and with good instrument design, these safety issues can be minimized. Indeed, as pointed out by D. Stark, the risk-to-benefit ratio of the MR exam is very low. This approach has been used in thousands of cases in the world and has proved to be of tremendous benefit to patients in the evaluation of their medical condition. Thus, it seems that the real safety issues in MR lie more in the further applications in which we wish to use higher magnetic fields, more RF energy, and fast gradient switching times. Clearly, we must move cautiously in these new and exciting applications to assure that the risk-to-benefit ratio does not significantly decrease to the point where these studies would be inappropriate.

Closing Remarks

BERTIL PERSSON

Department of Radiation Physics
University of Lund
S-221 85 Lund, Sweden

On behalf of the organizers and my cochairmen, Robert Liburdy and Richard Magin, I wish to thank all the scientists and supporters who have contributed so much to this conference. I wish to thank particularly the New York Academy of Sciences and their committed staff for organizing this conference and making all practical arrangements. The large number of people attending the conference clearly indicates that the topic of "Biological Effects and Safety Aspects of Nuclear Magnetic Resonance Imaging and Spectroscopy" is of great concern among authorities, users (physicists and physicians), and industries.

The biological effects are important to consider for the safety of patients, operating staff, and third parties. There are no reports so far of real biological detriment among those operating the MR machines. In the future developments of ultra high fields and ultra fast gradient switching, it will be necessary to consider both physical effects and nonthermal effects observed in animal studies that might put limits on the extent of exposure of the staff.

For the patients, however, the technical development is already approaching the edge where the biological and physiological effects put limits on the exposure. The experience reported at the conference shows that there are many investigations available that can be used in setting safe operating limits. The reports presented at the conference about physical and biological interactions will hopefully be used when setting standards for the function and use of MR imaging and spectroscopy machines in the future. It has been a great pleasure to have representatives from the IEC as well as the FDA and other organizations present at the conference. Their active participation in the discussions has been very valuable and is greatly appreciated.

The hazard of greatest concern for the patients undergoing MR examination is the interaction with electronic devices implanted in the patients that are of vital importance to the patient's life. Also, metallic implants might be considered as a risk, particularly if they are manufactured from ferromagnetic materials. An important problem is how to ensure that patients with such devices do not enter the examination room without full knowledge about these devices. The knowledge about these hazards is important for developing new types of materials and equipment and to give guidelines in how to protect the patients carrying such devices.

The risk to third parties occurs if uninformed people enter the magnet room with equipment that can affect the machine (equipment made of iron and steel) or that can be magnetized and malfunction (cameras and magnetic memory). Therefore, an unlocked MR examination room should never be left unattended. Warning signs that clearly indicate that the magnet is on must always be present.

The aim of this conference has been to collect enough knowledge about risks and about how to minimize or avoid risks to the patient, staff, and third parties.

This conference will hopefully be looked upon in the future as an important milestone in the development of clinical MR as a safe and successful diagnostic method. The information gathered here in this volume will for a long time be the fundamental reference for the safe development of MR in clinical examinations.

Thanks once again to everybody.

Comparison of the Effect of ELF on c-myc Oncogene Expression in Normal and Transformed Human Cells

EWA CZERSKA,[a] JON CASAMENTO,[a] JOHN NING,[a]
MAYS SWICORD,[a] HEBA AL-BARAZI,[b]
CHRISTOPHER DAVIS,[b] AND EDWARD ELSON[c]

[a] Center for Devices and Radiological Health
Food and Drug Administration
Rockville, Maryland 20857

[b] Department of Electrical Engineering
University of Maryland
College Park, Maryland 20742

[c] Department of Microwave Research
Walter Reed Army Institute of Research
Washington, District of Columbia 20307

INTRODUCTION

The effects of extremely low frequency (ELF) electromagnetic field exposure on c-myc oncogene expression have been reported in HL-60 cells in which quantitative levels of c-myc transcripts were analyzed by dot blot hybridization analysis.[1] To further characterize the effect of ELF exposure on c-myc oncogene expression, we assessed the effects of exposure on two transformed human cell lines, HL-60 and Daudi, as well as normal peripheral human lymphocytes by Northern hybridization analysis.[2]

MATERIALS AND METHODS

HL-60, a human promyelogenous leukemia cell line, and Daudi, a human lymphoma cell line, were obtained from ATCC and were cultured in RPMI-1640 medium supplemented with 20% fetal bovine serum. Normal peripheral human lymphocytes were cultured in chromosome medium containing 2.5 μg/mL phytohemagglutinin (PHA). Equal numbers of cells in suspension were placed in 10-mL Corning T75 tissue culture flasks containing fresh medium one hour prior to exposure. Cells were exposed for 30, 45, 60, or 180 min to 60-Hz continuous waves at 1 gauss in a 5% CO_2 incubator at 37 °C. After exposure, total RNA was immediately extracted with guanidinium isothiocyanate and the RNA was pelleted through a CsCl step gradient ultracentrifugation. The purified total RNA was then run in a denaturing formaldehyde agarose gel and transferred to polymer membrane. A nick-translated human c-myc exon 3 probe and a beta-actin probe were used to hybridize against the Northern blots. Washing was carried out under stringent conditions and autoradiography was carried out at −70 °C for 2–3 days. The intensity of hybridization to c-myc and beta-actin probes was quantitated using a laser scanning densitometer.

RESULTS

Northern analysis (FIGURE 1) indicates that c-myc oncogene expression was increased 1.78-fold with ELF exposure for 60 min in Daudi lymphoma cells. No

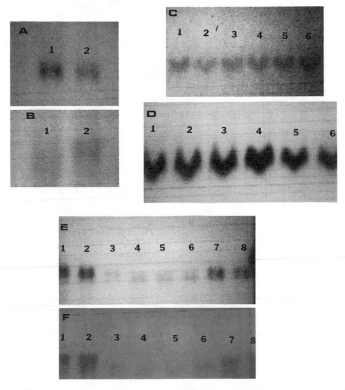

FIGURE 1. Effect of 60-Hz continuous wave exposure on c-myc gene expression in Daudi, HL-60, and human peripheral lymphocytes. Key—A: Daudi probed with c-myc, lane 1 = exposed 60 min, lane 2 = control 60 min; B: Daudi probed with beta-actin, lane 1 = exposed 60 min, lane 2 = control 60 min; C: HL-60 probed with c-myc, lane 1 = exposed 30 min, lane 2 = control 30 min, lane 3 = exposed 60 min, lane 4 = control 60 min, lane 5 = exposed 180 min, lane 6 = control 180 min; D: HL-60 probed with beta-actin, lane 1 = exposed 30 min, lane 2 = control 30 min, lane 3 = exposed 60 min, lane 4 = control 60 min, lane 5 = exposed 180 min, lane 6 = control 180 min; E: human lymphocyte probed with c-myc, lane 1 = sham exposed 30 min, lane 2 = sham control 30 min, lane 3 = exposed 45 min, lane 4 = control 45 min, lane 5 = exposed 60 min, lane 6 = control 60 min, lane 7 = exposed 180 min, lane 8 = control 180 min; F: human lymphocyte probed with beta-actin, lane 1 = sham exposed 30 min, lane 2 = sham control 30 min, lane 3 = exposed 45 min, lane 4 = control 45 min, lane 5 = exposed 60 min, lane 6 = control 60 min, lane 7 = exposed 180 min, lane 8 = control 180 min.

TABLE 1. Laser Densitometric Quantitation of c-myc Expression in FIGURE 1[a]

Cell Type	Exposure Time (min)	Ratio Exposed/Control
Daudi	60	1.78
HL-60	30	1.04
HL-60	60	0.98
HL-60	180	0.61
lymph	30 (sham)	1.19
lymph	45	1.16
lymph	60	1.20
lymph	180	0.89

[a]Each c-myc hybridization is normalized with its hybridization to beta-actin to compensate for differences in sample loading.

appreciable changes in c-myc oncogene expression were observed with ELF exposure in HL-60 cells or in PHA-stimulated normal peripheral human lymphocytes; however, c-myc expression appeared to decrease at 180 min (TABLE 1).

DISCUSSION

Northern hybridization analyses have been run several times with similar results. Discrepancies between our data and results reported in the literature may be due to the different exposure conditions employed.[3] Another plausible explanation may relate to the presence of a translocation involving the c-myc locus on the chromosome on lymphoma cell lines.[4] The structurally altered c-myc gene may interact and respond to ELF differently than the intact c-myc gene.[5] Experiments are under way to test this possibility.

REFERENCES

1. WEI, L., R. GOODMAN & A. HENDERSON. 1990. Changes in levels of c-myc and histone H2B following exposure of cells to low-frequency sinusoidal electromagnetic fields: evidence for a window effect. Bioelectromagnetics 11: 269.
2. LEHRACH, H., et al. 1977. RNA molecular weight determinations by gel electrophoresis under denaturing conditions: a critical reexamination. Biochemistry 16: 4743.
3. MCLEOD, B., A. PILLA & M. SAMPSELL. 1983. Electromagnetic fields induced by Helmholtz coils inside saline filled boundaries. Bioelectromagnetics 4: 357.
4. WIMAN, K., et al. 1984. Activation of a translocated c-myc gene: role of structural alterations in the upstream region. Proc. Natl. Acad. Sci. U.S.A. 81: 6798.
5. MCMANAWAY, W., et al. 1990. Tumour-specific inhibition of lymphoma growth by an antisense oligodeoxynucleotide. Lancet 335: 808.

MRI Can Cause Focal Heating

PETER L. DAVIS, YULIN SHANG, AND
LALITH TALAGALA

Department of Radiology
University of Pittsburgh Medical Center
Pittsburgh, Pennsylvania 15213

INTRODUCTION

MRI uses radio-frequency fields that are known to cause tissue heating. However, the body is not a uniform electrical conductor. Organ shapes and highly resistive fat planes can disrupt the path of the induced electrical currents. In theory, this disruption of the current paths can lead to focal heating. We test in a phantom model whether substantial focal heating can be caused by an MR imager.

MATERIALS AND METHODS

Two phantoms were each made from agar mixed in five liters of saline. The first "uniform" phantom was made by pouring the agar mixture into a 27-cm-diameter cylindrical plastic container. The second "bridge" phantom was similarly prepared, but a 1.5-cm-narrow bridge of agar was created by inserting a styrofoam cup 1.5 cm from the edge of the container. Temperature in the phantoms was measured by a fluoroptic thermometer. RF heating was performed with a 1.5-T MR imager. The average power entering the transmission line was approximately 140 W. The magnetic gradients were turned off.

To test the radial distribution of heat deposition, the uniform phantom was heated for 95 minutes with the temperature probes at 0.0, 4.5, 9.0, and 13.0 cm from the center of the phantom. The bridge phantom was heated three times for approximately 150 minutes each. The temperature probes were placed at the narrow bridge, at the diametrically opposite periphery, and at the center.

RESULTS

In the uniform phantom, the SARs were 0.78, 1.34, 3.31, and 4.68 W/kg at radial distances of 0.0, 4.5, 9.0, and 13.0 cm, respectively. The average SAR for the entire phantom was 3.17 W/kg. For the bridge phantom, the uniform periphery had an average SAR of 5.11 W/kg, but the narrow path had an average SAR of 16.8 W/kg. The heating between the uniform periphery and the narrow path was significantly different (FIGURE 1).

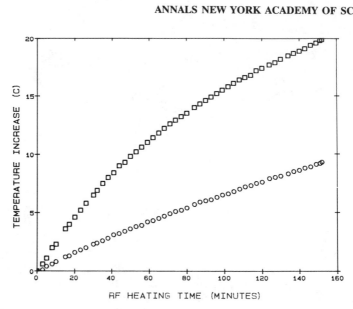

FIGURE 1. Graph of RF heating time (minutes) versus temperature increase (°C) for the bridge phantom. The temperature increase was more rapid for the narrow path (squares) than for the opposite uniform periphery (circles).

DISCUSSION

According to theory and as shown in the uniform phantom, greater current induction and therefore greater heating will occur at the periphery of a uniform object than at its center. However, the shape of organs in the human body and their separation by higher impedance fat planes can disrupt the path of the induced electrical current and can cause current path narrowing, which in turn will cause focal heating. In the bridge phantom, the SAR at the narrow bridge was over three times the SAR at the more uniform periphery and over five times the average SAR of the uniform phantom. Hence, if the current conduction conditions are appropriate, significant focal heating can occur. Computer modeling by Orcutt and Gandhi[1] of the human body using parameters consistent with MR imagers operating at 1.5 T demonstrated that such focal heating may occur in the paraspinal muscles. Considering the higher RF depositions of some MR techniques, such as magnetization transfer, focal heating should be considered in addition to average SAR.

REFERENCE

1.   ORCUTT, N. & O. P. GANDHI. 1988. IEEE Trans. Biomed. Eng. 31: 577.

Permeability of the Blood-Brain Barrier of the Rat Is Not Significantly Altered by NMR Exposure[a]

R. P. LIBURDY,[b] D. J. DE MANINCOR,[b]
M. S. ROOS,[c] AND K. M. BRENNAN[d]

[b]Bioelectromagnetics Research Group
[c]NMR Research Group
[d]Research Medicine and Radiation Biophysics Division
Lawrence Berkeley Laboratory
University of California at Berkeley
Berkeley, California 94720

INTRODUCTION

Several studies have reported recently that NMR fields may[1-3] or may not[4,5] act to influence the permeability of the blood-brain barrier (BBB). In comparing these studies, a common denominator is that Sprague-Dawley rats were employed. Otherwise, there are differences in experimental design among these studies that could contribute to the conflicting findings.

In the present study, we have incorporated what we believe to be the best design features from the above investigations. Thus, the present study has a combination of features that set it apart from previous studies: acoustic controls were employed because the NMR environment is associated with significant acoustic noise; a protein marker normally found in plasma was employed, namely, bovine serum albumin (BSA), to avoid the possibility that horseradish peroxidase, which has been used in the past as a BBB permeability marker, might induce systemic inflammatory or anaphylactic reactions in the animals;[4] *in situ* perfusion of the brain was performed immediately after NMR field treatment to eliminate confounding effects of residual marker isotope in the vasculature; a ketamine-based anesthesia was substituted for pentobarbital because the latter has been shown to significantly reduce blood flow.[6,7] Ketamine operates by a different mechanism and increases blood flow.[6,7] Because solutes such as BSA, which are not subject to transport, show increased permeability when blood flow is increased, ketamine has the potential to improve the sensitivity of the study.

Using these design features, the findings from our study support the conclusion that 2.35-T NMR does not alter BBB permeability in the rat.

METHODS

Adult male Sprague-Dawley rats of an average weight of 230 g were employed. This type of rat was used in the previous studies.[1-4] Rats were anesthetized using

[a]This research was supported in part by the Department of Energy, Office of Health and Environmental Research, under Contract No. DE-AC-3-76SF00098.

345

ketamine (45 mg/kg), xylazine (4.5 mg/kg), and acepromazine (0.09 mg/kg) intraperitoneally and the femoral artery was catheterized. At time zero, 10 μCi of ^{125}I-labeled BSA was injected via the catheter. The NMR or acoustic treatment was started at 5 minutes thereafter. At 90 minutes, the animal was anesthetized (im) and, 30 minutes later, the animal was removed from the magnet, the contralateral femoral artery was exposed, a catheter was inserted, and a blood sample was taken. The animal was then immediately perfused via the femoral artery with 70 mL of phosphate-buffered saline (5 minutes, 14 mL/min). Samples of perfusate and liver were taken to ascertain the quality of perfusion. The brain was harvested and ratios of the activities (cpm/g tissue) of cerebral hemispheres and the cerebellum to activity of the blood were determined.

NMR exposures of 120 minutes were performed in a 2.35-T Bruker imaging spectrometer. The 40-cm bore of this magnet enabled up to four rats to be placed in Lucite restraining tubes that were mechanically isolated from the bore using foam pedestals during exposures. The magnet bore temperature was 25.0 $\pm$ 2.0 °C. Animals were placed such that the brain experienced a switched gradient field of $B_{peak} = 1$ mT, $dB/dt = 1$ T/s. The RF field was a pulsed 100-MHz carrier wave of 64-μT intensity. This NMR environment is described in detail in the article in this symposium dealing with biological interactions of cellular systems with time-varying magnetic fields.[8] Acoustic exposures were carried out such that both the spectral intensity and frequency content of the NMR acoustic environment were simulated in an NMR-field-free laboratory.

RESULTS AND DISCUSSION

We determined the input function for ^{125}I-BSA employed in these studies to establish the time course of clearance of the tracer from the circulation during a typical NMR exposure. This is critical to understanding how tracer concentration varies in the blood during NMR treatment: constant tracer concentration is desirable during experimental treatment. These data were collected by anesthetizing an animal, inserting a femoral artery catheter, injecting tracer, and (at times thereafter) withdrawing blood samples for isotope counting while replacing this volume with isotonic saline.

FIGURE 1 illustrates a typical input function curve for ^{125}I-BSA for the rat. We observed that a significant amount of tracer remains in the circulation over the 120-minute period associated with our NMR treatments. The shape of this curve is consistent with the presence of a compound in the blood whose concentration is reasonably constant and does not rapidly decline during NMR treatment; sucrose, mannitol, and small molecular weight DTPA derivatives, which have been used in previous studies,[2-5] are rapidly removed from the circulation via glomerular filtration.

A series of experiments were performed in which NMR or acoustic exposure treatments were administered to groups of three or more rats per exposure group. The results of these experiments are shown in FIGURE 2, in which data from identical treatment groups from different days have been pooled; n refers to the number of rats in the pooled groups. The results of a paired t-test in which data from cerebral hemispheres are compared for matched NMR versus acoustic treatments indicate that no significant alterations were detected. Tracer uptake in the cerebellum appears slightly greater than that observed in the cerebrum for the acoustic control treatment group and this is consistent with the fact that the cerebellum is apparently more highly vascularized than the cerebrum. The cerebellum, however, shows no significant difference between matched NMR and acoustic treatments. These findings indicate that these studies did not detect alterations in the BBB permeability associated with NMR.

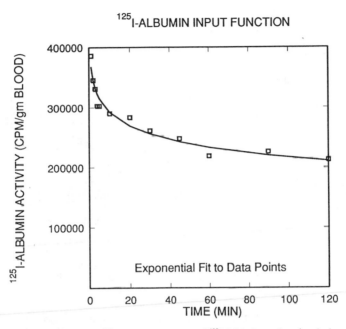

FIGURE 1. Input function for ^{125}I-BSA. Clearance of ^{125}I-BSA from the circulation of the rat was assessed after injection via the femoral artery. Plotted are typical values for ^{125}I-BSA obtained over a 120-minute period simulating the NMR exposure time. Plasma concentration of ^{125}I-BSA is relatively constant, indicating that this protein marker is not rapidly removed from the circulation within 120 minutes.

The experimental design modifications that we employed in these studies represent an effort to combine the best aspects of previous studies. These modifications represent changes that should be considered in future studies and are as follows:

(1) We did not use pentobarbital, which has been reported to decrease blood flow.[6,7] Ketamine was substituted, which increases blood flow and has the potential to improve the sensitivity of the study. Pentobarbital was employed in four previous studies.[1-4]

(2) We employed a tracer compound, BSA, that has a zero BBB permeability. It also represents a plasma protein normally found in the circulation that is not actively transported across the BBB. Previous studies have employed mannitol[3] and sucrose,[4] which are relatively small compounds.

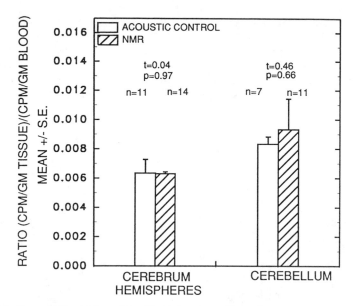

FIGURE 2. Permeability of the rat blood-brain barrier to ^{125}I-BSA during NMR exposure. Rats were exposed to an NMR imaging environment (2.35 T, dB/dt = 1 T/s, 100-MHz RF) or to an acoustic simulation outside the NMR environment for 120 minutes. No differences were detected between treatment groups at the $p \leq 0.05$ level for either cerebrum or cerebellum tissue.

(3) The plasma protein tracer, ^{125}I-BSA, displays an input function that is relatively constant over most of the NMR exposure period. In contrast, tracer compounds such as mannitol,[3] sucrose,[4] and other relatively small molecular weight DTPA derivatives[2] are cleared rapidly from the circulation mainly via glomerular filtration.

(4) We avoided using horseradish peroxidase (HRP), which is cited as a possible factor in a systemic anaphylactic reaction to compromise BBB integrity;[4] HRP was employed in one previous BBB study.[1]

(5) Because the NMR environment has a significant acoustic noise component, we deemed it important to employ acoustic treatment controls; acoustic treatment controls were not employed[3,4] nor referred to by previous investigators[1,5] except in one study.[2] Personal communication with F. Prato confirms, however, that acoustic controls were employed in his 1987 study.[1]

REFERENCES

1. SHIVERS, R. R., M. KAVALIERS, G. C. TESKEY, F. S. PRATO & R. M. PELLETIER. 1987. Magnetic resonance imaging temporarily alters blood-brain barrier permeability in the rat. Neurosci. Lett. **76:** 25–31.
2. PRATO, F. S., R. J. H. FRAPPIER, R. R. SHIVERS, M. KAVALIERS, P. ZABEL, D. DROST & T. Y. LEE. 1990. Magnetic resonance imaging increases the blood-brain barrier permeability to 153-gadolinium diethylenetriaminepentaacetic acid in rats. Brain Res. **523:** 301–304.

3. GARBER, H. J., W. H. OLDENDORF, L. D. BRAUN & R. B. LUFKIN. 1989. MRI gradient fields increase brain mannitol space. Magn. Reson. Imag. **7:** 605–610.
4. PRESTON, E., K. BUTLER & N. HAAS. 1989. Does magnetic resonance imaging compromise integrity of the blood-brain barrier? Neurosci. Lett. **101:** 46–50.
5. ADZAMLI, I. K., F. A. JOLESZ & M. BLAU. 1989. An assessment of blood-brain barrier integrity under MRI conditions: brain uptake of radiolabeled Gd-DTPA and In-DTPA-IgG. J. Nucl. Med. **30:** 839 (abstract).
6. SAIJA, A., P. PRINCI, R. DE PASQUALE & G. COSTA. 1989. Modifications of the permeability of the blood-brain barrier and local cerebral metabolism in pentobarbital and ketamine anesthetized rats. Neuropharmacology **28:** 997–1002.
7. GJEDDE, A. & M. RASMUSSEN. 1980. Pentobarbital anesthesia reduces blood-brain glucose transfer in the rat. J. Neurochem. **35:** 1382–1387.
8. LIBURDY, R. P. 1992. Biological interactions of cellular systems with time-varying magnetic fields. This volume.

The Effects of a Single Intraoperative Immersion in Various Chemical Agents and Electromagnetic Field Exposure on Onlay Bone Grafts to the Facial Skeleton

JOHN T. NING AND ISAAC L. WORNOM III

Plastic and Reconstructive Surgery
Medical College of Virginia
Virginia Commonwealth University
Richmond, Virginia 23298

INTRODUCTION

Bone grafts are used extensively in craniomaxillofacial surgery. When used as onlay bone grafts to alter facial contour, the volume of graft maintained is unpredictable. Any intervention making their survival more predictable and permanent would find wide application in plastic and reconstructive surgery. Electrical stimulation of onlay bone grafts has been reported to decrease graft resorption,[1] but it inherently has several disadvantages when compared with electromagnetic field exposure. All electrodes are subject to some electrolysis, which has deleterious effect on osteogenesis.[2] In addition, the electrode-stimulated bone formation is spatially limited due to the small size of the electrode compared to the repair site and would necessitate open reduction with its attendant surgical hazards and complications. We therefore examined the effect of extremely low frequency (ELF) electromagnetic field exposure on onlay bone grafts to the facial skeleton in the rabbit model. Concurrently, we also assessed the effectiveness of a single intraoperative immersion of onlay bone grafts to stable chemical inducers of various second messengers known to be involved in osteogenesis in *in vitro* bone culture systems.[3,4]

MATERIALS AND METHODS

Twelve adult male New Zealand white rabbits were used in this pilot study with two rabbits in each treatment group. Each rabbit underwent harvest of two iliac crest (endochondral bone) and two calvarial (membranous bone) grafts of known volume, measured directly by a caliper. The grafts then were implanted subperiosteally onto the rabbit snout after a single 15-min immersion in Dulbecco Modified Eagle's Medium (DMEM) with one of the following agents: 0.1 μM forskolin, 0.5 μM phorbol 12-myristate 13-acetate, 10 μM calcium ionophore A23187, or 0.4 μM beta-glycerol phosphate. The control grafts were immersed in DMEM alone for 15 min. Grafts in the ELF experiment were immersed in phosphate-buffered saline for 15 min and were exposed for 2 to 6 hours per day, 5 days per week for 12 weeks, to 60-Hz continuous waves at 1 gauss in a plastic cage placed inside the Helmholtz coils.

TABLE 1. Percent Onlay Graft Volume (in mm^3) Remaining at 12 Weeks after Subperiosteal Implantation on the Rabbit Snout

Treatment Group	Iliac Crest	Calvarium
control	3.7	45.1
forskolin	60.6	172.8
phorbol myristate acetate	21.4	109.8
beta-glycerol phosphate	70.0	205.0
calcium ionophore A23187	64.0	139.2
60 Hz, CW, 1 gauss, 2–6 h/day	18.4	112.4

All rabbits received food and water ad libitum and had alternating 12-h light and dark cycles in temperature- and humidity-controlled animal facilities. At the end of 12 weeks, the rabbits were sacrificed and both the final graft volume and the percentage of graft remaining were calculated.

RESULTS

In all treatment groups, the resorption of membranous bone grafts was much less than that of endochondral bone grafts (TABLE 1). All treatment groups had a greater percent of graft volume remaining at the end of 12 weeks than control grafts. The treated membranous grafts all exhibited final volumes greater than initial graft volumes, with beta-glycerol phosphate treatment having the biggest effect on final

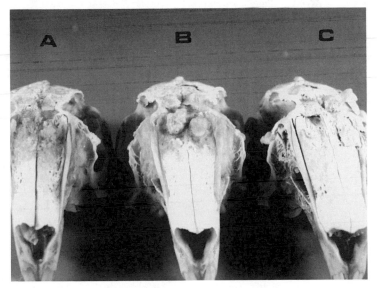

FIGURE 1. Apparent dose-response relationship between the amount of ELF exposure and the volume of surviving onlay bone grafts to the facial skeleton in the rabbit snout: (A) control, (B) 6-h/day ELF exposure, (C) 2-h/day ELF exposure.

graft volume. ELF-exposed grafts appeared to exhibit a dose-response relationship between the final graft volume and the amount of ELF exposure (FIGURE 1).

DISCUSSION

The resorption of membranous bone grafts was less than that of endochondral bone grafts in our rabbit model and this is in agreement with the literature.[5] It is interesting to note that membranous bone grafts in most treatment groups have appreciably larger final graft volumes than the original volumes, indicating that *de novo* bone deposition has occurred. A repeat of this study is under way to verify that the addition of a simple 15-min intraoperative immersion step or an ELF exposure postimplantation can increase the volume of surviving onlay bone grafts in the rabbit model.

REFERENCES

1. STALNECKER, M., L. WHITAKER & C. BRIGHTON. 1988. Electrical stimulation of onlay bone grafts. Plast. Reconstr. Surg. **82:** 580.
2. BASSETT, C., R. PAWLUK & A. PILLA. 1976. *In vivo* effects of direct current in the mandible. J. Dent. Res. **55:** 383.
3. MOLLER, J., *et al.* 1989. Immunodeficiency after allogeneic bone marrow transplantation in man: effect of phorbol ester and calcium ionophore *in vitro.* Scand. J. Immunol. **30:** 441.
4. TURKSEN, K., *et al.* 1990. Forskolin has biphasic effects on osteoprogenitor cell differentiation *in vitro.* J. Cell. Physiol. **142:** 61.
5. ZINS, J. & L. WHITHER. 1983. Membranous versus endochondral bone: implications for craniofacial reconstruction. Plast. Reconstr. Surg. **72:** 778.

Comparison of the Effect of ELF on Total RNA Content in Normal and Transformed Human Cells

JOHN NING,[a] JON CASAMENTO,[a] EWA CZERSKA,[a]
MAYS SWICORD,[a] HEBA AL-BARAZI,[b]
CHRISTOPHER DAVIS,[b] AND EDWARD ELSON[c]

[a] Center for Devices and Radiological Health
Food and Drug Administration
Rockville, Maryland 20857

[b] Department of Electrical Engineering
University of Maryland
College Park, Maryland 20742

[c] Department of Microwave Research
Walter Reed Army Institute of Research
Washington, District of Columbia 20307

INTRODUCTION

Various reports in the literature have indicated that extremely low frequency (ELF) electromagnetic radiation exposure can have differing effects on gene transcription in human cells *in vitro*.[1-3] Therefore, we investigated the effect of ELF on cellular transcription by flow cytometry on intact human cells. Flow cytometry enables us to estimate simultaneously with high accuracy the relative quantities of a variety of cellular constituents, including total RNA content.[4]

MATERIALS AND METHODS

HL-60, a human promyelogenous leukemia cell line, and Daudi, a human lymphoma cell line, were obtained from ATCC and were routinely cultured in RPMI-1640 medium supplemented with 20% fetal bovine serum. Normal peripheral human lymphocytes were routinely cultured in chromosome medium containing 2.5 μg/mL phytohemagglutinin (PHA). Equal numbers of cells in suspension were placed in 10-mL Corning T75 tissue culture flasks containing fresh medium one hour prior to exposure. Cells in a 5% CO_2 incubator at 37 °C were exposed for 30 and 60 min to 60-Hz continuous waves at 1 gauss or to pulsed electromagnetic fields (PEMF) produced by an EBI generator. After exposure, the cells were immediately fixed in 50% ethanol, incubated with acridine orange,[5] and processed for flow cytometric analysis. For each analysis of data, 10,000 cells were counted and their RNA fluorescence was displayed as a histogram.

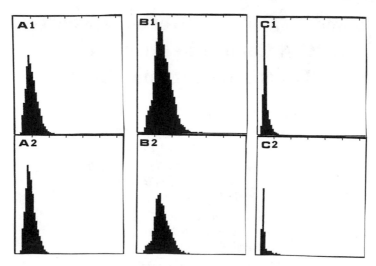

FIGURE 1. Effect of 60-Hz continuous wave exposure for 30 min on the total RNA fluorescence of Daudi, HL-60, and human peripheral lymphocytes. Increasing RNA fluorescence corresponds to a shift to the right on the abscissa—A1: HL-60 exposed, A2: HL-60 control; B1: Daudi exposed, B2: Daudi control; C1: lymph exposed, C2: lymph control.

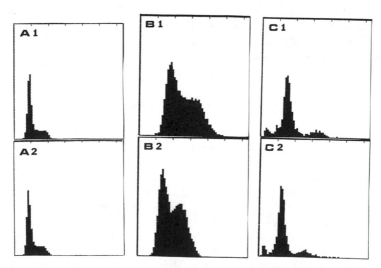

FIGURE 2. Effect of PEMF exposure for 30 min on the total RNA fluorescence of Daudi, HL-60, and peripheral human lymphocytes. Increasing RNA fluorescence corresponds to a shift to the right on the abscissa—A1: HL-60 exposed, A2: HL-60 control; B1: Daudi exposed, B2: Daudi control; C1: lymph exposed, C2: lymph control.

RESULTS

Total RNA fluorescence increased for PHA-stimulated normal peripheral human lymphocytes and Daudi lymphoma cells that were exposed to PEMF. However, no appreciable effects on total RNA fluorescence were seen in HL-60 promyelogenous leukemia cells exposed to PEMF. The magnitude of the RNA fluorescence increase was greater in cells exposed to PEMF than in those exposed to 60 Hz.

DISCUSSION

It is interesting to note that ELF exposure apparently has different effects on HL-60 and Daudi cells. These experiments have been repeated several times with similar results, suggesting that the observed difference is real. Further experiments are needed to examine more closely the different effects of ELF on Daudi and HL-60 cellular transcription.

REFERENCES

1. GREENE, J., *et al.* 1991. Delineation of electric and magnetic field effects of extremely low frequency electromagnetic radiation on transcription. Biochem. Biophys. Res. Commun. **174:** 742.
2. LITOVITZ, T., *et al.* 1990. Amplitude windows and transiently augmented transcription from exposure to electromagnetic fields. Bioelectromagnetics **11:** 297.
3. GOODMAN, R. & A. HENDERSON. 1986. Sine waves enhance cellular transcription. Bioelectromagnetics **7:** 23.
4. DARZYNKIEWICZ, Z., *et al.* 1979. Relationship between RNA content and progression of lymphocytes through the S phase of the cell cycle. Proc. Natl. Acad. Sci. U.S.A. **76:** 358.
5. DARZYNKIEWICZ, Z., *et al.* 1978. Discrimination of cycling and non-cycling lymphocytes by BUdR-suppressed acridine orange fluorescence in a flow cytometric system. Exp. Cell Res. **115:** 31.

Increased Permeability of the Blood-Brain Barrier Induced by Magnetic and Electromagnetic Fields

BERTIL R. R. PERSSON,[a] LEIF G. SALFORD,[b]
ARNE BRUN,[c] JACOB L. EBERHARDT,[a]
AND LARS MALMGREN[a]

[a]Department of Medical Radiation Physics
[b]Division of Experimental Neuro-oncology
Department of Neurosurgery
[c]Department of Neuropathology
Lund University Hospital
S-221 85 Lund, Sweden

The mammal brain is protected from potentially harmful compounds in the blood by the so-called blood-brain barrier (BBB), a selectively permeable, hydrophobic barrier. The intact BBB protects the brain from damage, whereas a dysfunctioning BBB allows influx of normally excluded hydrophilic molecules into the brain tissue. This might lead to cerebral edema, increased intracranial pressure, and (in the worst case) irreversible brain damage.

The normal selective permeability of the blood-brain barrier can be altered in several neuropathological conditions and experimental situations such as in severe trauma to the skull, in epileptic seizures, and during X-ray irradiation.

Several investigators have reported that electromagnetic exposure alters BBB permeability. Others have reported difficulties in confirming this finding.

We first studied the permeability of the blood-brain barrier after exposure to the components of the MRI electromagnetic fields: static magnetic fields (SMF), low frequency pulsed magnetic fields (TVMF), radio-frequency electromagnetic fields (RF), and a combination of these three types of fields.[1]

Anesthetized Sprague-Dawley rats, male and female, weighing 175–225 g were exposed for two hours in the MRI machine. We found an increase in the extravasation of Evan's Blue in all fields (SMF, TVMF, RF) (see TABLE 1). The most significant effect was found after exposure to RF electromagnetic fields and to the combined NMR sequence. Extravasation of the dye was seen in the fluorescence microscope as a red halo immediately outside the vessels, sometimes with the appearance of hairy protrusions.

We have also studied leakage of endogenous albumin and fibrinogen during exposure to microwaves of 915 MHz that are continuous wave (CW) and modulated at various low frequencies (8–215 Hz).[1] Fischer 344 rats, male and female, weighing about 175–225 g were used in these experiments. The rats were not anesthetized during the exposure. The exposure of the rats took place in a TEM-cell tuned to 915 MHz.

We found albumin leakage in 3 out of 20 control animals and in most of the

TABLE 1. Results for Evan's Blue of Histopathological Evaluation of Exposed and Control Animals[a]

	Unexposed Controls	SMF 0.08 T	TVMF 1.5 T/s	RF 0.2 W, 400–800 ms, 1 Hz	MRI Exposed
	*	***	***	***	***
	*	***	***	***	***
	0	**	**	***	***
	0	**	**	***	***
	0	*	*	***	***
			*		**
no. of animals	5	5	6	5	6
mean no. of asterisks	0.4	2.2	2.0	3.0	2.8
Mann-Whitney difference from control (p value)		0.02	0.02	0.007	0.005

[a]Key: *** = extensive extravasation, ** = moderate extravasation, * = minor extravasation, 0 = no extravasation.

animals exposed to 915-MHz microwaves. Continuous wave exposure resulted in 11 positive findings out of 23 ($p = 0.03$). With pulsed 915-MHz microwaves at modulation frequencies of 215, 50, 16, and 8 Hz, 28 out of 35 were positive ($p < 0.0001$) (see TABLE 2). The results indicate that pulsed electromagnetic fields especially have the potency to open the BBB for albumin passage.

We also studied the effect of a spin-echo MRI examination in a 2.35-tesla machine during one hour. The comparison between 4 exposed and 4 control animals (Fischer 344 rats) revealed no opening of the blood-brain barrier.

Our conclusion is that radio-frequency radiation has the effect of increasing permeability of the BBB. The effect was found for continuous radiation, but was even more pronounced for pulsed radio-frequency radiation at 8–215 Hz. The effect of high field MRI examinations on the blood-brain barrier could not be confirmed by

TABLE 2. Results of Positive Signs of Penetration of Albumin through the Blood-Brain Barrier after Exposure to 915-MHz Electromagnetic Fields (Continuous and Modulated at Various Frequencies)

Type of Experiment	Number of Rats	Ratio: Positive/Total (%)	Significance Test (chi-squares or Fischer's test)
control	20	3/20 (15%)	
CW (3 W)	23	11/23 (48%)	CW/control: $p = 0.027$
Σ modulated 8–215 Hz, pulse length 0.6–4 ms, effect 1–10 W/pulse	35	28/35 (80%)	Σ modulated/control: $p < 0.0001$ Σ modulated/CW: $p = 0.023$
exposed	58	39/58 (67%)	exposed/control: $p < 0.0001$

us. The question of whether the opening of the blood-brain barrier constitutes a health hazard demands further investigation.

REFERENCE

1. SALFORD, L. G., A. BRUN, L. MALMGREN, B. R. R. PERSSON, S. STRÖMBLAD & K. STURESSON. 1989. Increased permeability of the blood-brain barrier during magnetic resonance imaging. Presented at the Meeting on Interaction of Mechanisms of Low-Level Electromagnetic Fields in Living Systems—Resonant Phenomena, held at the Royal Swedish Academy of Sciences, Stockholm.

Potential Health Risk due to Cardiac Applications of Echo Planar Imaging

MICHAEL B. SMITH, ROSALIE F. TASSONE, AND
TIMOTHY J. MOSHER

Center for NMR Research
Departments of Radiology, Cellular and Molecular Physiology,
and Biological Chemistry
Pennsylvania State University College of Medicine
Milton S. Hershey Medical Center
Hershey, Pennsylvania 17033

INTRODUCTION

Current-induced muscle contraction generated by the fast switching, high amplitude gradients used for echo planar imaging is a growing concern.[1] Gradient strengths as large as 4–20 G/cm are presently used in animals and humans.[2,3] We have prepared a finite-element model of the human chest suitable to predict current densities in the body under a variety of gradient intensities and frequencies used for echo planar imaging. The unique behavior of the tissue properties for conductivity and permittivity at frequencies around 100–1000 Hz has produced interesting results.[4]

METHODS

If a conductive material is placed in the presence of an oscillating magnetic field, eddy currents and displacement currents are generated in the conductor. The induced currents circulate orthogonal to the oscillating magnetic field. The effect of induced currents depends on their location and on their direction with respect to the source current. Induced currents and magnetic fields can be calculated by solving for A and ϕ in equation 1:

$$\nabla x (1/\mu)\nabla x A = (\sigma + j\omega\epsilon)\,(-j\omega A - \nabla\phi), \tag{1}$$

where A is the magnetic vector potential, ϕ is the electric scalar potential, μ is the magnetic permeability, ω is the angular frequency at which all quantities are oscillating, σ is the conductivity, ϵ is the permittivity, and ∇x is the curl operator.

The right-hand side of equation 1 is in the form of complex conductivity $(\sigma + j\omega\epsilon)$ multiplied by the complex value of E $(-j\omega A - \nabla\phi)$, which equals the complex current density. The current density can be divided into source $(-\sigma\nabla\phi)$, induced eddy $(-j\omega\sigma A)$, and displacement $(-j\omega\epsilon\nabla\phi + \omega^2\epsilon A)$ densities. The total current density is the sum of these components. The $j\omega$ term in the eddy and displacement components indicates that they are frequency-dependent and are more significant at higher frequencies.

The human chest has been modeled at the level of the ninth thoracic vertebra using finite-element software from the Ansoft Corporation. FIGURE 1 represents a cross section of the chest that extends infinitely into space in both directions. Specific regions for blood, bone, cardiac muscle, smooth muscle, spinal cord, fat, lung, and skeletal muscle are shown. A total of 2200 triangles were used to generate the

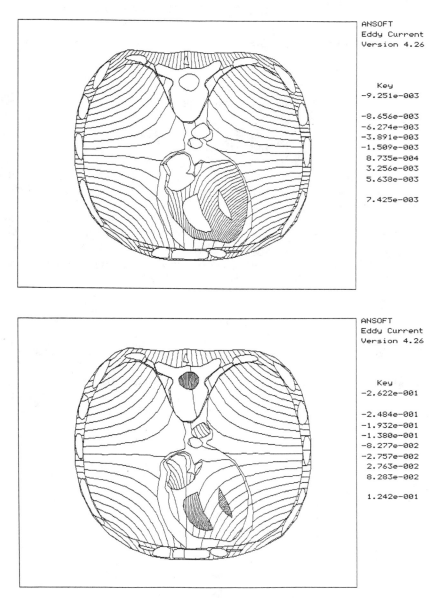

FIGURE 1. Model of the human chest at the ninth thoracic vertebra demonstrating uniform lines of total current density (A/m²) for (top) 0° and (bottom) 90° phase.

finite-element mesh. The chest is centered between a set of coils that produce a linear field gradient of 10 G/cm oscillating sinusoidally at 1 kHz.

RESULTS AND DISCUSSION

Eddy and displacement currents manifest themselves differently depending on phase. Maximum values for eddy and displacement currents occur 90° out of phase with respect to one another. FIGURE 1 shows plots of the uniform lines of the total current density (A/m^2) in the chest model in which the current phase is shifted by 90°.

The top panel in FIGURE 1 at 0° phase is dominated by displacement currents. The current density is nonuniform because the density is very sensitive to the magnitude of the tissue dielectric constant. Note the absence of current lines in the regions of bone and blood. At 1 kHz, the dielectric constant or the permittivity of the heart tissue is 310,000 as compared to a blood permittivity of 2000. Because the heart muscle has the highest permittivity, even greater than skeletal muscle (130,000), the highest displacement current density is measured there. A high current gradient exists on all surfaces of the heart under these conditions.

The bottom panel in FIGURE 1 shows the plot of the total current density at 90° phase in which eddy currents dominate the current distribution. Because the conductivity of the chest is reasonably uniform, except for blood, the current density is uniform and decreases smoothly with distance from the gradient coil windings. However, the regions corresponding to blood now contain the highest current densities due to their higher conductivity. A high current gradient is present between blood and heart tissue.

In this example, the maximum current density determined in the apex of the heart is 6.4×10^{-2} A/m^2 for eddy currents and 9.2×10^{-3} A/m^2 for displacement currents. This is below the 10 A/m^2 needed to cause stimulation of cardiac cells.[5] Threshold currents for heart fibrillation range from 1 to 10 A/m^2 over a frequency range of 6 to 1000 Hz. The magnitude of the current density is spatially dependent because the magnetic gradient is zero at the isocenter and increases with distance along the gradient axis. The current density produced in the heart will increase substantially as it is placed more asymmetrically within the gradient set.

A second calculation was performed using the same gradient set, but substituting a circular cross section for the human heart. The circular cross section (12-cm diameter) was defined with the same permittivity and conductivity as cardiac muscle for each frequency used in the calculation. FIGURE 2 displays a plot showing the maximum (a) total current (82°), (b) displacement current (0°), and (c) eddy current (90°) densities generated in simulated heart muscle at frequencies between 100 and 10,000 Hz. The phase angle given for each current indicates where the maximum current density was found. Both eddy and displacement currents are significant contributors to the current density, but the eddy current is always larger in magnitude. The current reaches a maximum value of 0.2 A/m^2 at about 10,000 Hz. This is well above the gradient switching frequencies used for echo planar imaging, but is approaching current densities capable of stimulating heart muscle. At the highest echo planar frequencies near 1000–2000 Hz, significant current densities (0.015–0.034 A/m^2) are produced. Budinger *et al.*[1] have shown normal stimulation (mild

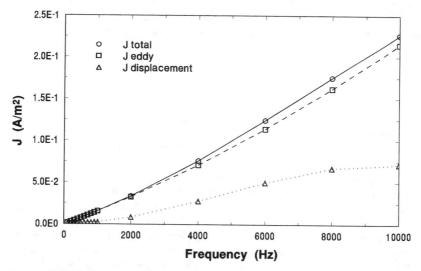

FIGURE 2. Current density versus frequency in simulated heart tissue.

electrical shock) at 60 T/s at oscillation frequencies of 1270 Hz, which are an order of magnitude below the values modeled in this study. Neural stimulation occurs at energies far below cardiac stimulation.

REFERENCES

1. BUDINGER, T. F., H. FISCHER, D. HENTSCHEL, H. E. REINFELDER & F. SCHMITT. 1990. Neural stimulation dB/dt thresholds for frequency and number of oscillations using sinusoidal magnetic gradient fields. *In* SMRM Ninth Annual Meeting, p. 276.
2. LEBIHAN, D., R. TURNER & P. DOUEK. 1990. Is water diffusion restricted in human brain? *In* SMRM Ninth Annual Meeting, p. 377.
3. MINTOROVITCH, J., J. KUCHARCZYK, M. E. MOSELEY, N. DERUGIN, S. ROCKLAGE & D. NORMAN. 1990. Correlation of T_2-weighted and echo planar magnetic susceptibility enhanced MRI of acute stroke in cats. *In* SMRM Ninth Annual Meeting, p. 1133.
4. DURNEY, C. H., H. MASSOUDI & M. F. ISKANDER. 1986. Radiofrequency Radiation Dosimetry Handbook (Fourth Edition). Electrical Engineering Department, University of Utah. Salt Lake City, Utah.
5. PERSSON, B. R. R. & F. STAHLBERG, Eds. 1989. Health and Safety of Clinical NMR Examinations, p. 51. CRC Press. Boca Raton, Florida.

Magnetic Resonance Imaging and X-ray Effects on Eye Development in C57BL/6J Mice

D. A. TYNDALL

Department of Diagnostic Sciences
School of Dentistry
University of North Carolina at Chapel Hill
Chapel Hill, North Carolina 27599-7450

Magnetic resonance imaging (MRI) techniques feature very powerful static magnetic fields, time-varying gradient magnetic fields, and radio-frequency (RF) fields. MRI techniques are gaining rapid acceptance in diagnostic medicine and dentistry. The fact that MRI is growing in usage and the fact that very few studies have been published evaluating its teratogenic potential at organ-specific sensitive stages of development provided the rationale for this investigation. A recently convened NIH Consensus Development Conference highlighted the inadequacy of the scientific literature addressing MRI teratogenicity. In addition, the area of MRI interactive effects with X-irradiation has been largely ignored. The aims of this study were (1) to determine if MRI fields increase the eye malformation rates of C57BL/6J mice (13% in controls) and (2) to determine if MRI and X-ray (30 cGy) exposures combine to produce interactive effects regarding elevated eye malformation rates.

Experimental or sham control procedures were performed on 10-week-old C57BL/6J mice on day 7 of gestation. Day 7 was chosen because this is the most susceptible stage of development for the eye. Dams ($N = 15$) were subjected to T_2-weighted spin-echo (TR = 2100 ms, TE = 50 ms) MRI fields at the isocenter (MAG I group) and entrance (MAG II group) to the magnet where field strengths were 1.5 and 0.4 tesla, respectively. The radio-frequency utilized was 64 MHz. Two other groups were exposed to X-irradiation (30 cGy) alone and in combination with MRI fields at the isocenter. Preexposure and postexposure colonic temperatures revealed no evidence of core hyperthermia. Sham controls were part of the experimental protocol as well. Concepti were removed at day 14 and were photographed under uniform magnification conditions. Quantification of eye malformations was performed by two methods. In one, a veterinary ophthalmologist scored eyes as normal or abnormal (microphthalmia, coloboma, or both) and, in the other, a computerized morphometric analysis system measured eye (globe) area for each eye of each fetus. Any eye measuring two standard deviations below the control was judged to be abnormal. All comparisons were made between concepti of the same anatomically determined developmental stage. All data were then combined to yield a percentage affected fetuses score (FIGURE 1). Pairwise statistical comparisons were made using the Kruskal-Wallis test.

The data revealed, for the first time, the potential teratogenicity of clinically realistic MRI exposures in a (strain-specific) mouse model. There is a clear suggestion that MRI exposure may induce a higher-than-normal rate of eye malformation in a genetically predisposed mouse strain (C57BL/6J) (FIGURE 1). That these data were created under MRI exposures typical for humans is important. Traditionally, studies designed to evaluate teratogenicity have utilized "doses" of the suspected agent at levels greater than those employed in humans.

Also, previous studies utilized albino mice, where eye defects are more difficult to detect. Although it is significant that the potential for MRI teratogenicity exists at the isocenter, it is somewhat surprising that animals placed at the entrance to the magnet exhibited signs of elevated abnormal eye development. The reasons for this are speculative. Whereas static and RF field strengths are less at the entrance, there

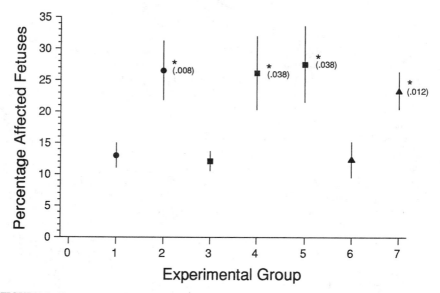

FIGURE 1. Percentage affected fetuses score. Experimental groups: (1) X-ray sham control, (2) 30 cGy group, (3) MRI sham control, (4) MAG I (isocenter), (5) MAG II (magnet entrance), (6) X/MRI sham control, and (7) X/MRI exposed (30 cGy). An asterisk denotes $p \leq 0.05$ for pairwise comparison with respective control groups. For group 7 versus group 2, $p = 0.662$.

is a high gradient of magnetic field differences at the lumen of any magnet due to convergence of the magnetic field lines. At the isocenter, these lines are relatively parallel, whereas at the lumen entrance the field lines converge, creating a gradient across the mice bodies. These gradients could have caused microlocalized heating and/or electrical effects, thus accounting for the malformations. The interesting inference from these data is that individuals near the magnetic entrance such as operating personnel and family members, if pregnant, may be placing the conceptus at risk. The data do not indicate MRI enhancement of X-ray teratogenesis, but X-ray teratogenesis at 30 cGy has been confirmed.

Possible mechanisms of damage include a microlocalized hyperthermia resulting in cell death or in changes in cell cycle cytokinetics, disruption of cell migration, and bioelectrical effects produced by blood flow perpendicular to the magnetic field. Although direct extrapolation of data from laboratory mammals to humans is not possible, a comparison of the results of controlled animal investigations with human epidemiologic data suggests that the qualitative effects of ionizing radiations may be extrapolated because the developmental processes are so similar. It could be that this is also true for some forms of nonionizing radiation fields.

In conclusion, these data suggest a potential for MRI teratogenicity in a strain of mouse predisposed to eye malformations. Only after further studies have been completed can the relationship between MRI, a diagnostically powerful imaging tool, and the developing human be ascertained, hence establishing the system's ultimate safety.

Magnetic Stimulation of the Human Brain

S. UENO AND T. MATSUDA

Department of Electronics
Kyushu University
Fukuoka 812, Japan

We have developed a method of focal magnetic stimulation of the brain to stimulate a localized area of the cortex within a 5-mm resolution.[1-4] The basic idea is to concentrate induced eddy currents locally in the vicinity of a target by a pair of opposing pulsed magnetic fields that can be produced by a figure-of-eight coil. Spatial distributions of induced eddy currents have been calculated in cubical and spherical volume conductor models by a finite element method. A computer simulation shows that the current density at the target attains a peak that is 2–3 times higher than current densities in the surrounding regions. Because the concentrated eddy currents at the target beneath the intersection of the figure-of-eight coil flow in the direction parallel to the tangent of both circular coils, vectorial stimulation can be achieved. Based upon this focal and vectorial magnetic stimulation, the various parts in the motor cortex have been stimulated by the figure-of-eight coil and we have obtained functional maps related to the hand and foot areas. The amplitude of stimulating magnetic fields was 1.0–2.0 T peak at the center of each coil and the pulse duration was 100 μs. We have observed that an optimal direction of stimulating currents for neural excitation exists in each functional area in the cortex. We have also observed that the functional maps of the cortex vary with the orientation of the stimulating current. To explain the mechanism responsible for producing this anisotropic response to brain stimulation, we have developed a model of neural excitation elicited by magnetic stimulation. The model is based on the assumption that a nerve axon is excited easily when the magnetically induced eddy currents flow in the direction parallel to the nerve axon. We have simulated the neural excitation as a function of the angle between the figure-of-eight coil and the nerve fiber. The model explains our observation that the induced current vectors reflect both functional and anatomical organization of neural fibers in the brain.

Magnetic brain stimulation was carried out in the central areas of both the left and right hemispheres. The electromyographic (EMG) signals from both the right and left abductor digiti minimi muscles (ADMs) were measured simultaneously.

FIGURE 1 shows the optimal directions for neural excitation at points A, B, and C in the human motor cortex related to the foot areas. The *Y* axis runs parallel to the nasion-inion axis and the zero point is *Cz* of the international 10–20 system. The solid-line arrows represent the inferred directions of neural fibers that innervate the left ADM and the dotted-line arrows represent the inferred directions of neural fibers that innervate the right ADM. The results at point A verified that ipsilateral neural innervation exists in the motor cortex related to the foot region. The

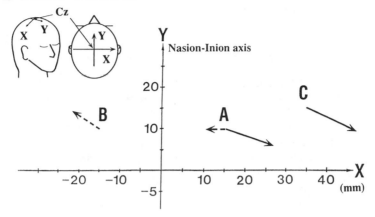

FIGURE 1. Optimal directions for neural excitation at points A, B, and C. The solid-line arrows represent the inferred directions of neural fibers that innervate the left abductor digiti minimi muscle (ADM) and the dotted-line arrows represent the inferred directions of neural fibers that innervate the right ADM.

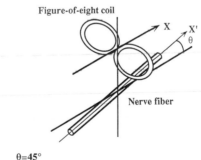

FIGURE 2. Simulation of nerve excitation elicited by magnetically induced eddy currents. See text for full details.

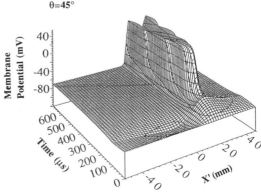

excitation of neural fibers was dependent on the direction of induced eddy currents. This vector map may reflect the anatomical structures of neural fibers.

FIGURE 2 shows an example of computer simulation of nerve excitation elicited by magnetically induced eddy currents. The X axis orientates parallel to the direction of the tangent of both circular coils. In this simulation, currents in the coil flow along the $-X$ axis at the intersection; thereby, currents induced in the body flow along the X axis. The X' axis lies in a direction parallel to the nerve fiber. The coil size is 50 mm in diameter and the distance between the coil and the nerve is 10 mm. When the angle between the figure-of-eight coil and the nerve is 45°, as shown in FIGURE 2, the nerve is excited at point $X' = 20$ mm and the excitation propagates to both sides of the nerve fiber. In contrast, when the angle between the figure-of-eight coil and the nerve is −45°, the nerve fiber is not excited.

REFERENCES

1. UENO, S., *et al.* 1988. J. Appl. Phys. **64:** 5862–5864.
2. UENO, S., *et al.* 1989 (March). Dig. Intermagn. Conf. (GD-10), Washington, District of Columbia.
3. UENO, S., *et al.* 1989. *In* Advances in Biomagnetism. S. J. Williamson *et al.*, Eds.: 529–532. Plenum. New York.
4. UENO, S., T. MATSUDA & M. FUJIKI. 1990. IEEE Trans. Magn. **MAG-26**(no. 5): 1539–1544.

Safety Problems of $d\text{B}/dt$ Associated with Echo Planar Imaging

S. UENO,[a] O. HIWAKI,[a] T. MATSUDA,[a] H. YAMAGATA,[b]
S. KUHARA,[c] Y. SEO,[b] K. SATO,[c] AND T. TANOUE[b]

[a]Department of Electronics
Kyushu University
Fukuoka 812, Japan

[b]Medical Engineering Laboratory
TOSHIBA
Otawara 32926, Japan

[c]Research and Development Center
TOSHIBA
Kawasaki 210, Japan

In designing high-speed MRI systems such as echo planar imaging (EPI) systems, it is imperative to assess the potential hazards of stimulatory effects on excitable tissues by magnetically induced electrical currents.[1-3] No experimental studies on the effects of trapezoidal gradient magnetic fields have been reported. In the present study, we first made a comparison of the thresholds for peripheral nerve stimulation elicited by trapezoidal and sinusoidal pulse trains for readout gradient pulses of EPI. A figure-of-eight coil[4-6] was used to stimulate a localized area and to delineate the differences of the thresholds for nerve excitation. The coil size was 60 mm in inside diameter and 80 mm in outside diameter. The coil was positioned on the right clavicle to stimulate plexus brachialis. We evaluated the thresholds in a blind manner, changing the coil current that gave rise to nerve excitation around the clavicle. The rise time t_p and plateau t_s of the trapezoid were $t_p = 100$ μs and $t_s = 200$ μs for a period of 800 μs and $t_p = 100$ μs and $t_s = 512$ μs for a period of 1424 μs (FIGURE 1). Eleven volunteers were examined. The results showed that, at the same power level, the threshold of trapezoidal pulses was the same as in the case of sinusoidal pulses; the threshold of $d\text{B}/dt$ for nerve excitation was 300–400 T/s (FIGURE 2). We simulated the nerve excitation elicited by trapezoidal and sinusoidal magnetic fields.

We also evaluated the thresholds for sensation of the somatosensory systems of the human head. We designed a miniature coil system that could produce gradient magnetic fields in MRI systems. The miniature cylinder on which the gradient coil was positioned was 240 mm in diameter and 460 mm in length. The coil was driven by a train of 64 trapezoidal pulsed currents ($t_p = 100$ μs, $t_s = 200$ μs) to produce gradient time-varying magnetic fields. We, as volunteers, inserted our heads into the cylinder. We did sense somatosensory sensation at the middle of the forehead. The threshold for the sensation was 80–100 T/s.

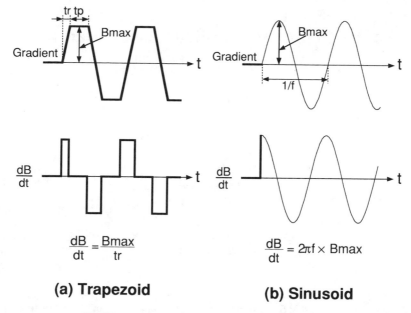

FIGURE 1. Waveforms of the gradient and its $d\text{B}/dt$.

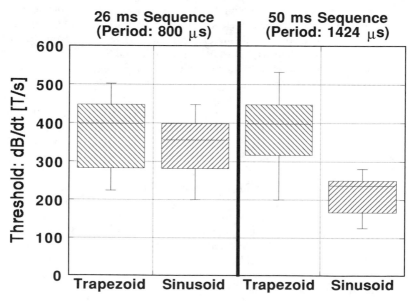

FIGURE 2. Comparison of the thresholds for sensation.

REFERENCES

1. COHEN, M. S., R. M. WEISSKOFF, R. R. RZEDZIAN & H. L. KANTOR. 1990. Sensory stimulation by time-varying magnetic fields. Magn. Reson. Med. **14**(no. 3): 409–414.
2. REILLY, J. P. 1989. Peripheral nerve stimulation by induced electric currents: exposure to time-varying magnetic fields. Med. Biol. Eng. Comput. **27**: 101–110.
3. EGERTER, D. E. 1990. MR nerve stimulation: new safety concern? *In* Diagnostic Imaging, p. 127–131.
4. UENO, S., T. TASHIRO & K. HARADA. 1988. Localized stimulation of neural tissues in the brain by means of paired configuration of time-varying magnetic fields. J. Appl. Phys. **64**: 5862–5864.
5. UENO, S., T. MATSUDA & M. FUJIKI. 1989. Localized stimulation of the human brain by a pair of opposing magnetic fields. *In* Advances in Biomagnetism. S. J. Williamson *et al.*, Eds.: 529–532. Plenum. New York.
6. UENO, S., T. MATSUDA & O. HIWAKI. 1990. Localized stimulation of the human brain and spinal cord by a pair of opposing pulsed magnetic fields. J. Appl. Phys. **67**: 5838–5840.

APPENDIX[a]

Principles for the Protection of Patients and Volunteers during Clinical Magnetic Resonance Diagnostic Procedures[b]

SCOPE

The Board has the responsibility for advising the Department of Health on acceptable limits of exposure of patients and volunteers to magnetic fields encountered during clinical diagnosis by magnetic resonance (MR) systems for imaging (MRI) or spectroscopy (MRS). Such examinations may last up to about 1 h and result in exposure to static, extremely low frequency (ELF) gradient, and radiofrequency (RF) magnetic fields. Previous advice was issued in 1984.[1] The following revised recommendations are based on a reassessment of the possible effects on human health derived from new information from studies of the experimental exposure of humans and animals to electromagnetic fields and from extensive operational experience. These recommendations consider both whole-body and partial-body exposure and the implications of heterogeneous patterns of energy deposition. Restrictions on staff exposure to time-varying magnetic fields (including ELF and RF fields) are covered by separate guidance;[2] this advice is presently under revision and will include restrictions on exposure to static magnetic fields.

PRINCIPLES

The data available at present are insufficient to allow thresholds for adverse effects of acute exposure of humans to electromagnetic fields to be accurately defined. As an interim measure, a two-tier system of restriction is recommended: a lower level identifies exposures considered to be safe and which may be exceeded under certain controlled circumstances; an upper level identifies exposures which present evidence suggests it would be inadvisable to exceed. The adoption of a two-tier standard is to provide some flexibility and to allow the cautious development of MR diagnostic techniques in which humans may be exposed to magnetic fields greater than those commonly used at present. Any effects of exposure between the lower and upper levels are expected to be small, although such exposure should be under carefully controlled conditions. The assessment of patient responses at exposures between these two levels of restriction and the publication of these data will provide valuable information for future revision of this advice.

Restrictions on exposure to *static magnetic fields* are intended to prevent the possibility of adverse health effects resulting from reduced aortic blood flow,

[a]This appendix combines various statements that provide information on the current standards used to determine safe exposure levels for the electric and magnetic fields associated with MR imaging systems.

[b]Statement by the National Radiological Protection Board: 1991. *Documents of the NRPB.* Volume 2, number 1. NRPB. Chilton, United Kingdom.

increased blood pressure, cardiac arrhythmia, and impaired mental function. These effects have been observed experimentally or predicted at high levels of exposure, but are not well established. A degree of caution in patient and volunteer exposure is therefore needed until further operational experience becomes available.

Restrictions on *gradient (ELF) magnetic field* exposure are intended to prevent the stimulation of peripheral nerves and muscles, particularly cardiac muscle, by magnetically induced electric currents. Threshold current densities for peripheral nerve or cardiac muscle stimulation are estimated to be similar at low frequencies. Both can be avoided by setting a basic restriction on induced current densities to below threshold values for these responses. Relaxation of this restriction can be envisaged for short periods of magnetic field change due to the progressively shorter time available for the accumulation of the electric charge necessary for stimulation of the nerve cell membrane. The threshold for cardiac muscle stimulation rises at longer wavelengths (or lower frequencies) of magnetic field change than do thresholds for peripheral nerve stimulation. Thus, in this region, stimulation of peripheral nerves should give adequate warning of cardiac stimulation. Restrictions intended to avoid the stimulation of cardiac muscle, but not peripheral nerves, should be exceeded only under controlled conditions. Secondary restrictions on the rate of change of magnetic flux density can be derived from these basic restrictions, but may be exceeded where it can be shown that the basic restrictions will not be exceeded.

Heating is a major consequence of exposure to the *RF frequencies* used in MR. Restrictions on RF magnetic field exposure are intended to prevent adverse responses to increased heat load and elevated body temperature. These responses include increased cardiac output, associated with elevated skin blood flow, and sweating, and may be contraindicated in patients with decreased thermoregulatory ability or cardiovascular problems. Increased body temperature is also associated with decreased mental function and with other physiological changes. These adverse effects of whole-body heat load can be adequately avoided by setting basic restrictions on the rise in body temperature. Secondary restrictions on the specific energy absorption rate (SAR)[c] averaged over the whole body can be derived from these basic restrictions and may be exceeded provided that the appropriate restriction on rise in body temperature is not exceeded. Despite the effects of cooling, body temperature increases with an increase in the total amount of RF energy absorbed, at least for the first 30 min of exposure, so that, for a given rise in body temperature, progressively higher rates of energy absorption (SARs) can be applied for decreasing periods of exposure.

In practice, exposure to RF magnetic fields during MRI and particularly during MRS is predominantly to a region of the body such as the head or abdomen. In addition, the distribution of RF absorption and the rise in tissue temperature within the exposed region will be nonuniform due to tissue inhomogeneities and variation in blood flow. Restrictions on this localized absorption of RF energy are intended to prevent adverse effects on tissues and organs resulting from elevated temperatures. Basic restrictions are needed for the maximum temperature in different regions of

[c]The specific energy absorption rate (SAR) represents the rate of absorption of electromagnetic energy, for example, by tissue, normalized to the mass under consideration and is expressed in watts per kilogram (W/kg). In terms of thermal loading, the SAR can be equated with the rate of metabolic heat production.

the body. The head and, in pregnant women, the embryo or fetus are regarded as particularly vulnerable to elevated temperature; tissues in the trunk and limbs are regarded as less sensitive. Secondary restrictions on localized SAR are intended to prevent tissue temperatures exceeding basic restrictions.

Patients with certain medical disorders or under medication may be at some risk from exposure above the lower advised levels of static, ELF, or RF magnetic fields. In particular, patients with compromised thermoregulatory abilities may be particularly susceptible to RF heating; such patients may well include those with cardiac problems or with a fever and those taking certain drugs. In addition, infants, pregnant women, and old people may be considered compromised in this respect. In these circumstances, the doctor in charge must make this judgement and weigh the benefit of diagnosis against any possible risk. Since the potentially sensitive categories of patient are not well defined, it is advised that all patients exposed above the lower level of restriction have simple physiological parameters, such as body temperature, blood pressure, and heart rate, routinely monitored.

Patients should be exposed only with the approval of a registered medical practitioner who should be satisfied either that the exposure is likely to result in a net benefit to the patient or that it is part of a research project which has been approved by a local research ethical committee.

The exposure of volunteers participating in experimental trials of MR imaging or spectroscopic techniques should be approved by a local ethical committee. Volunteers should be medically assessed for general fitness. They should be freely consenting and fully informed. Additional guidance is given in WHO Technical Report No. 611.[3]

Although there is no good evidence that mammalian embryos are sensitive to the magnetic fields encountered in magnetic resonance systems, it is prudent, until further information becomes available, to exclude pregnant women during the first three months of pregnancy. However, MR diagnostic procedures should be considered where the only reasonable alternative to MR diagnosis requires the use of X-ray procedures. There is no need to exclude women for whom a termination of pregnancy has been indicated. It is advised that pregnant women should not be exposed above the advised lower levels of restriction.

Metallic implants may present a hazard because of RF induced heating. In addition, implants made of ferromagnetic material will experience a force exerted on them by the static magnetic field which may result in movement of the implant and local tissue damage. In general, exposure is contraindicated unless a careful evaluation has been carried out. The exposure of persons with large metallic implants such as hip prostheses should be stopped immediately if any discomfort is experienced.

Pacemakers and other electrically, mechanically, or magnetically activated implants may be subject to electromagnetic interference, heating, and a mechanical force if made of magnetic material; persons fitted with such implants should not be exposed unless the particular implant has been demonstrated to be unperturbed by MR fields.

REFERENCES

1. NRPB. 1984. Advice on acceptable limits of exposure to nuclear magnetic resonance clinical imaging. National Radiological Protection Board, ASP5. HMSO. London.

2. NRPB. 1989. Guidance as to restrictions on exposure to time-varying electromagnetic fields and the 1988 recommendations of the International Non-Ionizing Radiation Committee. National Radiological Protection Board, NRPB-GS11. HMSO. London.
3. WHO. 1977. Use of ionizing radiation and radionuclides on human beings for medical research, training, and nonmedical purposes. Report of a WHO Expert Committee. Technical Report Series No. 611. World Health Organization. Geneva.

Limits on Patient and Volunteer Exposure during Clinical Magnetic Resonance Diagnostic Procedures

Recommendations for the Practical Application of the Board's Statement[a]

INTRODUCTION

The Board has the responsibility for advising on acceptable limits of exposure of patients and volunteers to the static, gradient, and radio-frequency magnetic fields encountered during clinical diagnosis by magnetic resonance (MR) systems. The purpose of the advice is to offer to clinicians guidance on the degree of risk presented to patients by exposure to the magnetic fields generated by MR. In addition, guidance on operational limitations is provided for manufacturers and those with responsibilities for the safe operation of these systems. The advice[1] issued in 1984 by the Board has been revised. The revised advice takes into account advances in the understanding of the biological effects of these magnetic fields during MR imaging (MRI) and/or spectroscopy (MRS) and the substantial experience gained since 1984 of patient and volunteer exposure.

BIOLOGICAL BASIS FOR ADVICE

Static Magnetic Fields

Static (time-invariant) magnetic fields exert a weak force on molecules and on moving charged particles such as ions; their possible effects on humans have been comprehensively reviewed elsewhere.[2,3]

Human Studies

Most experiments with human volunteers show that body temperature, heart rate, and blood pressure are unaffected by acute exposure to fields up to about 1–5 tesla (T),[4-6] although one experiment reports a slight drop in heart rate in humans exposed to 2 T.[7] The existence of flow potentials is well established, but their significance is not clear; estimated[8,9] maximum values across the human aorta range between 7 and 16 millivolts per tesla (mV/T). The peak flow potential in man during exposure to 2.5 T is calculated to be 40 mV, the depolarization threshold for stimulation of myocardial cells. However, only a small fraction of this potential will be expressed across individual cells.

---

[a]Statement by the National Radiological Protection Board: 1991. *Documents of the NRPB.* Volume 2, number 1. NRPB. Chilton, United Kingdom.

In addition, the magnetic field will exert a force on the flow of blood resulting in a reduction in blood flow and an increase in blood pressure;[8] the effect is expected to be greatest in large diameter blood vessels. However, this has not been tested experimentally.

Workers, but not patients, have apparently experienced vertigo, occasionally followed by nausea and headaches, when working around a 4-T magnet.[10] In addition, visual sensations (magnetic phosphenes) and a metallic taste were experienced on moving the eyes or head. These effects are probably related to electric currents induced in the head during movement.

Animal and Cell Studies

There is no unequivocal evidence from animal studies that prolonged exposure to static magnetic fields of 1–2 T over days to years has any adverse effect on body weight, hematological profile, or immunological response. Experiments with mammals, including two primate species, confirm the observation in humans of a lack of effect on cardiac function of acute exposure to fields of less than about 2 T.[11-14] In particular, there were no significant changes in heart rate or arterial blood pressure in monkeys exposed to 1.5 T, although this exposure was sufficient to generate measurable flow potentials. Irregularities in heart rate (cardiac arrhythmia) and a temporary slowing were observed in one experiment in which squirrel monkeys were acutely exposed to fields mainly between 4 and 7 T, although no threshold was identified.[15] Exposures to more intense static fields (up to 9.7 T) have been reported to disrupt animal behavior. Two studies[16,17] report that the performance of learned tasks by squirrel monkeys was reduced during exposure to static fields in excess of about 4.6 T.

Exposure of mice to about 1 T *in utero* has had no significant effect on prenatal or postnatal development.[18,19] There was no effect of exposure to fields of up to about 1 T on dominant lethal frequency in male germ cells irradiated *in vivo*[20] nor on the frequency of chromosome aberrations and sister chromatid exchanges in cells exposed *in vitro*.[21,22] Tumor growth in mice was unaffected by exposure to fields of up to about 1 T.[23,24]

Conclusions

The evidence suggests that the acute exposure of humans to static magnetic fields below about 2.5 T is unlikely to have any adverse effect on health. In addition, there have been no reports of adverse effects from MR systems operating at 2.35 T. Short-term exposure to fields above about 4 T may produce significant detrimental health effects, including vertigo and nausea, reduced aortic blood flow, and increased blood pressure; experiments with primates suggest increased cardiac arrhythmia and reduced mental function above 4–5 T. These effects are not well established, but suggest a degree of caution should be exercised in the exposure of patients to fields above 2.5 T.

The prolonged exposure of animals and cells to static fields of about 1 T had no effect on prenatal or postnatal development and did not result in damage to chromosomes in germ cells or in somatic cells. Thus, developmental and genetic (including hereditary) effects are unlikely.

Gradient Magnetic Fields

Time-varying magnetic fields induce electric fields and circulating eddy currents in biological systems which may affect normal cell function, particularly the function of electrically excitable nerve and muscle cells; the possible effects of exposure have been comprehensively reviewed elsewhere.[2,25]

Human Studies

Experiments with volunteers suggest that the most sensitive response to ELF magnetic fields is the occurrence of magnetic phosphenes, faint flickering sensations in the periphery of the visual field, resulting from induced currents affecting cells in the retina. They were first reported by D'Arsonval[26] in 1896 and have subsequently been confirmed and further investigated by many authors. They are not considered to be hazardous *per se*. The threshold for magnetic phosphenes is about 5–10 mT at 20 Hz, rising at lower and higher frequencies.[27–29] Intense magnetic fields of up to 100 mT at 50–60 Hz are reported to have no effect on the electroencephalogram, electrocardiogram, or blood pressure of volunteers, although some unexplained changes occurred in the visual evoked potential response.[30–32] In addition, volunteers complained of headaches during exposure to fields above 60 mT.

Stimulation of peripheral nerves and muscles by magnetically induced electric current requires exposure to much more rapidly changing magnetic fields which, in many experiments, have been generated only as one short pulse or as a few short pulses. A threshold of perception of about 2×10^3 T/s has been described[33] in human volunteers whose forearms were exposed to a damped sinusoidal magnetic field. The current induced in the peripheral tissues was calculated to be approximately 5 A/m². Very short (180 μs) pulses with a rate of change of magnetic flux density of about 10^4 T/s have been used[34] to stimulate the median nerve of the forearm. In addition, the direct stimulation of the motor cortex of volunteers has been reported[35,36] using very short (<1 ms) magnetic pulses. More recently, the sensation of muscular twitches has been reported in two volunteers exposed to 1.4 kHz sinusoidal fields[37] in gradient coils developed for rapid imaging techniques; rms (root mean square) rates of change of magnetic flux density were 61 T/s. Another study[38] reported a mean neural stimulation threshold in ten volunteers of about 60 T/s (peak) for 1.27 kHz sinusoidal fields.

Electrophysiological Considerations

There is not sufficient information in these experiments to define a safe level of restriction for exposure to intense extremely low frequency (ELF) magnetic fields. There is, however, an extensive literature on the effect of electric currents applied directly to the body via external electrodes, from which insight into the possible health risks can be gained. These data have been extensively reviewed[39-41] and a threshold electric field strength in tissue of 6.2 V/m, corresponding to an induced current density of 1.2 A/m^2 (assuming a tissue conductivity of 0.2 S/m), has been derived for both peripheral nerve and cardiac muscle stimulation at low frequencies (< 100 Hz).[39,41] Thus, both tissues appear equally sensitive to induced electric fields and currents; however, threshold rates of change of magnetic flux density vary slightly because of the different locations of both tissues within the body. With uniform exposure of the entire body, Reilly[41] quotes threshold peak rates of change for peripheral nerve stimulation to vary between about 40 and 60 T/s, depending on the orientation of the magnetic field vector relative to the body. The lowest threshold occurred when the magnetic field vector was orthogonal to the long axis of the body, a reflection of the larger inductive current loop radius. These predicted thresholds for peripheral nerve stimulation have received some corroboration from the two recent volunteer experiments[37,38] described above. Cardiac stimulation thresholds were predicted[41] to vary between about 45 and 70 T/s. Thus, both peripheral nerve and cardiac muscle stimulation can be adequately avoided by restricting exposure to sinusoidal or pulsed magnetic fields in any orientation to less than 20 T/s.

It is well understood that electrical stimulation thresholds rise as the current pulse width decreases below the nerve or muscle cell membrane time-constant (the product of electric resistance and capacitance). This is due to the progressively shorter time available for the accumulation of the electric charge necessary for depolarization of the nerve cell membrane. The rise in threshold is predicted to be exponential, but can be approximated by maintaining the product of the pulse width and threshold current density constant. Cardiac muscle fibers have a longer membrane time-constant (3 ms) than peripheral nerve fibers (120 μs). Thus, for pulses shorter than 3 ms, cardiac muscle fiber stimulation can still be avoided if the restriction on the rate of change of magnetic flux density (dB/dt) of 20 T/s is relaxed in proportion to the inverse of the period of magnetic field change.[41] For periods of magnetic field change shorter than 120 μs, peripheral nerve stimulation can still be avoided if the restriction on dB/dt is similarly relaxed. For continuous sinusoidal stimulation, it has been predicted that cardiac stimulation thresholds will begin to rise at around 120 Hz; for peripheral nerve stimulation, this figure is around 5.4 kHz.

Further relaxation can be envisaged for gradient fields which undergo a phase change over the volume of the body under consideration, such as the transverse gradients in MR systems where the main static magnetic field vector is orientated parallel to the long axis of the body.[42] In this case, the induction of current is reduced because of the smaller effective current loop radius.

It is clear from these data that the threshold rate of change of magnetic flux density for peripheral nerve stimulation is much lower than that for cardiac stimulation only for periods of magnetic field change shorter than 3 ms; for longer periods, peripheral nerve stimulation does not provide an adequate warning for preventing cardiac stimulation. It is not clear, however, whether there are groups of people within the population, possibly those taking neuroactive medication such as certain stimulants or with neurological disorders such as epilepsy, that may be particularly sensitive to induced currents. This possibility should be further investigated.

In theory, as the period of gradient magnetic field change decreases below about

5 μs, the effects of heating begin to predominate and restrictions on SAR[b] become more appropriate. Power dissipation (SAR) can be equated with the flow of current through a conductive medium. Thus, making certain assumptions, the restrictions on SAR identified in the following section can be applied to induced currents and therefore to rates of change of magnetic flux density. It can be calculated that an SAR of 1 or 2 W/kg will be induced in the peripheral tissues by a peak rate of change of magnetic flux density of about 700–1100 or 1000–1700 T/s, respectively, depending on tissue conductivity (which varies with frequency) and inductive loop radius. However, gradient field switching rates are unlikely to exceed 10 kHz.

Animal and Cell Studies

There is some limited evidence that suggests that weak electric currents can affect early embryogenesis. Several groups[43-46] have reported the abnormal development of chick embryos exposed for the first two days after fertilization to pulsed or sinusoidal magnetic fields greater than 1.2 μT at frequencies between 10 and 1000 Hz. However, other research groups[47-49] reported a lack of statistically significant effects after the exposure of chick embryos to pulsed or sawtooth magnetic fields at frequencies of up to 20 kHz. Thus, the evidence is equivocal and the direct relevance to humans unclear. Several studies[50-53] have examined the effects on mammalian development of exposure to extremely low frequency magnetic fields; the results have generally been negative. It would seem that it is unlikely that mammalian development is affected by exposure to time-varying magnetic fields below 100 kHz, but this is not unequivocally established.

Few studies of possible mutagenic and carcinogenic responses to ELF magnetic field exposure have been carried out; much available data indicate a lack of effect *in vivo*. No significant effects of 60 Hz magnetic fields have been seen on sister chromatid exchange rates in human lymphocytes exposed to up to 220 μT[54,55] nor on point mutation frequency in Chinese hamster ovary cells exposed to up to 50 μT.[56] The lack of effect on chromosome structure has suggested that ELF magnetic fields are unlikely to act as carcinogens. Several *in vitro* studies have reported increased DNA synthesis in human fibroblasts exposed to 15 Hz–4 kHz fields of 2.3–560 μT[57] and enhanced DNA transcription and altered levels of protein synthesis in dipteran salivary glands after exposure to 1–72 Hz pulsed and sinusoidal magnetic fields of about 0.5–3.5 mT.[58-61] However, altered transcription, translation, or DNA synthesis does not necessarily demonstrate that ELF magnetic fields promote the appearance of cancer; it is possible that they reflect changes to other aspects of cell metabolism. Their implications for acute human exposure are not clear.

Conclusions

Human nerve and muscle cells can be stimulated by rates of change of gradient magnetic flux density which induce current densities sufficient to stimulate electri-

---

[b]The specific energy absorption rate (SAR) represents the rate of absorption of electromagnetic energy, for example, by tissue, normalized to the mass under consideration and is expressed in watts per kilogram (W/kg). In terms of thermal loading, the SAR can be equated with the rate of metabolic heat production.

cally excitable tissue. Threshold current densities for peripheral nerve or cardiac muscle stimulation are about 1.2 A/m^2 at stimulation frequencies below about 100 Hz. Both can be avoided adequately by restricting induced current densities to less than 400 mA/m^2. In most cases, this can be achieved by restricting exposure to rates of change of magnetic flux density to less than 20 T/s; some relaxation can be considered for gradient fields orthogonal to the static field vector. In addition, relaxation of this value can be envisaged for short periods of magnetic field change (<3 ms for cardiac stimulation and <120 μs for peripheral nerve stimulation). It should be noted that, for periods of flux density change longer than 3 ms, peripheral sensation does not adequately protect against cardiac stimulation. Individuals are likely to vary in their sensitivity to induced currents; some, under neuroactive medication or with neurological disorders, may be particularly sensitive, although this is not well established. It would seem reasonable to monitor people exposed above the lower level of restriction until further information becomes available.

There is some equivocal data suggesting that the developing chick embryo is sensitive to prolonged exposure to weak ELF magnetic fields. The results from mammalian studies are mostly negative; it seems prudent, however, to avoid exposure of pregnant women during organogenesis (the first trimester) until the consequences are more clearly established. Such exposure does not seem to affect chromosome structure and is therefore unlikely to have mutagenic or hereditary effects.

Radio-Frequency Magnetic Fields

The effects of heating begin to predominate over electrical excitation above 100 kHz; thus, heating is a major consequence of the RF frequencies used in MR which are usually greater than 1 MHz. Much evidence from experiments with animals and cell cultures suggests that many established effects of acute exposure to RF which may be considered adverse result from heat.[62] However, a number of authors (see, for example, reference 63) challenge the assumption that the effects in this region are only those of heating; however, the physiological consequences of these proposed athermal interactions are not yet clear.

The overall heat load can be related to the average, whole-body SAR; in practice, the SAR within an exposed animal or human varies considerably and may result in localized heating. Localized heat is rapidly dissipated by the blood and lost to the environment by various thermoregulatory mechanisms. However, in simple terms, neglecting the effects of cooling, an SAR of 1 W/kg applied for an hour would result in a temperature rise of about 1 °C.

Human Studies

The tolerance by humans of moderate increases in body temperature and the ensuing risks of adverse effects are not clearly understood,[64] although it is known that mental performance declines as heat load increases. An upper limit threshold value of 1 °C rise in body temperature has been proposed[65,66] for industrial workers in hot environments. However, even in people lying at rest, a short-term rise in body temperature of this magnitude will induce large increases in cardiac output and skin blood flow, coupled with a decrease in mean arterial pressure and blood flow through other tissues.[67,68] It has been estimated[69] in a review of dosimetric and thermoregulatory models that an SAR of 2–3 W/kg would cause this rise within 1 h in a lightly clothed man seated in a comfortable environment (ambient temperature 25 °C, relative humidity 50%, and air velocity 0.13 m/s). However, it is important to note that some people are less heat tolerant than others; pre-employment tests of heat tolerance are common in industries involving work in hot environments.[64] Physiological and physical correlates which are associated with a decreased ability to adapt to an increased heat load include old age, obesity, and hypertension.[70] Various drugs, such as diuretics, tranquilizers and sedatives, and vasodilators, decrease heat tolerance.[71] In addition, the thermoregulatory ability of infants is not well developed; pregnant women may also be compromised in their ability to dissipate heat. In this context, it is worth noting that heat loss from the embryo and fetus across the placental barrier may be less efficient than heat dissipation in other well-vascularized tissues.

The whole-body thermoregulatory response of humans exposed to magnetic resonance imaging has been mathematically modeled.[72] The authors concluded that the body temperature of a lightly clothed patient whose thermoregulatory ability was unimpaired would rise by up to 0.6 °C, depending on environmental conditions, during exposure at whole-body SARs of up to 4 W/kg. Skin blood flow was estimated to rise to maximum values at higher SARs, requiring increased cardiac output. The authors note that the health of patients with impaired cardiac function could be compromised under these circumstances. More recent calculation[73] suggests that patients with moderately impaired skin blood flow (60–70% impairment) would experience small rises in body temperature (< 1 °C) at whole-body SARs of up to 4 W/kg for up to 40 min under moderate ambient conditions; more severe impairment was considered to contraindicate exposure greater than 3 W/kg for more than 20 min.

These calculations are fairly well supported by the limited studies of thermoregulatory responses of patients and volunteers exposed to RF fields in magnetic resonance systems. Heart rate was reported to increase by a mean value of three beats per minute in volunteers exposed for 17 min at 0.8 W/kg; blood pressure was minimally affected.[74] Another study,[75] in which volunteers were exposed at a whole-body SAR of 3 W/kg for 20 min, reported increases in heart rate of up to 45% (mean increase of 30%); rectal temperatures rose by up to 0.7 °C (mean rise of 0.3 °C). In contrast, two studies reported minimal changes in body temperature and heart rate in volunteers exposed at 2.7–4 W/kg for 20–30 min.[76–78]

The thermoregulatory responses of patients, some with conditions (unspecified) associated with impaired temperature regulation, have also been investigated. The mean body temperature of 50 patients exposed at SARs between 0.41 and 1.2 W/kg (mostly at SARs in the lower part of this range) for 15 min was reported[79] to rise by 0.2 °C; individual responses varied by up to 0.5 °C. However, average heart rate and blood pressure were unaffected, but several subjects felt warm and 60% had visible signs of perspiration. A subsequent study[80] investigated the responses of 35 patients to magnetic resonance imaging of the brain. No changes were found in body temperature after exposure at an average whole-body SAR of 0.06 W/kg. However, local SARs (presumably in the head) were estimated at 2.5 W/kg and 40% of the patients had visible signs of sweating on their foreheads. In contrast, there is one report[81] of cardiac patients, or patients with compromised sweat glands, experiencing discomfort within 10 min at a whole-body SAR of 2 W/kg.

These data describing whole-body responses to average, whole-body SARs provide no information about the distribution of SAR within the body or of the responses to high, localized SARs. The average whole-body SARs quoted in magnetic resonance studies will have resulted from much higher, localized SARs distributed around the RF coil. Simple calculation, assuming a uniform magnetic field and a homogeneous, cylindrical human phantom, suggests that SAR is maximal in the superficial tissues.[82,83] However, cooling is also greatest at the body surface—indeed, skin temperatures are notoriously labile—and so maximum temperatures will not necessarily exist on the skin surface.[84] Recent calculations based on a heterogeneous mathematical model of the human body[85,86] suggest that localized SARs within the body could be up to ten or even seventy times greater over small volumes compared to the whole-body average SAR.[86,87] However, these relative increases are reduced to a factor of between two and four when the localized SAR is averaged over individual body organs.[87,88] It is clear that appropriate averaging volumes are not well established, although they are central to restrictions on localized SAR. Further investigation should be carried out.

It has been suggested by Czerski and Athey[89] that localized temperatures of up to about 38 °C in the head, 39 °C in the trunk, and 40 °C in the extremities are unlikely to produce adverse effects. Simple calculation[90] relating localized heating in the eye to SAR in the head suggests that exposure resulting in an SAR to the head of 3 W/kg is unlikely to raise the temperature of the eye by more than 1.6 °C; brain temperatures are unlikely to rise by more than 1 °C under these conditions. It seems probable that higher SARs, averaged over the exposed part of the body, are acceptable for the trunk and limbs provided that whole-body heat loads are not exceeded.

Animal Studies

Experiments with animals have reported various effects which result from induced heating. A number of studies have reported threshold SARs of 0.5–5 W/kg in rodents[91,92] and primates[93] for thermoregulatory responses or various stratagems for minimizing total heat load (such as reduced metabolic heat production). Threshold SARs for vasodilation and sweating of 0.3–3 W/kg, depending on ambient temperature, have been reported in primates.[94,95] Behavioral thermoregulation, in which animals select cooler environmental temperatures or shorter durations of infrared heating, has also been described in rodents[96] and primates;[97] threshold SARs were estimated as about 1 W/kg in both cases. These responses reflect normal adjustments to slightly altered heat loads or environmental conditions. It is worth noting, however, that exposure which results in increased heating of the deeper tissues is less effective in eliciting appropriate thermoregulatory responses than exposure at frequencies where RF power absorption occurs predominantly in superficial tissues.[95,98] This is thought to result from the less effective stimulation of the superficial temperature receptors by the more deeply penetrating radiation.

Increased heat loads have resulted in decreased mental function; the performance of learned (operant) tasks by primates was significantly decreased by exposure at 2.5–5 W/kg for 1 h[99–101] and rectal temperatures rose by about 1 °C. Similar responses have been described in rodents.[102–105] Other physiological effects consistent with responses to increased body temperatures or heat stress include increased plasma cortisol/corticosterone levels,[106,107] increased cardiac output coupled with decreased peripheral resistance,[108–110] and decreased barbiturate-induced sleeping time.[111,112]

A large number of studies of effects of microwaves and RF on the immune responses of hemopoietic tissues have been carried out,[113–118] but the observed changes have been transient; the immune system has considerable redundancy[119] and small, transient changes may be of little long-term consequence.

Some tissues may be particularly sensitive to RF radiation. The lens of the eye is regarded as potentially sensitive because of its lack of a blood supply and its tendency to accumulate damage and cellular debris. High local temperatures induced by exposure of the head to microwave frequencies will induce cataracts (opacities) in the lens of anesthetized rabbit eyes.[120–123] The most effective frequencies appear to lie between 1 and 10 GHz.[124] The threshold temperature in the lens for prolonged (> 140 min) exposure is between about 41 and 43 °C; the corresponding local SAR is about 100 W/kg. However, primate eyes appear to be less susceptible to heating by microwave radiation,[123] due probably to anatomical differences; opacities have not been produced experimentally.

The testis is also regarded as heat-sensitive. Testicular temperatures are normally several degrees below body temperature and male germ cells, particularly those undergoing meiosis (rather than the recycling stem cell population), are adversely affected by elevated temperatures. They can be readily depleted by acute exposure to microwaves at SARs in excess of 30 W/kg in anesthetized mice[125] and at SARs in excess of 8–10 W/kg in anesthetized rats.[126] In contrast, the acute or chronic exposure of conscious mice[127] to up to 20 W/kg and rats[128] to up to 9 W/kg did not affect testicular function. However, two studies[129,130] reported that chronic exposure of male rats at about 6 W/kg resulted in a transient decrease in fertility; body temperatures are estimated to have risen by 1–3 °C.

Heat has been shown to be teratogenic in various animal species including primates and has been implicated in central nervous system and facial defects in children whose mothers developed prolonged, severe hyperthermia (> 39 °C), especially during the first trimester of pregnancy.[131] A number of behavioral and skeletal abnormalities were induced in the offspring of marmosets whose body temperatures were raised to 41.5 °C for 1 h per day for five consecutive days between days 25 and 50 of gestation.[132] Many studies have shown that exposure to microwave or radio-frequency radiation sufficient to cause significant maternal heating is also associated with increased abnormalities.[133,134] For example, exposure of rats at 11 W/kg, raising maternal temperature to 43 °C, was sufficient to induce embryo and fetal death and developmental abnormalities;[135–137] chronic exposure of rats at 6–7 W/kg during pregnancy was reported[138,139] as inducing growth retardation and subtle behavioral changes postnatally. In general, exposure at less than 4 W/kg had no effect.[140–143] Similar effects were found in mice, but at higher SARs. It has been concluded[134] that heat causes birth defects and prenatal mortality when the temperature of the pregnant mother reaches 40–44 °C; exposure that increases maternal core temperature to 39–41 °C generally does not result in gross structural malformations, but may significantly increase the incidence of prenatal mortality, result in lower body weight, cause histological or physiological change, or alter the behavior of exposed offspring. Thus, only exposures that result in appreciable heating are likely to affect human embryos adversely.

Much experimental evidence suggests that acute or chronic exposure to microwave radiation does not result in an increase in mutation or chromosome aberration frequency in male germ cells when temperatures are maintained within physiological limits.[129,144,145] Similarly, most experimental evidence suggests that microwave and RF radiation have no clastogenic effect on somatic cells either *in vitro* or *in vivo*. No effect on sister chromatid exchange rates, a sensitive index of mutagenesis, was reported in murine bone marrow cells after the chronic exposure of mice[146] at 21 W/kg or in human lymphocytes acutely exposed *in vitro* to up to 200 W/kg under mildly hyperthermic conditions.[147] Some of the positive effects reported in early papers have been attributed to excessive temperature rises.

The lack of evidence for a mutagenic effect of microwaves and RF suggests that these frequencies of electromagnetic radiation are unlikely to be carcinogenic. One study[148] has shown evidence of an increased progression of spontaneous or chemically induced tumors in mice exposed chronically (over months) at 2–8 W/kg; similar responses were noted with increased levels of stress caused by overcrowding. However, the relevance of studies on tumor progression to the process of cancer induction is questionable. *In vitro* studies[149,150] have reported increased transformation rates in mouse fibroblast ($10T_{1/2}$) cells after microwave exposure at 4.4 W/kg for 24 h, with or without X-radiation, followed by treatment with the chemical promoter TPA. However, the data were not always consistent between experiments. It is not clear from these studies whether acute exposure will affect the process of cancer initiation or promotion.

Conclusions

The main adverse effects likely to result from acute exposure to RF magnetic fields can be associated with responses to the heat load and the effects of induced rise in body or tissue temperature. It can be concluded that exposure of resting humans in moderate environmental conditions to RF magnetic fields at SARs of 1 W/kg to up to 4 W/kg for short periods will result in a tolerable heat load and a rise in body temperature of less than 1 °C. It is also clear that some people are less heat tolerant than others; it is advised that the rise in body temperature for such people should be restricted to less than 0.5 °C and that whole-body SARs should be restricted to a lower part of the above range. It may be prudent to monitor blood pressure, heart rate, and body temperature during exposure above the lower level of restriction because the less heat tolerant group is not well defined.

Exposure to RF magnetic fields during MRI and particularly during MRS is predominantly to a region of the body such as the head or abdomen. The heat generated in tissues within this region is dissipated to the rest of the body. Whilst the whole-body SAR gives an indication of the overall heat load, it seems reasonable to restrict maximum temperatures resulting from the nonuniform distribution of SAR within the exposed region. Some regions of the body such as the head may be particularly vulnerable to raised temperature. Simple calculation suggests that restrictions on SAR in any kilogram of the head to 2 W/kg, relaxing to 4 W/kg for short periods, will limit temperatures in any tissue in the head to less than 38 °C. The developing embryo or fetus should be regarded as particularly sensitive to raised temperatures; however, tissues in the trunk and limbs are considered less sensitive.

Much animal data indicate that adverse effects of acute exposure are unlikely provided that body temperatures are not increased by more than 1 °C. In particular, acute exposure is unlikely to affect the lens unless temperatures rise to at least 41 °C. A transient reduction in male fertility has been observed after RF exposure, but only from prolonged exposure sufficient to raise body temperature by about 1–3 °C. Adverse effects on embryo and fetal development will be avoided if temperatures in these tissues do not exceed 38 °C, although other factors, such as maternal tolerance of the increased heat load, should be taken into account in this context. The data suggest that acute exposure is unlikely to result in damage to chromosomes provided that temperatures are kept within physiological limits. There is no convincing evidence that acute exposure to RF fields will affect the process of carcinogenesis; such considerations are seen as more relevant to occupational exposures.

OTHER SAFETY CONSIDERATIONS

Information concerning the potential hazards resulting from the exposure of patients with ferromagnetic splinters, metallic implants, aneurysm clips, and activated implants such as pacemakers has been published elsewhere.[151–154] In addition, these authors have considered various other potential hazards such as those arising from the magnetically induced movement of ferromagnetic materials in the vicinity of the MR system and the occurrence of burns resulting when conductive loops are inadvertently created between conducting leads, such as electrocardiogram leads, and the patient's skin.

Detailed advice on the avoidance of these problems is beyond the scope of this review. However, the following points are mentioned briefly.

Ferromagnetic implants and materials are regarded as contraindications for MR because of the potential risks associated with their movement or displacement. A recent review of several studies of the deflection forces induced by static fields of up to 4.7 T on 127 such implants concluded that 95 (75%) did not preclude safe MR examination.[151] However, the author concluded that the potential risk to patients who have metallic implants or who have objects made from unknown materials should be evaluated before MR imaging is performed. Another study[152] reported that, although adverse effects might conceivably result from electric currents and heating induced in metallic implants, the temperature changes associated with imaging small metallic implants and several large orthopedic prostheses were negligible.

The risks associated with exposing patients with cardiac pacemakers are related to the possibility of movement, of reed switch closure or damage, of programming changes, of inhibition or reversion to an asynchronous mode, and of electromagnetic interference, and even to the possibility of induced currents in lead wires pacing the heart at the frequency of the applied MR pulses.[153,154] It can be assumed that other electrically, magnetically, or mechanically activated devices, such as cochlear implants and epidural nerve stimulators, are also likely to pose risks during exposure unless there is information to the contrary. In addition, it has been reported[155] that static magnetic fields of 1.7–4.7 mT caused the reversion of some demand pacemakers to an asynchronous pacing mode. Some consideration should be given to wearers of pacemakers in the vicinity of MR equipment.

RECOMMENDATIONS

Restrictions on Exposure

The following restrictions on exposure of patients and volunteers to the static, gradient, and RF magnetic fields experienced during magnetic resonance imaging or spectroscopy are recommended. In situations where more than one set of restrictions applies, then the appropriate values are those resulting in the lowest exposure.

Static Magnetic Fields

Until further information becomes available, exposure should be such as to avoid any possible adverse effect on mental alertness or on cardiac function and aortic

TABLE 1. Static Magnetic Fields: Restrictions on Magnetic Flux Density

Part of Body	Uncontrolled Level (T)	Upper Level (T)
trunk and head	2.5	4.0
limbs	4.0	4.0

blood flow. This possibility will be avoided if the static magnetic flux density to the head and trunk does not exceed 2.5 T. The limbs may be exposed to up to 4 T (see TABLE 1). Relaxation of the restriction on head and trunk exposure to up to 4 T may be allowed under controlled conditions (see subsection entitled SUPERVISION OF EXPOSED PERSONS).

Gradient Magnetic Fields

Exposure should be such as to avoid the stimulation of peripheral nerves and muscles, particularly cardiac muscle, by magnetically induced electric currents. It is considered that peripheral nerve and muscle (including cardiac muscle) stimulation will be avoided if the induced current density is restricted to less than 400 mA/m^2 at any body location for induced current pulse widths exceeding 120 µs. This should be achieved for all magnetic field orientations by restricting exposures to periods of magnetic flux density change exceeding 120 µs to peak rates of change of less than 20 T/s (see TABLE 2). When the waveform is sinusoidal rather than pulsed, the period of change represents the half-period of the sine wave.

For shorter current pulse widths, the induced current density should be restricted according to the relationship $It < 48 \times 10^{-3}$, where I is the value of the induced current density expressed in mA/m^2 and t is the duration of the induced current pulse in seconds. This will be achieved for all magnetic field orientations if the relationship $(dB/dt)t < 2.4 \times 10^{-3}$ is observed, where dB/dt is the peak value of the rate of change of magnetic flux density in any part of the body in T/s and t is the duration of the change of magnetic flux density in seconds. For periods of magnetic field change of less than 3 ms, relaxation of this restriction is allowed under controlled conditions (see later), provided that the relationship $(dB/dt)t < 60 \times 10^{-3}$ is observed. This is in order to avoid cardiac muscle stimulation (but not peripheral nerve stimulation) and is based on restricting the induced current density for induced current pulse widths of less than 3 ms according to the relationship $It < 1.2$.

It should be noted that, for periods of flux density change longer than 3 ms, thresholds for peripheral nerve and cardiac muscle stimulation are similar; peripheral sensation does not provide an adequate warning against this more hazardous response. In these circumstances, the exposure of patients with cardiac problems to peak rates of change of flux density approaching 20 T/s should be carefully assessed.

TABLE 2. Gradient Magnetic Fields: Restrictions on Peak Rates of Change of Magnetic Flux Density

Duration of Field Change	Uncontrolled Level (T/s)	Upper Level (T/s)
$t > 3$ ms	20	20
120 µs $< t <$ 3 ms	20	$60 \times 10^{-3}/t$
45 µs $< t <$ 120 µs	$2.4 \times 10^{-3}/t$	$60 \times 10^{-3}/t$
2.5 µs $< t <$ 45 µs	$2.4 \times 10^{-3}/t$	1300^a (2 W/kg)
$t < 2.5$ µs	950^a (1 W/kg)	1300^a (2 W/kg)

^{a}Peak dB/dt values calculated assuming a tissue electric conductivity of 0.4 S/m and an inductive loop radius of 0.15 m.

In theory, as the period of gradient field change decreases below about 5 µs (or as sinusoidal gradient field frequencies increase above 100 kHz), the effects of heating begin to predominate over electrical excitation. In practice, however, even very rapid gradient field switching is unlikely to exceed 10 kHz. Should more rapid gradient field switching be envisaged, then users will have to demonstrate by calculation that restrictions on specific energy absorption rate (SAR) described below are not exceeded by the sum of the SAR resulting from the gradient and RF fields.

The derived (secondary) restrictions on rate of change of magnetic flux density can be exceeded if it can be shown that the basic restriction on induced current density is not exceeded.

Radio-Frequency Fields

Exposure should be such as to avoid a rise of more than 0.5 °C in the body temperature of patients (and volunteers), including those compromised with respect to their thermoregulatory ability. This basic restriction will be ensured for patients and volunteers exposed for periods longer than 30 min under moderate environmen-

TABLE 3a. RF Magnetic Fields: Restrictions on Whole-Body Temperature Rise

	Uncontrolled Level	Upper Level
Whole-body temperature rise (°C)	0.5	1.0

tal conditions (relative humidity < 50% and ambient temperature < 22 °C) by restricting the whole-body SAR to an average of 1 W/kg (see TABLES 3a–d). For periods of less than 30 min, restriction of the whole-body SAR can be relaxed in proportion to the decrease in exposure duration to a maximum of 2 W/kg averaged over a 15-min period. A relaxation of the basic restriction on rise in body temperature to 1 °C can be envisaged under the controlled conditions described in the next subsection. For exposures longer than 30 min, the whole-body SAR should be restricted to an average of 2 W/kg and can be progressively relaxed for shorter periods up to a maximum of 4 W/kg averaged over a 15-min period.

Exposure to RF magnetic fields during MR imaging or spectroscopy is mostly to the part of the body under examination. In addition, during spectroscopy, RF magnetic fields may be confined to small regions of the body. Restrictions on the average SAR in different regions of the body should be such as to prevent a local rise in temperature above 38 °C in any tissue in the head and fetus, 39 °C in any tissue in the trunk, and 40 °C in any tissue in the limbs (see TABLES 3a–d). These basic restrictions should be ensured for patients and volunteers exposed for periods longer than 30 min by restricting the SAR, averaged over any one kilogram and over any 6-min period, to 2 W/kg in the head (and fetus, in the case of a pregnant woman), to 4 W/kg in the trunk, and to 6 W/kg in the limbs. For exposure periods of less than 30 min, these restrictions can be progressively relaxed in proportion to the decrease in exposure duration to maximum values, averaged over a period of 6 min, of 4 W/kg for the head, 8 W/kg for the trunk, and 12 W/kg for the limbs.

Tissue inhomogeneities can create localized peaks in RF power absorption leading to potential hot spots; there may also be localized heating in the proximity of the RF antenna. It is considered that excessive localized heating will be avoided by the restrictions on SAR described above. However, the distribution of SAR within patients undergoing MR examination and the relationship between localized peak SAR values and temperature are not well understood at present and more detailed dosimetric calculation and thermoregulatory modeling are required.

The derived (secondary) restrictions on SAR can be exceeded if it can be shown that the basic restriction on temperature or temperature rise is not exceeded.

Supervision of Exposed Persons

Patients with certain medical disorders or under medication may be at some risk from exposure at levels above the lower advised levels of static, ELF, or RF magnetic

TABLE 3b. RF Magnetic Fields: Restrictions on Maximum Local Tissue Temperature

	Head	Trunk	Limbs
Maximum local tissue temperature (°C)	38	39	40

TABLE 3c. RF Magnetic Fields: Restrictions on Whole-Body SAR

Duration of Exposure	Uncontrolled Level[a]	Upper Level[a]
> 30 min	1 W/kg	2 W/kg
15–30 min	30 W · min/kg	60 W · min/kg
< 15 min	2 W/kg	4 W/kg

[a]Averaged over any 15-min period.

fields. In particular, patients with compromised thermoregulatory abilities may be particularly susceptible to RF heating; such patients may well include those with cardiac and circulatory problems or with a fever and those taking certain drugs. In addition, infants, pregnant women, and old people are likely to be considered compromised in this respect. In these circumstances, the doctor in charge of the patient must make this judgment and must weigh the benefit of diagnosis against any possible risk. Since the potentially sensitive categories of patient are not well defined, it is advised that all patients exposed above the lower level of restriction have simple physiological parameters, such as body temperature, blood pressure, and heart rate, routinely monitored.

Patients should be exposed only with the approval of a registered medical practitioner who should be satisfied either that the exposure is likely to contribute to the treatment of the patient or that it is part of a research project which has been approved by a local research ethical committee.

The exposure of volunteers participating in experimental trials of MR imaging or spectroscopic techniques should be approved by a local ethical committee. Volunteers should be medically assessed and pronounced suitable candidates before exposure. They should be freely consenting and fully informed. Additional guidance is given in WHO Technical Report No. 611.[156]

Although there is no good evidence that mammalian embryos are sensitive to the magnetic fields encountered in magnetic resonance systems, it is prudent, until further information becomes available, to exclude pregnant women during the first three months of pregnancy. However, MR diagnostic procedures should be considered where the only reasonable alternative to MR diagnosis requires the use of X-ray procedures. There is no need to exclude women for whom a termination of pregnancy has been indicated. It is advised that pregnant women should not be exposed above the lower advised levels of restriction.

Other Considerations

Metallic clips, particularly those used to treat aneurysms, and other metallic implants may present a hazard, especially if they are made of ferromagnetic

TABLE 3d. RF Magnetic Fields: Restrictions on Part-Body SAR

Duration of Exposure	Peak SARs in Any 1 kg[a]		
	Head	Trunk	Limbs
> 30 min	2 W/kg	4 W/kg	6 W/kg
15–30 min	60 W · min/kg	120 W · min/kg	180 W · min/kg
< 15 min	4 W/kg	8 W/kg	12 W/kg

[a]Averaged over any 6-min period.

materials; this would also apply to metallic foreign bodies. In general, exposure would be contraindicated unless careful evaluation is made on an individual basis with respect to the composition of the material of the implant or body and of its anatomical location. Information of value to this assessment is published elsewhere.[151,152] The exposure of individuals with large metallic implants, such as hip prostheses, should be stopped immediately if discomfort is experienced around the site of the implant.

Pacemakers and other electrically, mechanically, or magnetically activated implants may be subject to electromagnetic interference, heating, and a mechanical force if made of magnetic material; persons fitted with such implants should not be exposed unless the particular implant has been demonstrated to be unperturbed by MR fields. More detailed information is published elsewhere.[153,154]

REFERENCES

1. NRPB. 1984. Advice on acceptable limits of exposure to nuclear magnetic resonance clinical imaging. National Radiological Protection Board, ASP5. HMSO. London.
2. WHO. 1987. Magnetic fields. Environmental Health Criteria 69. World Health Organization. Geneva.
3. KOWALCZUK, C. I., Z. J. SIENKIEWICZ & R. D. SAUNDERS. 1991. Biological effects of exposure to non-ionising electromagnetic fields and radiation: I. Static electric and magnetic fields. NRPB-R238. HMSO. London.
4. SHELLOCK, F. G., D. J. SCHAEFER & C. J. GORDON. 1986. Effect of a 1.5 T static magnetic field on body temperature of man. Magn. Reson. Imag. 3: 644–647.
5. VOGL, T., K. KRIMMEL, D. DOPMEIER, M. SEIDERER & J. LISSNER. 1986. Influence of MR imaging on the central body temperature and peripheral temperature in humans. Radiology 161(P): 281.
6. VOGL, T., K. KRIMMEL, A. FUCHS & J. LISSNER. 1988. Influence of magnetic resonance imaging on human body core and intravascular temperature. Med. Phys. 15: 562–566.
7. JEHENSON, P., D. DUBOC, T. LAVERGNE, L. GUIZE, F. GUERIN, M. DEGEORGES & A. SYROTA. 1988. Change in human cardiac rhythm induced by a 2-T static magnetic field. Radiology 166: 227–230.
8. TENFORDE, T. S. & T. F. BUDINGER. 1986. Biological effects and physical safety aspects of NMR imaging and in vivo spectroscopy. In NMR in Medicine: Instrumentation and Clinical Applications. American Association of Physicists in Medicine Monograph No. 14. S. R. Thomas & R. L. Dixon, Eds.: 493–548. New York.
9. SAUNDERS, R. D. & J. S. ORR. 1983. Biologic effects of NMR. In Nuclear Magnetic Resonance (NMR) Imaging. C. L. Partain, A. E. James, F. D. Rollo & R. R. Price, Eds.: 383–396. Saunders. Philadelphia.
10. REDINGTON, R. W., C. L. DUMOULIN, J. F. SCHENCK, P. B. ROEMER, S. P. SOUZA, O. M. MUELLER, D. R. EISNER, J. E. PIEL & W. A. EDELSTEIN. 1988. MR imaging and bio-effects in a whole-body 4.0 tesla imaging system. Abstract, Society for Magnetic Resonance in Medicine (August 1988), p. 20.
11. GAFFEY, C. T. & T. S. TENFORDE. 1979. Changes in the electrocardiograms of rats and dogs exposed to DC magnetic fields. Lawrence Berkeley Laboratory (LBL-9085), University of California, Berkeley.
12. GAFFEY, C. T. & T. S. TENFORDE. 1981. Alterations in the rat electrocardiogram induced by stationary magnetic fields. Bioelectromagnetics 1: 357–370.
13. GAFFEY, C. T., T. S. TENFORDE & E. E. DEAN. 1980. Alterations in the electrocardiograms of baboons exposed to DC magnetic fields. Bioelectromagnetics 1: 209.
14. TENFORDE, T. S., C. T. GAFFEY, B. R. MOYER & T. F. BUDINGER. 1983. Cardiovascular alterations in Macaca monkeys exposed to stationary magnetic fields: experimental observations and theoretical analysis. Bioelectromagnetics 4: 1–9.
15. BEISCHER, D. E. & J. C. KNEPTON, JR. 1964. Influence of strong magnetic fields on the electrocardiogram of squirrel monkeys (Samiri sciureus). Aerosp. Med. 35: 939–944.

16. THACH, J. S., JR. 1968. A behavioral effect of intense DC electromagnetic fields. *In* Use of Non-human Primates in Drug Evaluation. H. Vagtborg, Ed.: 347–356. University of Texas Press. Austin, Texas.

17. DE LORGE, J. 1979. Effects of magnetic fields on behavior in nonhuman primates. *In* Magnetic Field Effects on Biological Systems. T. S. Tenforde, Ed.: 37–38. Plenum. New York.

18. SIKOV, M. R., D. D. MAHLUM, L. D. MONTGOMERY & J. R. DECKER. 1979. Development of mice after intrauterine exposure to direct-current magnetic fields. *In* Biological Effects of Extremely Low Frequency Electromagnetic Fields. Eighteenth Hanford Life Sciences Symposium, Richland, Washington (October 1978). R. D. Phillips, M. F. Gillis, W. T. Kaune & D. D. Mahlum, Eds.: 462–473. United States Department of Energy, National Technical Information Service. Springfield, Virginia.

19. KONERMANN, G. & H. MONIG. 1986. Studies on the influence of static magnetic fields on prenatal development of mice. Radiologe **26:** 490–497.

20. MAHLUM, D. D., M. R. SIKOV & J. R. DECKER. 1979. Dominant lethal studies in mice exposed to direct-current magnetic fields. *In* Biological Effects of Extremely Low Frequency Electromagnetic Fields. Eighteenth Hanford Life Sciences Symposium, Richland, Washington (October 1978). R. D. Phillips, M. F. Gillis, W. T. Kaune & D. D. Mahlum, Eds.: 474–484. United States Department of Energy, National Technical Information Service. Springfield, Virginia.

21. WOLFF, S., L. E. CROOKS, P. BROWN, R. HOWARD & R. B. PAINTER. 1980. Tests for DNA and chromosomal damage by nuclear magnetic resonance imaging. Body Comput. Tomogr. NMR **136:** 707–710.

22. COOKE, P. & P. G. MORRIS. 1981. The effects of exposure on living organisms. II. A genetic study of human lymphocytes. Br. J. Radiol. **54:** 622–625.

23. BELLOSSI, A. 1984. The effect of a static uniform magnetic field on mice—a study of methylcholanthrene carcinogenesis. Radiat. Environ. Biophys. **23:** 107–109.

24. BELLOSSI, A. 1986. The effect of a static non-uniform magnetic field on mice—a study of Lewis tumour graft. Radiat. Environ. Biophys. **25:** 231–234.

25. SIENKIEWICZ, Z. J., R. D. SAUNDERS & C. I. KOWALCZUK. 1991. Biological effects of exposure to non-ionising electromagnetic fields and radiation: II. Extremely low frequency electric and magnetic fields. NRPB-R239. HMSO. London.

26. D'ARSONVAL, A. 1896. Dispositifs pour la mesure des courants alternatifs de toutes frequences. C. R. Soc. Biol. (Paris) **48:** 450–451.

27. LOVSUND, P., P. A. OBERG & S. E. G. NILSSON. 1979. Qualitative determination of the thresholds of magnetophosphenes. Radio Sci. **14:** 199–200.

28. LOVSUND, P., P. A. OBERG & S. E. G. NILSSON. 1980. Magneto- and electro-phosphenes: a comparative study. Med. Biol. Eng. Comput. **18:** 758–764.

29. LOVSUND, P., P. A. OBERG, S. E. G. NILSSON & T. REUTER. 1980. Magnetophosphenes: a qualitative analysis of thresholds. Med. Biol. Eng. Comput. **18:** 326–334.

30. SILNY, J. 1981. Influence of low-frequency magnetic field (LMF) on the organism. Proc. EMC (Zurich), p. 175–180.

31. SILNY, J. 1985. Effects of low-frequency, high intensity magnetic field on the organism. *In* IEE International Conference on Electric and Magnetic Fields in Medicine and Biology (London, December 1985), p. 103–107. London. IEE.

32. SILNY, J. 1986. The influence threshold of the time-varying magnetic field in the human organism. *In* Biological Effects of Static and Extremely Low Frequency Magnetic Fields (Neuherberg, May 1985). BGA Schriften 3/86. J. H. Bernhardt, Ed.: 105–112. MMV Medizin Verlag. Munich.

33. MCROBBIE, D. & M. A. FOSTER. 1984. Thresholds for biological effects of time-varying magnetic fields. Clin. Phys. Physiol. Meas. **5:** 67–78.

34. POLSON, M. J. R., A. T. BARKER & I. L. FREESTON. 1982. Stimulation of nerve trunks with time-varying magnetic fields. Med. Biol. Eng. Comput. **20:** 243–244.

35. BARKER, A. T., R. JALINOUS & I. L. FREESTON. 1985. Non-invasive magnetic stimulation of human motor cortex. Lancet **8437:** 1106–1107.

36. BARKER, A. T., I. L. FREESTON, R. JALINOUS & J. A. JARRATT. 1986. Clinical evaluation of conduction time measurements in central motor pathways using magnetic stimulation of human brain. Lancet **8493:** 1325–1326.

37. COHEN, M. S., R. M. WEISSKOFF, R. R. RZEDZIAN & H. L. KANTOR. 1990. Sensory stimulation by time-varying magnetic fields. Magn. Reson. Med. **14:** 409–414.

38. BUDINGER, T. F., D. FISCHER, D. HENTSCHEL, H-E. REINFELDER & F. SCHMITT. 1990. Neural stimulation dB/dt thresholds for frequency and number of oscillations using sinusoidal magnetic gradient fields. Abstract, Society for Magnetic Resonance in Medicine (August 1985), p. 916–917.

39. REILLY, J. P. 1988. Electrical models for neural excitation studies. Johns Hopkins APL Tech. Dig. **9:** 44–59.

40. REILLY, J. P. 1989. Peripheral nerve stimulation by induced electric currents: exposure to time-varying magnetic fields. Med. Biol. Eng. Comput. **27:** 101–110.

41. REILLY, J. P. 1990. Peripheral nerve and cardiac excitation by time-varying magnetic fields: a comparison of thresholds. Report No. MT 90-100, prepared for the Center for Devices and Radiological Health, Food and Drug Administration (Rockville, Maryland), by Metatec Associates (Silver Spring).

42. MANSFIELD, P. & P. G. MORRIS. 1982. NMR Imaging in Biomedicine. Academic Press. New York.

43. DELGADO, J. M. R., J. LEAL, J. L. MONTEAGUDO & M. G. GRACIA. 1982. Embryological changes induced by weak, extremely low frequency electromagnetic fields. J. Anat. **134:** 533–551.

44. UBEDA, A., J. LEAL, M. A. TRILLO, M. A. JIMENEZ & J. M. R. DELGADO. 1983. Pulse shape of magnetic fields influences chick embryogenesis. J. Anat. **137:** 513–536.

45. JUUTILAINEN, J., M. HARRI, K. SAALI & T. LAHTINEN. 1986. Effects of 100-Hz magnetic fields with various waveforms on the development of chick embryos. Radiat. Environ. Biophys. **25:** 65–74.

46. JUUTILAINEN, J., E. LAARA & K. SAALI. 1987. Relationship between field strength and abnormal development in chick embryos exposed to 50-Hz magnetic fields. Int. J. Radiat. Biol. **52:** 787–793.

47. MAFFEO, S., M. W. MILLER & E. L. CARSTENSEN. 1984. Lack of effect of weak low frequency electromagnetic fields on chick embryogenesis. J. Anat. **139:** 613–618.

48. SISKEN, B. F., I. FOWLER, C. MAYAUD, J. P. RYABY, J. RYABY & A. A. PILLA. 1986. Pulsed electromagnetic fields and normal chick development. J. Bioelectr. **5:** 25–34.

49. SANDSTROM, M., K. HANSSON-MILD & S. LOVTRUP. 1987. Effects of weak pulsed magnetic fields on chick embryogenesis. *In* Work with Display Units 86. B. Knave & P. G. Wideback, Eds.: 135–140. Elsevier. Amsterdam.

50. TRIBUKAIT, B., E. CEKAN & L-E. PAULSSON. 1987. Effects of pulsed magnetic fields on embryonic development in mice. *In* Work with Display Units 86. B. Knave & P. G. Wideback, Eds.: 129–134. Elsevier. Amsterdam.

51. FROLEN, H., B. M. SVEDENSTALL, P. BIERKE & H. FELLNER-FELDEGG. 1987. Repetition of a study of the effect of pulsed magnetic fields on the development of fetuses in mice. English language version of Concluding Report (June 1987), National Institute of Radiation Protection, Sweden. SSI Project No. 346,86.

52. STUCHLY, M. A., J. RUDDICK, D. VILLENEUVE, K. ROBINSON, B. REED, D. W. LECUYER, K. TAN & J. WONG. 1988. Teratological assessment of exposure to time-varying magnetic field. Teratology **38:** 461–466.

53. BRINKMANN, K., S. BUNTENKOTTER, E. ZITTLAU, R. ZWINGELBERG & H. J. REINHARD. 1988. A teratological study on rats exposed to 50-Hz magnetic fields. *In* Abstracts, Tenth Annual Meeting of the Bioelectromagnetics Society (June 1987, Stamford, Connecticut), p. 38.

54. COHEN, M. M., A. KUNSKA, J. A. ASTEMBORSKI, D. MCCULLOCH & D. A. PASKEWITZ. 1986. Effect of low-level, 60-Hz electromagnetic fields on human lymphoid cells: I. Mitotic rate and chromosome breakage in human peripheral lymphocytes. Bioelectromagnetics **7:** 415–423.

55. COHEN, M. M., A. KUNSKA, J. A. ASTEMBORSKI & D. MCCULLOCH. 1986. Effect of low-level, 60-Hz electromagnetic fields on human lymphoid cells: II. Sister-chromatid exchanges in peripheral lymphocytes and lymphoblastoid cell lines. Mutat. Res. **172:** 177–184.

56. FRAZIER, M. E., J. E. SAMUEL & W. T. KAUNE. 1987. Viabilities and mutation frequencies of CHO-K1 cells following exposure to 60-Hz electric fields. *In* Interaction of

Biological Systems with Static and ELF Electric and Magnetic Fields. Twenty-third Hanford Life Sciences Symposium, Richland, Washington (October 1984). L. E. Anderson, B. J. Kelman & R. J. Weigel, Eds.: 471–485. Pacific Northwest Laboratory. Richland, Washington.

57. LIBOFF, A. R., T. WILLIAMS, JR., D. M. STRONG & R. WISTAR. 1984. Time-varying magnetic fields: effect on DNA synthesis. Science 223: 818–820.

58. GOODMAN, R. & A. S. HENDERSON. 1986. Sine waves enhance cellular transcription. Bioelectromagnetics 7: 23–29.

59. GOODMAN, R. & A. S. HENDERSON. 1988. Exposure of salivary glands to low-frequency electromagnetic fields alters polypeptide synthesis. Proc. Natl. Acad. Sci. U.S.A. 85: 3928–3932.

60. GOODMAN, R., J. ABBOTT & A. S. HENDERSON. 1987. Transcriptional patterns in the X chromosome of Sciara coprophila following exposure to magnetic fields. Bioelectromagnetics 8: 1–7.

61. GOODMAN, R., L-H. WEI & A. S. HENDERSON. 1987. Induction of the expression of c-myc following exposure of cultured cells to low frequency electromagnetic fields. In Transactions of the Seventh Annual Meeting of the Bioelectrical Repair and Growth Society (October 1987, Toronto, Ontario). Vol. 7: 85.

62. SAUNDERS, R. D., C. I. KOWALCZUK & Z. J. SIENKIEWICZ. 1991. Biological effects of exposure to non-ionising electromagnetic fields and radiation: III. RF and microwave radiation. NRPB-R240. To be published.

63. ADEY, W. R. 1983. Biological effects of low-energy electromagnetic fields on the central nervous system. In Biological Effects and Dosimetry of Nonionizing Radiation, Radiofrequency, and Microwave Energies. M. Grandolfo, S. M. Michaelson & A. Rindi, Eds.: 359–391. Plenum. New York.

64. NIOSH. 1980. Proceedings of a NIOSH Workshop on Recommended Heat Stress Standards. F. N. Dukes-Dubos & A. Henschel, Eds. United States Department of Health and Human Services. DHHS (NIOSH) 81-108. Cincinnati, Ohio.

65. NIOSH. 1972. Criteria for a Recommended Standard: Occupational Exposure to Hot Environments. United States Department of Health, Education, and Welfare, National Institute for Occupational Safety and Health. HSM 72-10269 (NIOSH 73-11009).

66. ACGIH. 1983. TLVs: Threshold Limit Values for Chemical Substances and Physical Agents in the Work Environment with Intended Changes for 1983–84. American Conference of Governmental Industrial Hygienists. Cincinnati, Ohio.

67. ROWELL, L. B. 1974. Human cardiovascular adjustments to exercise and thermal stress. Physiol. Rev. 54: 75.

68. ROWELL, L. B. 1983. Cardiovascular aspects of human thermoregulation. Circ. Res. 52: 367.

69. TELL, R. A. & F. HARLEN. 1979. A review of selected biological effects and dosimetric data useful for development of radiofrequency safety standards for human exposure. J. Microwave Power 14: 405–424.

70. KENNEY, W. L. 1985. Physiological correlates of heat intolerance. Sports Med. 2: 279–286.

71. MINARD, D. 1980. Pre-employment and periodic medical examinations for workers on hot jobs. In Proceedings of a NIOSH Workshop on Recommended Heat Stress Standards. F. N. Dukes-Dubos & A. Henschel, Eds.: 61–70. United States Department of Health and Human Services. DHHS (NIOSH) 81-108. Cincinnati, Ohio.

72. ADAIR, E. R. & L. G. BERGLUND. 1986. On the thermoregulatory consequences of NMR imaging. Magn. Reson. Imag. 4: 321–333.

73. ADAIR, E. R. & L. G. BERGLUND. 1988. Thermoregulatory consequences of MR imaging when capacity for skin blood flow is reduced. Abstract, Society for Magnetic Resonance in Medicine (August 1988), p. 171.

74. KIDO, D. K., T. W. MORRIS, J. L. ERICKSON, D. B. PLEWES & J. H. SIMON. 1987. Physiologic changes during high field strength MR imaging. Am. J. Neuroradiol. 8: 263–266.

75. ABART, J., G. BRINKER, W. IRLBACHER & J. GREBMEIER. 1989. Temperature and heart

rate changes in MRI at SAR levels of up to 3 W/kg. Abstract, Society for Magnetic Resonance in Medicine (August 1989), p. 998.

76. SCHAEFER, D. J., B. J. BARBER, C. J. GORDON, J. ZIELONKA & J. HECKER. 1985. Thermal effects of magnetic resonance imaging (MRI). *In* Abstracts: Society of Magnetic Resonance in Medicine. Vol. 2: 925–926. Society of Magnetic Resonance in Medicine. Berkeley, California.

77. GORDON, C. J., D. J. SCHAEFER, J. ZIELONKA & J. HECKER. 1986. Thermoregulatory effects of magnetic resonance (MR) imaging. Fed. Proc. **45:** 1017 (abstract).

78. SHELLOCK, F. G., D. J. SCHAEFER & J. V. CRUES. 1989. Alterations in body and skin temperatures caused by magnetic resonance imaging: is the recommended exposure for radiofrequency radiation too conservative? Br. J. Radiol. **62:** 902–909.

79. SHELLOCK, F. G. & J. V. CRUES. 1987. Temperature, heart rate, and blood pressure changes associated with clinical MR imaging at 1.5 T. Radiology **163:** 259–262.

80. SHELLOCK, F. G. & J. V. CRUES. 1988. Temperature changes caused by MR imaging of the brain with a head coil. Am. J. Neuroradiol. **9:** 287–291.

81. BUDINGER, T. F., W. PAVLICEK, D. D. FAUL & A. W. GUY. 1985. RF heating at 1.5 tesla and above in proton NMR imaging. Abstract, Society for Magnetic Resonance in Medicine (August 1985), p. 276.

82. BOTTOMLEY, P. A. & E. R. ANDREW. 1978. RF magnetic field penetration, phase shift, and power dissipation in biological tissue: implications for NMR imaging. Phys. Med. Biol. **23:** 630–643.

83. BOTTOMLEY, P. A. & W. A. EDELSTEIN. 1981. Power deposition in whole-body NMR imaging. Med. Phys. **8:** 510–512.

84. ADAIR, E. R. 1983. Sensation, subtleties, and standards: synopsis of a panel discussion. *In* Microwaves and Thermoregulation. E. R. Adair, Ed.: 231–238. Academic Press. New York.

85. GANDHI, O. P., J. F. DEFORD & H. KANAI. 1984. Impedance method for calculation of power deposition patterns in magnetically induced hyperthermia. IEEE Trans. Biomed. Eng. **BME-31:** 644–651.

86. ORCUTT, N. & O. P. GANDHI. 1988. A 3-D impedance method to calculate power deposition in biological bodies subjected to time-varying magnetic fields. IEEE Trans. Biomed. Eng. **35:** 577–583.

87. GABRIEL, C. 1989. Localised SAR in people undergoing NMR imaging. Report prepared for the National Radiological Protection Board (Chilton, United Kingdom) by University Microwave (London).

88. GRANDOLFO, M., P. VECCHIA & O. P. GANDHI. 1990. Magnetic resonance imaging: calculation of rates of energy absorption by a human-torso model. Bioelectromagnetics **11:** 117–128.

89. CZERSKI, P. & T. W. ATHEY. 1987. Safety of magnetic resonance *in vivo* diagnostic examinations: theoretical and clinical considerations. Report, Center for Devices and Radiological Health, Rockville, Maryland.

90. ATHEY, T. W. 1989. A model of the temperature rise in the head due to magnetic resonance imaging procedures. Magn. Reson. Med. **9:** 177.

91. LOVELY, R. H., D. E. MYERS & A. W. GUY. 1977. Irradiation of rats by 918-MHz microwaves at 2.5 mW/cm^2: delineating the dose-response relationship. Radio Sci. **12:** 139–146.

92. LOVELY, R. H., S. J. Y. MIZUMORI, R. B. JOHNSON & A. W. GUY. 1983. Subtle consequences of exposure to weak microwave fields: are there nonthermal effects? *In* Microwaves and Thermoregulation. E. R. Adair, Ed.: 401–429. Academic Press. New York.

93. ADAIR, E. R. & B. W. ADAMS. 1982. Adjustments in metabolic heat production by squirrel monkeys exposed to microwaves. J. Appl. Physiol. Respir. Environ. Exercise Physiol. **52:** 1049–1058.

94. ADAIR, E. R. & B. W. ADAMS. 1980. Microwaves induce peripheral vasodilation in squirrel monkey. Science **207:** 1381–1383.

95. LOTZ, W. G. & J. L. SAXTON. 1987. Metabolic and vasomotor responses of rhesus monkeys exposed to 225-MHz radiofrequency energy. Bioelectromagnetics **8:** 73–89.

96. STERN, S., L. MARGOLIN, B. WEISS & S. M. MICHAELSON. 1979. Microwaves: effect on thermoregulatory behavior in rats. Science **206:** 1198–1201.

97. ADAIR, E. R. & B. W. ADAMS. 1980. Microwaves modify thermoregulatory behavior in squirrel monkey. Bioelectromagnetics **1:** 1–20.

98. ADAIR, E. R. & B. W. ADAMS. 1988. Microwave exposure at resonant frequency alters behavioral thermoregulation. *In* Abstracts, Tenth Annual Meeting of the Bioelectromagnetics Society (June 1988), p. 45.

99. DE LORGE, J. O. 1976. The effects of microwave radiation on behavior and temperature in rhesus monkeys. *In* Biological Effects of Electromagnetic Waves. Selected Papers of the USNC/URSI Annual Meeting, Boulder, Colorado (October 1975). Volume 1. C. C. Johnson & M. L. Shore, Eds.: 158–174. United States Department of Health, Education, and Welfare. HEW Publication (FDA) No. 77-8010. Rockville, Maryland.

100. DE LORGE, J. 1979. Operant behavior and rectal temperature of squirrel monkeys during 2.45-GHz microwave irradiation. Radio Sci. **14:** 217–225.

101. DE LORGE, J. O. 1984. Operant behavior and colonic temperature of *Macaca mulatta* exposed to radiofrequency fields at above resonant frequencies. Bioelectromagnetics **5:** 232–246.

102. JUSTESEN, D. R. & N. W. KING. 1970. Behavioral effects of low level microwave irradiation in the closed space situation. *In* Biological Effects and Health Implications of Microwave Radiation: Symposium Proceedings. S. F. Cleary, Ed.: 154–179. United States Department of Health, Education, and Welfare. BRH/DBE 70-2. Rockville, Maryland.

103. D'ANDREA, J. A., O. P. GANDHI & R. P. KESNER. 1976. Behavioral effects of resonant electromagnetic power absorption in rats. *In* Biological Effects of Electromagnetic Waves. Selected Papers of the USNC/URSI Annual Meeting, Boulder, Colorado (October 1975). Volume 1. C. C. Johnson & M. L. Shore, Eds.: 257–273. United States Department of Health, Education, and Welfare. HEW Publication (FDA) No. 77-8010. Rockville, Maryland.

104. D'ANDREA, J. A., O. P. GANDHI & J. L. LORDS. 1977. Behavioral and thermal effects of microwave radiation at resonant and nonresonant wavelengths. Radio Sci. **12:** 251–256.

105. SANZA, J. N. & J. DE LORGE. 1977. Fixed interval behavior of rats exposed to microwaves at low power densities. Radio Sci. **12:** 273–277.

106. LOTZ, W. G. & R. P. PODGORSKI. 1982. Temperature and adrenocortical responses in rhesus monkeys exposed to microwaves. J. Appl. Physiol. Respir. Environ. Exercise Physiol. **53:** 1565–1571.

107. LOTZ, W. G. & S. M. MICHAELSON. 1978. Temperature and corticosterone relationships in microwave-exposed rats. J. Appl. Physiol. Respir. Environ. Exercise Physiol. **44:** 438–445.

108. COOPER, T., T. PINAKATT & A. W. RICHARDSON. 1961. Effect of microwave-induced hyperthermia on the cardiac output of the rat. Physiologist **4:** 21 (abstract).

109. PINAKATT, T., T. COOPER & A. W. RICHARDSON. 1963. Effect of ouabain on the circulatory response to microwave hyperthermia in rat. Aerosp. Med. **34:** 497–499.

110. CHOU, C-K., L. F. HAN & A. W. GUY. 1980. Microwave radiation and heart-beat rate of rabbits. J. Microwave Power **15:** 87–93.

111. BLACKWELL, R. P. 1980. Effects of microwave exposure on anesthesia in the mouse. *In* Proceedings of the International Symposium on Electromagnetic Waves and Biology (Jouy en Josas, June/July 1980), p. 71–73. URSI/CNFRS. Paris.

112. CLEARY, S. F. & R. T. WANGEMANN. 1976. Effect of microwave radiation on pentobarbital-induced sleeping time. *In* Biological Effects of Electromagnetic Fields. Selected Papers of the USNC/URSI Annual Meeting, Boulder, Colorado (October 1975). Volume 1. C. C. Johnson & M. L. Shore, Eds.: 311–323. United States Department of Health, Education, and Welfare. HEW Publication (FDA) No. 77-8010. Rockville, Maryland.

113. LIBURDY, R. P. 1977. Effects of radio-frequency radiation on inflammation. Radio Sci. **12:** 179–183.

114. LIBURDY, R. P. 1979. Radiofrequency radiation alters the immune system: modification

of T- and B-lymphocyte levels and cell-mediated immunocompetence by hyperthermic radiation. Radiat. Res. **77**: 34–46.

115. DEICHMANN, W. B., J. MIALE & K. LANDEEN. 1964. Effect of microwave radiation on the hemopoietic system of the rat. Toxicol. Appl. Pharmacol. **6**: 71–77.

116. RAMA RAO, G., C. A. CAIN, J. LOCKWOOD & W. A. F. TOMPKINS. 1983. Effects of microwave exposure on the hamster immune system. II. Peritoneal macrophage function. Bioelectromagnetics **4**: 141–155.

117. YANG, H. K., C. A. CAIN, J. LOCKWOOD & W. A. F. TOMPKINS. 1983. Effects of microwave exposure on the hamster immune system. I. Natural killer cell activity. Bioelectromagnetics **4**: 123–139.

118. SMIALOWICZ, R. J., R. R. ROGERS, R. J. GARNER, M. M. RIDDLE, R. W. LUEBKE & D. G. ROWE. 1983. Microwaves (2450 MHz) suppress murine natural killer cell activity. Bioelectromagnetics **4**: 371–381.

119. SZMIGIELSKI, S., M. BIELEC, S. LIPSKI & G. SOKOLSKA. 1988. Immunologic and cancer-related aspects of exposure to low-level microwave and radiofrequency fields. *In* Modern Bioelectricity. A. A. Marino, Ed.: 861–925. Dekker. New York.

120. CARPENTER, R. L., D. K. BIDDLE & C. A. VAN UMMERSON. 1960. Opacities in the lens of the eye experimentally induced by exposure to microwave radiation. IRE Trans. Med. Electron. **ME-7**: 152–157.

121. CARPENTER, R. L., D. K. BIDDLE & C. A. VAN UMMERSON. 1960. Biological effects of microwave radiation with particular reference to the eye. *In* Proceedings of the Third International Conference on Medical Electronics, p. 401–408. International Federation for Medical Electronics. London.

122. GUY, A. W., J. C. LIN, P. O. KRAMAR & A. F. EMERY. 1975. Effect of 2450-MHz radiation on the rabbit eye. IEEE Trans. Microwave Theory Tech. **MTT-23**: 492–498.

123. KRAMAR, P., C. HARRIS, A. F. EMERY & A. W. GUY. 1978. Acute microwave irradiation and cataract formation in rabbits and monkeys. J. Microwave Power **13**: 239–249.

124. ELDER, J. A. 1984. Special senses. *In* Biological Effects of Radiofrequency Radiation. J. A. Elder & D. F. Cahill, Eds.: 5-64 to 5-78. Health Effect Research Laboratory, United States Environmental Protection Agency. EPA-600/8-83-026F. North Carolina.

125. SAUNDERS, R. D. & C. I. KOWALCZUK. 1981. Effects of 2.45 GHz microwave radiation and heat on mouse spermatogenic epithelium. Int. J. Radiat. Biol. **40**: 623–632.

126. LEBOVITZ, R. M., L. JOHNSON & W. K. SAMSON. 1987. Effects of pulse-modulated microwave radiation and conventional heating on potential of microwaves. Mutat. Res. **123**: 31–46.

127. CAIRNIE, A. B. & R. K. HARDING. 1981. Cytological studies in mouse testis irradiated with 2.45-GHz continuous-wave microwaves. Radiat. Res. **87**: 100–108.

128. LEBOVITZ, R. M. & L. JOHNSON. 1987. Acute, whole body microwave exposure and testicular function of rats. Bioelectromagnetics **8**: 37–43.

129. BERMAN, E., H. B. CARTER & D. HOUSE. 1980. Tests for mutagenesis and reproduction in male rats exposed to 2450 MHz (CW) microwaves. Bioelectromagnetics **1**: 65–76.

130. JOHNSON, L., R. M. LEBOVITZ & W. K. SAMSON. 1984. Germ cell degeneration in normal and microwave irradiated rats. Potential sperm production rates at different developmental steps in spermatogenesis. Anat. Rec. **209**: 501–507.

131. PLEET, H., J. M. GRAHAM & D. W. SMITH. 1981. Central nervous system and facial defects associated with maternal hyperthermia at 4 to 14 weeks gestation. Paediatrics **67**: 785–789.

132. POSWILLO, D., H. NUNNERLY, D. SOPHER & J. KEITH. 1974. Hyperthermia as a teratogenic agent. Ann. R. Coll. Surg. Engl. **55**: 171–174.

133. O'CONNOR, M. E. 1980. Mammalian teratogenesis and radio-frequency fields. Proc. IEEE **68**: 56–60.

134. LARY, J. M. & D. L. CONOVER. 1987. Teratogenic effects of radiofrequency radiation. IEEE Eng. Med. Biol. Mag. **March**: 42–46.

135. LARY, J. M., D. L. CONOVER, E. D. FOLEY & P. L. HANSER. 1982. Teratogenic effects of 27.12-MHz radiofrequency radiation in rats. Teratology **26**: 299–309.

136. LARY, J. M., D. L. CONOVER, P. H. JOHNSON & J. R. BURG. 1983. Teratogenicity of

27.12-MHz radiation in rats is related to duration of hyperthermic exposure. Bioelectromagnetics **4:** 249–255.

137. LARY, J. M., D. L. CONOVER, P. H. JOHNSON & R. W. HORNUNG. 1986. Dose-response relationship between body temperature and birth defects in radiofrequency-irradiated rats. Bioelectromagnetics **7:** 141–149.

138. JENSH, R. P. 1984. Studies of the teratogenic potential of exposure of rats to 6000-MHz microwave radiation. I. Morphologic analysis at term. Radiat. Res. **97:** 272–281.

139. JENSH, R. P. 1984. Studies of the teratogenic potential of exposure of rats to 6000-MHz microwave radiation. II. Postnatal psychophysiologic evaluations. Radiat. Res. **97:** 282–301.

140. JENSH, R. P., W. H. VOGEL & R. L. BRENT. 1982. Postnatal functional analysis of prenatal exposure of rats to 915-MHz microwave radiation. J. Am. Coll. Toxicol. **1:** 73–90.

141. JENSH, R. P., I. WEINBERG & R. L. BRENT. 1982. Teratologic studies of prenatal exposure of rats to 915-MHz microwave radiation. Radiat. Res. **92:** 160–171.

142. JENSH, R. P., W. H. VOGEL & R. L. BRENT. 1983. An evaluation of the teratogenic potential of protracted exposure of pregnant rats to 2450-MHz microwave radiation. I. Morphologic analysis at term. J. Toxicol. Environ. Health **11:** 23–35.

143. JENSH, R. P., W. H. VOGEL & R. L. BRENT. 1983. An evaluation of the teratogenic potential of protracted exposure of pregnant rats to 2450-MHz microwave radiation. II. Postnatal psychophysiologic analysis. J. Toxicol. Environ. Health **11:** 37–59.

144. BEECHEY, C. V., D. BROOKER, C. I. KOWALCZUK, R. D. SAUNDERS & A. G. SEARLE. 1986. Cytogenetic effects of microwave irradiation on male germ cells of the mouse. Int. J. Radiat. Biol. **50:** 909–918.

145. SAUNDERS, R. D., C. I. KOWALCZUK, C. V. BEECHEY & R. DUNFORD. 1988. Studies of the induction of dominant lethals and translocations in male mice after chronic exposure to microwave radiation. Int. J. Radiat. Biol. **53:** 983–992.

146. MCREE, D. I., G. MACNICHOLS & G. K. LIVINGSTON. 1981. Incidence of sister chromatid exchange in bone marrow cells of the mouse following microwave exposure. Radiat. Res. **85:** 340–348.

147. LLOYD, D. C., R. D. SAUNDERS, J. E. MOQUET & C. I. KOWALCZUK. 1986. Absence of chromosomal damage in human lymphocytes exposed to microwave radiation with hyperthermia. Bioelectromagnetics **7:** 235–237.

148. SZMIGIELSKI, S., A. SZUDZINSKI, A. PIETRASZEK, M. BIELEC & J. K. WREMBEL. 1982. Accelerated development of spontaneous and benzopyrene-induced skin cancer in mice exposed to 2450-MHz microwave radiation. Bioelectromagnetics **3:** 179–191.

149. BALCER-KUBICZEK, E. K. & G. H. HARRISON. 1985. Evidence for microwave carcinogenesis *in vitro.* Carcinogenesis **6:** 859–864.

150. BALCER-KUBICZEK, E. K. & G. H. HARRISON. 1989. Induction of neoplastic transformation in C3H/10T$_{1/2}$ cells by 2.45-GHz microwaves and phorbol ester. Radiat. Res. **117:** 531–537.

151. SHELLOCK, F. G. 1988. MR imaging of metallic implants and materials: a compilation of the literature. Am. J. Radiol. **151:** 811–814.

152. SHELLOCK, F. G. & J. V. CRUES. 1988. High-field-strength MR imaging and metallic biomedical implants: an *ex vivo* evaluation of deflection forces. Am. J. Radiol. **151:** 389–392.

153. SHELLOCK, F. G. 1989. Biological effects and safety aspects of magnetic resonance imaging. Magn. Reson. Q. **5**(4): 243–261.

154. KANAL, E., F. G. SHELLOCK & L. TALAGALA. 1990. Safety considerations in MR imaging. Radiology **176:** 593–606.

155. PAVLICEK, W., M. GEISINGER, L. CASTLE, M. D. BORKOWSKI, T. F. MEANEY & J. H. GALLAGHER. 1983. The effects of nuclear magnetic resonance on patients with cardiac pacemakers. Radiology **147:** 149–153.

156. WHO. 1977. Use of ionizing radiation and radionuclides on human beings for medical research, training, and nonmedical purposes. Report of a WHO Expert Committee. Technical Report Series No. 611. World Health Organization. Geneva.

FDA Safety Parameter Action Levels[a]

The text herein describes the action levels for the following safety parameters: RF heating (SAR), rate of magnetic field strength change with time (dB/dt), static magnetic field strength (B_0), and acoustic noise. If levels cited in this section are to be exceeded, the manufacturer must provide valid scientific evidence to establish the safety of operating at intended levels.

STATIC MAGNETIC FIELD (B_0)

Static magnetic field strengths not exceeding 2.0 T are below the level of concern for the static magnetic field. Should the static magnetic field strength exceed 2.0 T, additional evidence of safety must be provided by the sponsor.

RATE OF MAGNETIC FIELD STRENGTH CHANGE WITH TIME (dB/dt)

Three alternate approaches are described. Option A is the level of concern below which there clearly is no apparent concern for the safety of the subject. This is the level that has been employed by the Agency in previous PMA submissions. Option B permits the sponsor to utilize values of dB/dt that may exceed the 6 T/s value, but evidence of the actual level achieved will undergo more stringent review. Option C permits the sponsor to use peripheral nerve stimulation as a basis for determination of dB/dt and will undergo close scrutiny. The pulse width (τ) is the width in microseconds of a rectangular pulse or the half-period of a sinusoidal dB/dt pulse.

Options

(A) Demonstrate that the maximum dB/dt of the system is 6 T/s or less: Below level of concern;
  OR
(B) For axial gradients:
  If $dB/dt < 20$ T/s for $\tau \geq 120$ μs, or
  if $dB/dt < 2400/\tau(\mu s)$ T/s for 12 μs $< \tau <$ 120 μs, or
  if $dB/dt < 200$ T/s for $\tau \leq 12$ μs;
  For transverse gradients:
  If dB/dt is less than three times the above limits for axial gradients: Below level of concern;
  OR
(C) Demonstrate with valid scientific evidence that the rate of change of magnetic field for the system is not sufficient to cause peripheral nerve

[a]From a Food and Drug Administration document (August 2, 1988): Guidance for content and review of a magnetic resonance diagnostic device 510(k) application—safety parameter action levels.

stimulation by an adequate margin of safety (at least a factor of three): Below level of concern.

The parameter dB/dt cited above must be shown to fall below either of the two levels of concern by presentation of valid scientific measurement, or sufficient calculational evidence must be provided to demonstrate that the time rate of magnetic field change (dB/dt) is of no concern.

RF HEATING (SAR)

The following are the levels of concern at which the reviewer shall exercise appropriate actions to ensure that the safety of the device is substantially equivalent to a predicate device.

Options

(A)   If SAR $\leq$ 0.4 W/kg whole body, and if SAR $\leq$ 8.0 W/kg spatial peak in any 1 gram of tissue, and if SAR $\leq$ 3.2 W/kg averaged over the head: Below level of concern;
OR

(B)   If exposure to radio-frequency magnetic fields insufficient to produce a core temperature increase in excess of 1 °C and localized heating to greater than 38 °C in the head, 39 °C in the trunk, and 40 °C in the extremities: Below level of concern.

The parameter of RF heating cited above must be shown to fall below either of the two levels of concern by presentation of valid scientific measurement or calculational evidence sufficient to demonstrate that RF heating effects (SAR) are of no concern.

ACOUSTIC NOISE

The acoustic noise levels associated with the device must be shown to be below the level of concern established by pertinent Federal Regulatory or other recognized standards-setting organizations. If the acoustic noise is not below the level of concern, the sponsor must recommend steps to reduce or alleviate the noise perceived by the patient.

Index of Contributors

Adair, E. R., 188–200
Al-Barazi, H., 340–342, 353–355
Athey, T. W., 242–257

Balaban, R. S., 335–337
Barnes, F. S., 69–73
Berglund, L. G., 188–200
Blackwell, G. G., 302–312
Boesiger, P., 160–165
Bottomley, P. A., 144–159
Brennan, K. M., 345–349
Brun, A., 356–358
Buchli, R., 160–165
Budinger, T. F., 1–18
Buettner, U. W., 59–66

Cao, G., 166–175
Carson, J. J. L., 44–58
Casamento, J., 340–342, 353–355
Chen, J-Y., 131–143
Cleary, S. F., 166–175
Czerska, E., 340–342, 353–355

Davis, C., 340–342, 353–355
Davis, P. L., 343–344
de Certaines, J. D., 35–43
de Manincor, D. J., 345–349
Drost, D. J., 44–58
Durney, C. H., 19–34

Eberhardt, J. L., 356–358
Elson, E., 340–342, 353–355

Fitzsimmons, J. R., 313–321
Frappier, J. R. H., 44–58

Gandhi, O. P., 131–143, 176–187
Goldstein, H. A., 322–331
Gordon, C. J., 273–284
Grandolfo, M., 176–187

Hiwaki, O., 369–371

Kanal, E., 204–224
Kashanian, F., 322–331
Kavaliers, M., 44–58
Kuhara, S., 369–371

Liburdy, R. P., 67–68, 74–95, 345–349
Liu, L-M., 166–175
Lotz, W. G., 201–203

Magin, R. L., ix–xi
Malmgren, L., 356–358
Matsuda, T., 366–368, 369–371
Meier, D., 160–165
Monahan, J. C., 258–259
Mosher, T. J., 359–362

Ning, J., 340–342, 350–352, 353–355

Olsen, R. G., 237–241
Ossenkopp, K-P., 44–58

Persson, B., 338–339, 356–358
Pohost, G. M., 302–312
Polichetti, A., 176–187
Prato, F. S., 44–58

Reilly, J. P., 96–117
Roemer, P. B., 144–159
Rohan, M. L., 118–128
Roos, M. S., 345–349
Rzedzian, R. R., 118–128

Salford, L. G., 356–358
Saner, M., 160–165
Sato, K., 369–371
Schaefer, D. J., 225–236
Schenck, J. F., 285–301
Seo, Y., 369–371
Shang, Y., 343–344
Shellock, F. G., 260–272, 302–312
Smith, M. B., 359–362
Stark, D. D., 332–334
Swicord, M., 340–342, 353–355

Talagala, L., 343–344
Tanoue, T., 369–371
Tassone, R. F., 359–362
Thomas, S. R., 129–130
Tyndall, D. A., 363–365

Ueno, S., 366–368, 369–371

Vecchia, P., 176–187

Weinreb, J. C., 258–259
Wiggins, J. R., 322–331
Wornom, I. L., III, 350–352

Yamagata, H., 369–371